McGraw-Hill Education

CCRN
REVIEW

McGraw-Hill Education

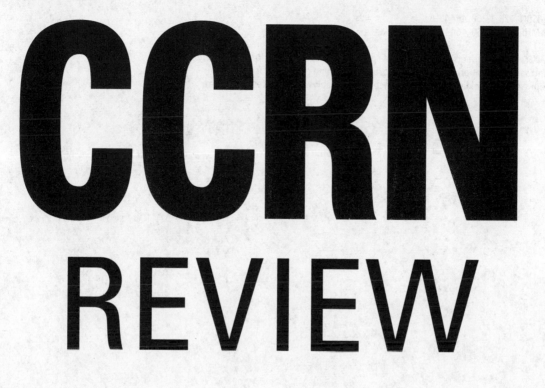

CCRN
REVIEW

MICHAEL REID, MSN, RN, CCRN

New York Chicago San Francisco Athens London Madrid
Mexico City Milan New Delhi Singapore Sydney Toronto

1 2 3 4 5 6 7 8 9   LHS   26 25 24 23 22 21

ISBN   978-1-260-46448-1
MHID   1-260-46448-2

e-ISBN 978-1-260-46449-8
e-MHID   1-260-46449-0

McGraw Hill products are available at special quantity discounts for use as premiums and sales promotions, or for use in corporate training programs. To contact a representative, please visit the Contact Us pages at www.mhprofessional.com.

Contents

Acknowledgments

First and foremost, I would like to commend and thank all of the nurses who worked during the COVID-19 crisis. Most of us had less than ideal situations to perform our jobs, but we nonetheless pushed through it and did what we do best. The majority of this book was written during the crisis as I worked in an ICU. This was an enormous challenge, but I hope you find benefit in this book as you push yourself to the next level of your career. You absolutely deserve it!

To my parents, Jane and Don Reid. I could not have done it without your support. To Edson, I love you.

About the Author

Michael Reid, MSN, RN, CCRN has been in critical care since entering the field of nursing many years ago. Initially being exposed to a cardiovascular surgical intensive care unit, Michael went on to work in medical, surgical, and trauma specialized intensive care units. He oversees the development of educational products for his company, *Nursology/The NCLEX Cure*, and as a consultant for companies and corporations. He is currently dividing his time between working in the ICU, teaching NCLEX and CCRN, writing books, and building new and exciting methods for education in nursing.

Introduction to the CCRN Exam

If you are reading this, you have likely reached a point in your career as a critical care nurse where you would like to take it to the next level. The CCRN certification does just that. It tells people around you that you have unique and specialized knowledge about critical care. It brings joy and confidence when working those long twelve-hour shifts. Depending on your institution, it may also result in a raise and potential job opportunities.

The American Association of Critical Care Nurses (AACN) creates the CCRN exam. This book is written for the adult critical care nursing certification and provides review on the entire test blueprint detailed in the following table. Certain areas are more important than others, so pay attention to where you spend your time studying. Practice makes perfect in so many things in life; with standardized tests such as this, I would agree.

Included in the Book

The CCRN exam blueprint was recently changed in early 2020. This book reflects this new update and includes **four** full-length practice tests, each brand new and made for the new blueprint. Each chapter has a detailed review of the testable areas and a quiz at the end to gauge retention.

Exam Structure

Kudos to you, critical care nurse! You have reached a point where you can take the CCRN certification exam. You have completed the requisite hours. Now is the time to put in the study hours and work to pass the exam itself. By reading this *McGraw-Hill Education CCRN Review*, you are on the right path to nailing this exam.

- Exam questions: 125 graded questions plus an additional 25 questions (not graded)
- Passing grade: 87 questions (70%) out of 125 questions required to pass

Adult CCRN Test Blueprint

TOPIC	NUMBER OF QUESTIONS (EXAM TOTAL: 125)	PERCENTAGE OF TEST
Clinical Judgment	**102 questions**	**80%**
Cardiovascular	21 questions	17%
Respiratory	19 questions	15%
Multisystem	17 questions	14%
Neurology	10 questions	8%
Gastrointestinal	8 questions	6%
Renal	8 questions	6%
Endocrinology	5 questions	4%
Behavioral/Psychosocial	5 questions	4%
Integumentary	3 questions	2%
Hematology/Immunology	3 questions	2%
Musculoskeletal	3 questions	2%
Professional Caring and Ethical Practice	**23 questions**	**20%**
Advocacy/Moral Agency	Questions roughly equal in weight for this section (~3% each)	
Caring Practices		
Response to Diversity		
Facilitation of Learning		
Collaboration		
Systems Thinking		
Clinical Inquiry		

If you have any questions regarding exam eligibility or the application itself, visit www.aacn.org.

Good Luck!
Michael Reid, MSN, RN, CCRN

CHAPTER 1

Critical Care Overview

This chapter includes catheter line access, hemodynamic monitoring, advanced electrocardiogram (ECG) interpretation, mechanical intubation, and sedation. These sections influence a variety of topic areas in this book and on the CCRN exam. By mastering these areas first, you will have a better idea of how the human body compensates or corrects issues visible to us through monitoring. Whether a patient has perforated the bowel, is experiencing a myocardial infarction, or has a severe allergic reaction, the data we assess is likely to show acute changes. Many questions on the CCRN exam will proceed assuming you know how to interpret all forms of hemodynamic information.

Catheter Line Access

There are two main forms of line access critical care nurses use on a daily basis, central lines and peripheral lines. There are many types of central lines; all require specialized training and care. Peripheral lines are covered in more detail in Chapter 7, "Integumentary," where infiltration is also covered.

Central Venous Catheter/Line (CAC)

- Catheter locations
  - Internal jugular (IJ-neck), subclavian (chest), and femoral (groin) lines
  - PICC lines and Midlines (arm)
  - Port-a-cath/Vas Cath/Perm-a-cath (chest)
- Clinical applications
  - Central venous pressure (CVP) monitoring
  - Medication (vasopressors, caustic meds)
  - Fluid administration
  - Total parenteral nutrition (TPN) administration
  - Long-term antibiotic needs
  - Dialysis (Shiley, Quinton)
  - Chemotherapy
- Risks
  - Pneumothorax, vascular damage, arrhythmias, or bleeding during placement
  - Infection (central line–associated bloodstream infection [CLABSI])

- Embolisms (thrombus formation, air embolism)
- Nursing considerations
  - Confirmation (x-ray) necessary before use
  - Never force flush clogged lumen (request alteplase)
  - Monitor coagulopathy
  - Always culture before antibiotics
  - Catheter tip sent to lab if pulled for CLABSI

Arterial Lines (A-line)

- Catheter locations
  - Radial or femoral (radial preferred; femoral carries larger infection risk)
- Clinical applications
  - Real-time blood pressure analysis
  - Arterial blood gas (ABG) draws
- Troubleshooting
  - Square Wave Test (zeroing of transducer)
  - Assess the patient first, then move toward technology
  - Overdamped: abnormally low reading (typically clots, kinks, or bad connections)
  - Underdamped: abnormally high reading (typically faulty set-up or transducer)
- Risks
  - Vasospasms during insertion → utilize lidocaine
  - Limb ischemia due to loss of collateral blood flow; always perform Allen's test to confirm adequate collateral blood flow.

Pulmonary Artery Catheter (PAC)

- Catheter locations
  - Pulmonary artery—the nurse may assist in the placement and be asked to inflate and deflate the balloon as the placement advances (see Figure 1-1)
  - Commonly called a *Swan-Ganz* catheter
- Clinical applications
  - Diagnostic assessment
    - Pulmonary pressure
    - Wedge pressures; read from the a-wave (little hill in the valley)
  - SvO_2 (mixed venous) blood draws/assessment
  - Monitor drug effects (pressors, inotropes, nitric oxide)
  - Treatment evaluations (balloon pumps, ventricular assistive devices)
- Troubleshooting
  - Square Wave Test
  - Overdamped (same as A-line)
  - Underdamped (same as A-line)
- Risks
  - Dysrhythmias during placement → monitor ECG for acute changes
  - Pneumothorax may occur during placement

- Catheter migration—it may slip out of position, monitor the waveform for changes
- Thrombosis formation—typically at the catheter tip. Never force flush.
- Pulmonary artery rupture (overinflated wedge) → never remove the balloon syringe from the port

Figure 1-1   Placement of PA Catheter: Pressure Analysis

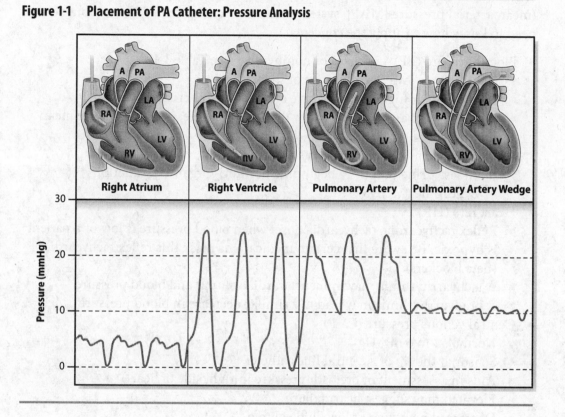

Dialysis Lines

Dialysis catheters are covered in more detail in Chapter 6, "Renal."

Hemodynamic Monitoring

On the CCRN exam, hemodynamic monitoring is included in questions for cardiovascular, pulmonary, and multisystem sections. It is most likely to arise in the cardiovascular section given the sheer number of questions in that test area. I have placed hemodynamic monitoring first in this book because of the vast importance to a number of critical care concepts.

Vital Signs/Hemodynamic Numbers

As a refresher, the following information shows vital signs and the general benchmarks. Changes occur to vital signs for a number of reasons. Aside from the disease process, vital signs may change due to treatments, medications, procedures, and complications. Being able to recognize an acute change from normal is essential. Advanced certification requires advanced reasoning. Luckily for you, the CCRN exam does not require you to memorize formulas for deducing numbers (mean arterial pressure [MAP], systemic vascular resistance [SVR], etc.), but you do need to know how to apply the concepts.

- Blood pressure (BP)—invasive or noninvasive (see Table 1-1)
  - 89 mmHg or lower is indicative of shock
  - 180 mmHg or higher is indicative of hypertensive crisis
  - Be cautious of an abnormally low diastolic pressure, it may influence mean arterial pressure and perfusion
  - MAP less than 60 often suggests a state of shock
    - Assess urine output → beginning of Multi-Organ Dysfunction Syndrome (MODS)
- Heart rate (HR)
  - Reflex tachycardia: tachycardia onset when blood pressure is low or a patient is hypoxic. Be aware that certain medications mask this reflex tachycardia (beta blockers).
  - A tachyarrhythmia may influence cardiac output and blood pressure
  - A bradyarrhythmia may lead to a similar decrease in blood pressure
- Central venous pressure (CVP)
  - Normal: 2 to 6 mmHg
  - Sensor at the tip of a central line catheter
  - Aids in assessment of preload (pressure in right side of heart)
  - Elevated may suggest heart failure
  - Decreased may suggest low fluid volume

Table 1-1   Quick A&P Review

BLOOD PRESSURE REGULATION

Baroreceptors	Chemoreceptors
• Aortic arch and carotid sinus	• Aortic arch and carotid sinus
• Artery walls stretch → vasodilation, decrease in HR (vagus nerve)	• O_2 and CO_2 sensitive
• Artery walls withdraw → vasoconstriction, increase in HR	• Decrease in oxygen → increase in HR and vasoconstriction (not in heart and brain)
	• Hydrogen ion (H^+) sensitive
Renin–Angiotensin–Aldosterone System (RAAS)	
• Renal blood flow regulates	
• Decrease in kidney perfusion → renin secretion	
• Na^+ and H_2O retention	
• Vasoconstriction	

Cardiac Output (CO)/Index

The amount of blood being pumped out of the heart will directly influence a number of processes. This is why CO is enormously important. Many factors influence CO, but the simplest way to understand CO is through the following equation: CO = HR × stroke volume (SV). Stroke volume equals the amount of blood ejected from the heart with every heartbeat.

- CO = HR × SV
- Cardiac output can change one of two ways:
  - Increase or decrease of heart rate
  - Changes to stroke volume (described below)
- Cardiac index (CI) is calculated by taking the CO and dividing it by body surface area (BSA): CI = CO/BSA

Stroke Volume

Changes to stroke volume affect a multitude of critical care areas—most noticeably, the cardiovascular system. What is the causative factor for a changing stroke volume? What signs and symptoms might be seen with changes in stroke volume? The following three terms are important; understand them well.

Preload
- Blood returning to the right side of the heart
- Central venous pressure (CVP): may show overall volume status and worsening right-sided compliance
- Pulmonary artery occlusion pressure (PAOP) is sometimes used when "wedging" the balloon on a PA catheter. It may show overall pressure from the left side of the heart → left-sided heart failure.
- Increasing preload may lead to ventricular failure and cardiomyopathy

Contractility
- The squeeze (contraction) of the heart
- Often manipulated via medications (inotropes)

Afterload
- The force with which the left ventricle must overcome to open valves and eject blood
- Systemic vascular resistance (SVR) affects left ventricle afterload
- Pulmonary vascular resistance (PVR) affects right ventricle afterload

Treatments for Hemodynamics

To be able to treat an abnormal hemodynamic value, you must first understand what normal is. Below are a series of treatment modalities for commonly seen abnormal hemodynamics.

Low Preload
- Patient may be hypovolemic (dehydrated)
- Often the first intervention to correct low BP issues

- Common saying to "fill up the tank"
- Administer
  - Crystalloids (normal saline and lactated Ringer's most common)
  - Colloids (albumin, blood products)

High Preload
- Patient may be fluid overloaded (edema)
- Administer
  - Diuretics (furosemide is common)
  - If the patient is too unstable for forced diuresis, an intravenous drip of bumetanide may be used to prevent rapid changes in fluid volume
  - In severely unstable patients who cannot tolerate even slight changes to volume status, continuous renal replacement therapy (CRRT) or continuous veno-venous hemofiltration (CVVH) may be used

Low Afterload
- Patient is likely vasodilated
- Often the sign of effective treatment such as intra-aortic balloon pump usage
- Expected finding in certain types of shock (septic, anaphylactic, neurogenic)
- Administer (if needed)
  - Norepinephrine (Levophed)
- Remember, if an afterload is abnormally low, it may be due to an overshoot or overly effective treatment. It is possible the primary treatment simply needs to be decreased.

High Afterload
- Patient is likely vasoconstricted (clamped down)
- Prolonged periods of high afterload may lead to heart failure
- Administer
  - Nitrates (nitroglycerin, nitroprusside) (SVR reduction)
  - Hydralazine and clonidine (SVR reduction)
  - Sildenafil or nitric oxide (PVR reduction)

Low Contractility
- Patient may have heart failure
- Administer
  - Inotropic agents
    - Digoxin
    - Dobutamine
    - Epinephrine
    - Dopamine (high dose)
    - Milrinone (right-sided heart failure)

High Contractility
- Patient may have heightened sympathetic nervous response (fight or flight) or metabolic issues (hyperthyroidism)
- Not typically dangerous unless sustained for long periods of time

- Administer
  - Beta blockers
  - Calcium-channel blockers
  - Fix the underlying problem (nervous system, metabolic pathways)

Hemodynamic Values

Learning all the key hemodynamic areas can certainly be tricky. Even more difficult is understanding what each direction may mean when one goes up or down. Begin with learning the normal hemodynamic ranges. To reiterate, Table 1-2 shows the most important hemodynamic numbers. The individual chapters of this book will explain why a certain hemodynamic change may happen due to a disease or disorder.

Table 1-2   Hemodynamic Values

HEMODYNAMIC/OXYGENATION VALUE	NORMAL PARAMETER
Mean arterial pressure (MAP)	70–110 mmHg • <60 mmHg considered shock (check urine output)
Cardiac output (CO)	4–8 L/min
Cardiac index (CI)	2.5–4.0 L/min/m²
Stroke volume (SV)	50–100 mL/beat
Stroke index	25–45 mL/beat/m²
Central venous pressure (CVP) Right atrial pressure (RAP)	2–6 mmHg
Pulmonary artery pressure	15–30 mmHg (systolic) 2–8 mmHg (diastolic)
Pulmonary artery wedge pressure (PAWP) Pulmonary artery occlusion pressure (PAOP)	6–12 mmHg
Systemic vascular resistance (SVR)	800–1200 dynes/s/cm⁻⁵
Pulmonary vascular resistance (PVR)	50–250 dynes/s/cm⁻⁵
Mixed venous oxygen saturation (SvO₂)	60–75%
Central venous oxygen saturation (ScvO₂)	Greater than 70%
Arterial oxygen saturation (SaO₂)	95–99% (room air) • Do not confuse with PaO₂ on arterial blood gases

Oxygenation Monitoring

By monitoring oxygenation throughout the body, the nurse may evaluate current levels, delivery, and consumption necessary for metabolic function. Changes in patient condition or evaluation of treatments may be assessed through monitoring oxygenation levels. These concepts are applied more specifically in the pulmonary chapter.

- Mixed venous oxygen saturation (SvO_2)
  - The amount of oxygen on hemoglobin returning to the lungs
  - Normal: 60% to 75%
    - Low: body using more oxygen (infection, low cardiac output, low SaO_2, anemia)
    - High: body using less oxygen (late septic shock, hypothermia)
- Central venous oxygen saturation ($ScvO_2$)
  - The amount of oxygen on hemoglobin returning to central access (IJ or subclavian line)
  - Normal: greater than 70%
  - Low or high for same reasons as SvO_2
- End-tidal carbon dioxide ($EtCO_2$)
  - The amount of partial pressure carbon dioxide at the end of exhalation
  - Capnography
  - Normal: 35 to 45 mmHg
  - Elevation of $EtCO_2$ displays retention and hypoventilation
  - Confirmation of endotracheal tube placement (colorimeter)
  - Assessment of CPR effectiveness
- Oxygen consumption (VO_2)
  - Normal: 250 to 350 mL/min
  - Consumption is low in septic shock
- Oxygen delivery (DO_2)
  - Normal: 900 to 1100 mL/min
  - Delivery is low in poor cardiac function

Advanced ECG Interpretation

One of the most difficult skills to master is the ability to read an ECG quickly, if at all. Many people struggle with being able to distinguish certain rhythms, especially since many of these rhythms may look similar. Supraventricular tachycardia may look a lot like atrial fibrillation with rapid ventricular response. The CCRN exam does not always have an ECG strip to analyze, so understand interventions for the rhythms and the full clinical picture. Certain things do pop up more often on the exam, such as pacing, QT prolongation, torsades, and implantable cardioverter-defibrillators (ICDs). Note that the exam assumes you understand advanced cardiovascular life support (ACLS) protocol and the basics of a code blue.

Applying Leads

Before placing leads, the nurse must know what kind of ECG is required. Understand a 3-lead, 5-lead, and 12-lead ECG. There are also circumstances where a reverse (right-sided) ECG may be requested by the physician. This is typically during a right-sided myocardial infarction. Remember the basic landmarks utilized when placing leads: the midclavicular line, mid-axillary line, and the ability to count intercostal spaces effectively.

- 3-lead ECG requires three bipolar leads: right arm, left arm, and left leg. It provides one angle of view on the heart.
- 5-lead ECG requires all four bipolar leads on the limbs. It also includes one precordial (unipolar) lead. The precordial lead is typically placed at the V_1 position, but it may be moved. It provides three angles of view on the heart.
- 12-lead ECG requires all four bipolar leads and six precordial leads.
- Right-sided ECG requires normal bipolar lead placement. The precordial leads are placed in the same V_1 through V_6 position, but mirrored or reversed:
  - V_1: fourth intercostal, right sternal border
  - V_2: fourth intercostal, left sternal border
  - V_3: halfway between V_2 and V_4
  - V_4: fifth intercostal, left midclavicular line
  - V_5: fifth intercostal, left anterior axillary line
  - V_6: fifth intercostal, left mid-axillary line

ECG Interpretation

Identifying a rhythm and how to react in each scenario is detailed next. A common strategy is to think about interventions from a "least invasive to most" mentality. This is how healthcare professionals commonly react in a hospital setting. Hopefully, a lot of this is review.

Normal Sinus Rhythm (NSR)

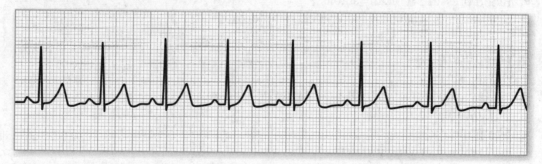

It is hard to understand what abnormal is without an understanding of normal. Here is a strip of NSR as a reference point. Note the consistency of the "p" waves with the corresponding skinny "QRS" complex and "T" wave.

Sinus Tachycardia

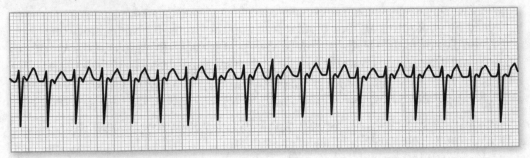

Interpretation
- 100 BPM or more

Causes
- Reflex tachycardia (hypovolemia, hypoxia)
- Stimulants (caffeine, drugs or medications, etc.)
- Pain or fear
- Hypoglycemia
- Hyperthyroidism

Signs and Symptoms
- Heart pounds or pacing (palpitations)
- Diaphoresis (sweating)
- Blood pressure typically stable
    - Dizziness: may be hypotensive (symptomatic)

Interventions
- Asymptomatic
    - Typically nothing; treat underlying problem
    - Continue to monitor
- Symptomatic
    - Treat underlying problem
    - Beta blocker

Sinus Bradycardia

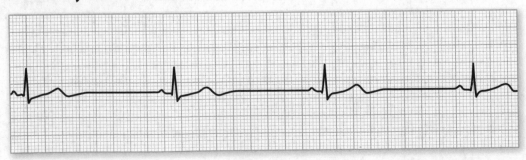

Interpretation
- 59 BPM or less

Causes
- Hypothyroidism
- Depressant medications
  - Alcohol
  - Benzodiazepines
  - Opioids
- Professional athletes

Signs and Symptoms
- Fatigue
- Hypotension causing dizziness (symptomatic)

Interventions
- Asymptomatic
  - Treat underlying problem
  - Continue to monitor
- Symptomatic
  - Treat underlying problem
  - Atropine if symptomatic
  - Pacing if nothing else works and patient condition warrants (unconscious, dangerously low BP)

Atrial Fibrillation without Rapid Ventricular Response (RVR)

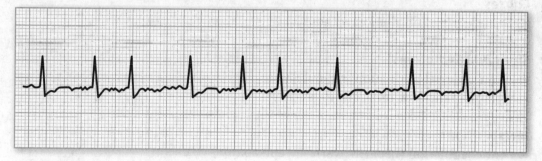

Interpretation
- Multiple atrial depolarizations with inconsistent "QRS" complexes
- 60–100 BPM

Causes
- Cardiovascular disease
- Heart failure
- Heart defect
- Heart surgery (especially when close to the SA node)
- Old age (chronic)

Signs and Symptoms
- Typically asymptomatic
- Severe if leading to embolism events (MI, PE, CVA)

Interventions
- Anticoagulant (heparin, warfarin, apixaban)
- If attempting to revert back to NSR
  - Cardizem (diltiazem)
  - Cardioversion may be used by physician request if the patient condition warrants and nothing else has worked
  - Catheter ablation (maze procedure)

Atrial Fibrillation with Rapid Ventricular Response (RVR)

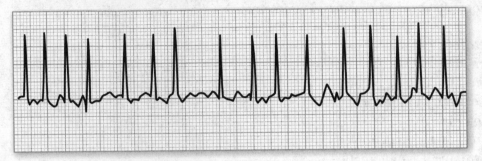

Interpretation
- Multiple atrial depolarizations with inconsistent "QRS" complexes
- 100 BPM or more

Causes
- Same as atrial fibrillation without RVR

Signs and Symptoms
- Same as atrial fibrillation without RVR
- Symptomatic (dizziness due to low BP)

Interventions
- Anticoagulation (heparin, warfarin, apixaban)
- Beta blocker
- Cardizem (diltiazem)
- Cardioversion may be used by physician request if the patient condition warrants and nothing else has worked
- Catheter ablation (maze procedure)

Atrial Flutter

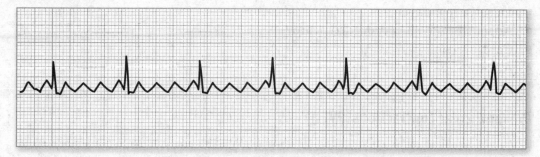

Atrial flutter has similar causes, signs and symptoms, and interventions to atrial fibrillation. It is typically spoken about in reference to the AV conduction. The above rhythm has a 4:1 conduction ratio. The sawtooth waves between "QRS" complexes are called "f" (flutter) waves.

Supraventricular Tachycardia (SVT)

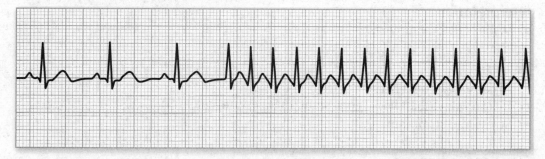

SVT is a type of reentry rhythm caused by an electrical loop moving around the atria at a fast rate. One of the easiest ways to differentiate between a sinus tachycardia and an SVT is by simply identifying the rate. Anything above 150 is fairly indicative of an SVT. This cannot be confirmed, however, without an ECG.

Interpretation
- 150 BPM or higher
- Skinny "QRS" complexes

Causes
- Often paroxysmal
- Atrial fibrillation or atrial flutter
- Wolff-Parkinson-White syndrome

Signs and Symptoms
- Palpitations
- Fatigue and shortness of breath
- Loss of blood pressure → unconscious

CCRN Tip

Wolf-Parkinson-White syndrome is an electrical conduction disorder. It typically leads to abnormally high heart rates with or without symptoms and may be diagnosed via short PR intervals and characteristic "delta" waves. If the condition is serious enough, radiofrequency ablation may be required.

Interventions

- Valsalva maneuver
- Adenosine (crash cart needed nearby)
- Cardioversion
- Ablation

Preventricular Contractions (PVCs)

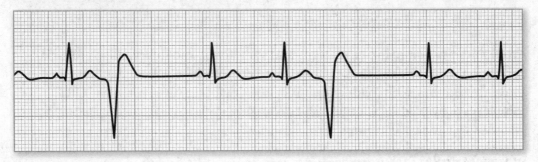

Interpretation

- Wide "QRS" complexes

Causes

- Myocardial damage (MI)
- Electrolyte imbalances (potassium, magnesium, calcium)
- Stress and stimulants

Signs and Symptoms

- Oftentimes none
- Feeling of skipped heartbeat

Interventions

- Telemetry monitoring
- Treat underlying problem
- Review chemistry panel
- Medications (amiodarone IV, lidocaine IV)

Intrinsic Automaticity

The underlying conduction system is fairly straightforward. Rhythms with a BPM above the intrinsic rate are typically called "accelerated." If they are significantly higher, the rhythm is called "tachycardia."

- SA node: 60 to 100 BPM
- AV node: 40 to 60 BPM
- Purkinje fibers: 20 to 40 BPM

Idioventricular Rhythm

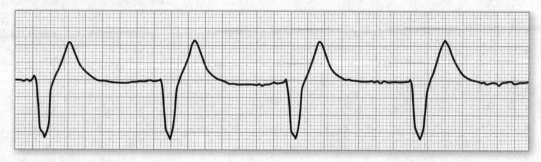

Interpretation
- Wide "QRS" complexes

Causes
- Diseases (infection, anemia)
- Drug toxicity
- Electrolyte imbalances
- Post reperfusion: this rhythm may be noticed transiently in ICU (accelerated idiopathic ventricular rhythm [AIVR])

Signs and Symptoms
- Often none (asymptomatic)
- Hypotension causing dizziness (symptomatic)

Interventions
- Treat the underlying problem
- Atropine
- Amiodarone or lidocaine
- Pacing

Ventricular Tachycardia (VT aka V-Tach)

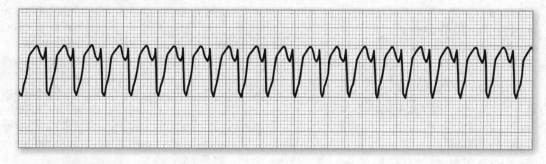

Interpretation
- Wide "QRS" complexes
- Typically 170 BPM or more

Causes
- Myocardial damage (MI)
- Hypotension/hypovolemia
- H's and T's

Signs and Symptoms
- Pulsed versus pulseless
- Conscious versus unconscious
- Diaphoretic and dizzy (symptomatic)

Interventions
- Pulseless electrical activity (PEA)
  - CPR, defibrillate, medications
  - Treat the underlying problem
- Asymptomatic
  - Treat the underlying problem
  - Monitor for progression to PEA

Torsades de Pointe

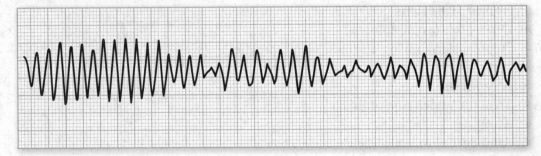

Interpretation
- Drastic variety of "QRS" complexes

Causes
- Hypomagnesemia
- QT prolongation

Signs and Symptoms
- Same as ventricular tachycardia

Interventions
- ACLS protocol
- Magnesium sulfate
- Treat the underlying problem

CCRN Tip

QT prolongation often occurs due to medications such as haloperidol or other antipsychotics. Some antibiotics and digitalis toxicity may also lead to QT prolongation. Less common causes are electrolyte imbalances.

Ventricular Fibrillation (VF aka V-Fib)

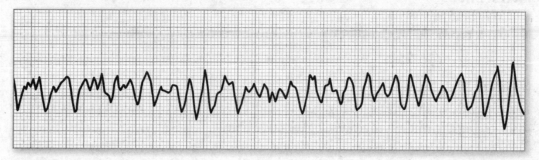

Interpretation
- Quivering or fibrillating waves

Causes
- H's and T's

Signs and Symptoms
- Pulseless
- Loss of blood pressure
- Unconscious

Interventions
- Code blue
- ACLS protocol

> **CCRN Tip**
>
> Any loss of perfusion to the brain longer than *5 minutes* may lead to brain damage.

Asystole

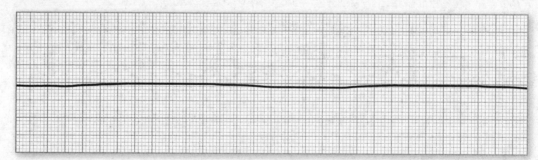

Interpretation
- Flat line

Causes
- H's and T's

Signs and Symptoms
- Pulseless
- Loss of blood pressure
- Unconscious

Interventions
- Code blue
- ACLS protocol: NOT a shockable rhythm

H's and T's

During code situations, utilizing the H's and T's is an effective way of potentially discovering the underlying cause of the code blue.

H's
- Hypovolemia
- Hypoxia
- Hydrogen ions (acidosis)
- Hypo/hyperkalemia
- Hypoglycemia
- Hypothermia

T's
- Tamponade
- Toxins
- Tension pneumothorax
- Thrombosis (heart or lungs)
- Trauma

First-Degree AV Block

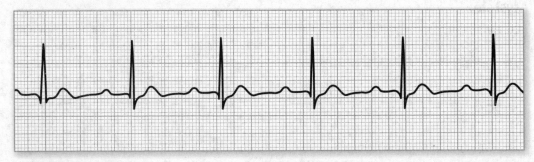

Interpretation
- Prolonged "PR" interval: longer than 0.20 seconds

Causes
- Node damage
- Myocardial damage
- Electrolytes and medication

Signs and Symptoms
- No symptoms

Interventions
- Correct underlying problem
- Benign → continue to monitor

Second-Degree Type 1 AV Block

Second-degree type 1 is also called a Mobitz type 1, or Wenckebach. Note the short PR interval that is followed by one or more longer intervals. Occasionally, the beat or "QRS" is completely dropped. It helps to say "short, longer, longer, drop." The causes, symptoms, and interventions are similar to the other first- and second-degree heart blocks.

Second-Degree Type 2 AV Block

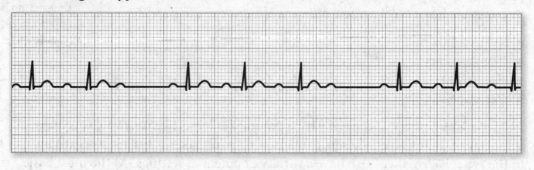

The manner in which a second-degree type 2 AV block is approached is similar to first-degree and second-degree type 1 AV blocks. Note the consistent distance of the PR interval. In a type 2, the "QRS" is dropped occasionally.

Third-Degree AV Block

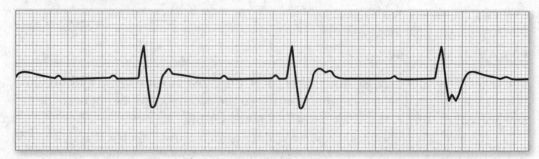

Third-degree AV block is certainly the most dangerous heart block. It is often called "complete" heart block given the complete noncommunication between the atria and the ventricles. The "p" waves are consistent and the "QRS" complexes are consistent, but not to each other.

Causes
- Myocardial damage (ischemia and infarction)
- Diseases and disorders

Signs and Symptoms
- Dizziness

Interventions
- Correct underlying condition
- Medications (positive chronotropes)
- Pacing

Pacing

There are many moments when pacing may be required in the ICU setting, but they all have a common theme. The rhythm of the patient is not conducive or adequate for patient survival. The most common indication for pacing is symptomatic bradycardia followed by complete heart block. A few different options exist to pace:

- Transcutaneous
- Transvenous
- Epicardial
- Permanent

CCRN Tip

Pacing is a fairly common subject on the CCRN exam in cardiology. Study this section here and in Chapter 2, "Cardiovascular."

Having an understanding of what a pacemaker looks like on an ECG is of equal importance. Being able to assess a functioning pacemaker is essential regardless of the type. Pacemakers also have a variety of potential settings. At the most basic, a pacemaker is either fixed at a rate or demand. Asynchronous settings (not listed below) are rarely used, it is not a good idea to override intrinsic electrical activity for too long. An "R on T" phenomenon may occur.

The common settings follow a basic pacemaker code with three letters. The first letter denotes the chamber paced. The second letter denotes the chamber sensed. The third letter denotes the response to the sensing.

- DDD: dual-chamber pacing
- VVI: ventricular demand
- AAI: atrial demand

The letter "I" symbolizes to inhibit. The pacer will sense any intrinsic rhythms and inhibit a stimulus. This is a common setting so the pacemaker does not override any normal rhythms. This is a type of "demand" setting.

The letter "D" symbolizes the pacer will sense an intrinsic electrical activity and fire a stimulus in response. The letter "O" symbolizes "none"—the pacer will do nothing in relation to that position letter. For example, if a setting is "VOO," the pacer will pace the ventricles asynchronously.

Atrial Pacing

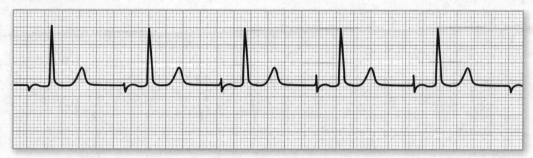

Interpretation
- Pacer spike before "p" waves

Ventricular Pacing

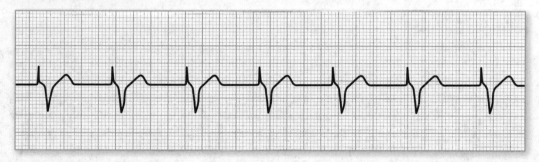

Interpretation
- Pacer spike before "QRS" complexes

Atrioventricular (AV) Pacing

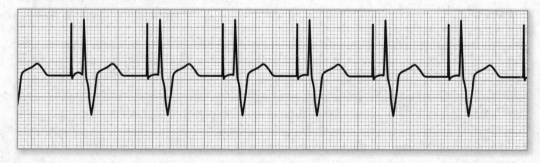

Interpretation
- Pacer spikes before "p" waves and "QRS" complexes
- Dual-chamber pacing

Failure to Pace

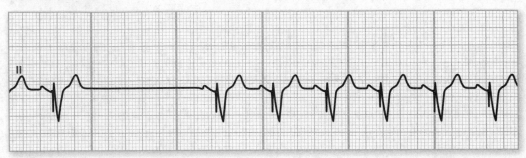

When there is a failure to pace, there is no spike at all. It often appears to be a simple flatline. This can be incredibly problematic for obvious reasons, especially if it lasts for too long (hypotension, orthostasis, syncope). Depending on the underlying rhythm, the patient may code.

Failure to Capture

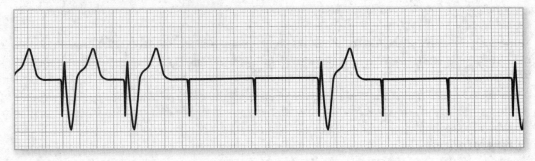

Interpretation
- Pacer spikes not followed by a depolarization (QRS)

Causes
- Low stimulus output
- Pacer dislodgement
- Scar tissue (fibrosis) buildup

Signs and Symptoms
- Typically none
- Possible hypotension if excessive

Interventions
- Increase stimulus power
- Confirm placement

Failure to Sense (Undersensing)

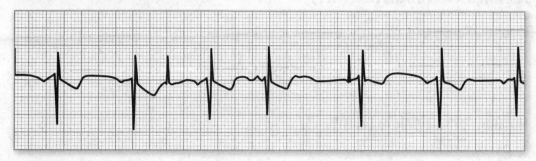

Interpretation
■ Pacer does not recognize intrinsic electrical activity of the heart
■ Asynchronized beats and pacer spikes

Causes
■ Pacer sensitivity too low
■ Malfunction
■ Lead displacement

Signs and Symptoms
■ Often none
■ Palpitations

Interventions
■ Increase pacer sensing
■ Check battery on pacer
■ Assess for underlying causative problems (electrolyte, etc.)

Defibrillation and ICDs

The two shockable rhythms—ventricular tachycardia and ventricular fibrillation—and how a nurse should behave in a code situation are covered by ACLS protocol. The CCRN exam expects an understanding of ACLS protocol—in *what order* actions are performed and *why* certain actions are performed. In the action of defibrillation, the pads are never placed over underlying technology, such as a pacemaker or ICD.

Most ICDs are placed due to a fatal dysrhythmia the patient may revert into (V-tach or V-fib). The majority of pacemakers, however, can also pace in addition to shocking. ICDs can send a rapid stimulus (burst) to override a tachyarrhythmia, the goal being to revert back to normal sinus. The ICD can also be programmed to pace and override a bradyarrhythmia.

Noninvasive Ventilation (NIV)

NIV is a useful tool for practitioners to assist patients with ventilation without intubation. Because intubation carries a number of risks, NIV is a preferable less-invasive measure to correct respiratory problems.

Nursing Considerations for NIV

- Mask should fit tightly
- Confirm rate and pressure with clinician
  - Inspiratory positive airway pressure (IPAP)
  - Expiratory positive airway pressure (EPAP)
- Confirm FiO_2 if required

Mechanical Intubation

There are a number of reasons why a patient may need to be intubated and mechanically ventilated. Most of these reasons are pulmonary in nature, but not all. Generally speaking, most situations begin by the use of noninvasive positive-pressure ventilation. As any ICU nurse knows, we have wonderful teams of respiratory therapists (RTs) to help manage the patient on a ventilator. While an RT is present on the unit, they may not always be available, so it is important to understand a variety of factors when dealing with a ventilated patient. *Review the reasons to intubate below:*

- Respiratory failure
  - Trauma
  - Pneumothorax
  - Acute respiratory distress syndrome (ARDS)
  - Alcohol/drug overdose
- Cardiac compromise
  - Cardiac arrest
  - Shock (loss of airway and breathing likely imminent)
- Airway obstruction
  - Burns to the airways (smoke inhalation)
  - Anaphylaxis
- Surgery

CCRN Tip

Malignant hyperthermia is a potentially fatal complication of neuromuscular blocking agents. Monitor for rapid-onset hyperthermia and muscle rigidity. The medication dantrolene is often used in this emergency.

Endotracheal Intubation

If the decision for intubating a patient has been made, collect the required equipment and notify the RT. Ensure an ambu-bag is in the room.

- Medications used during intubation → if the patient is conscious
  - Succinylcholine and rocuronium (**Caution:** Check potassium before giving the medication)
  - Etomidate
  - Propofol
- Endotracheal tube (ETT) placement confirmation
  - Observe color change on end-tidal CO_2
  - Observe bilateral lung rising
  - Auscultate lungs and stomach (no gurgling)
  - Chest x-ray
    - Carina (typically 3 cm above)
    - Tube may need to be manipulated
  - ABG analysis roughly 30 minutes after intubation

> **CCRN Tip**
>
> Height is a commonly used number to begin a baseline tidal volume before any ventilator changes may be made. Body mass is another tool commonly used. An average benchmark for tidal volume is 450–500 mL; 8–10 mL/kg is fairly standard.

Ventilator Modes

The art of mastering mode usage along with ventilator settings takes quite a bit of practice. In fact, there are entire books devoted solely to ventilators and their use. In general, most ICU ventilators begin at a predetermined setting upon intubation. Changes are made based on ABGs or patient presentation. An important thing to note is your ability as an RN to decide if an ABG is needed. If you are concerned about ventilator-related problems or changes in the patient oxygenation, relay that information and consult.

> **CCRN Tip**
>
> Understanding which mode and setting may be best for specific patients is often part of the CCRN exam. For example, a patient who is becoming exhausted in SIMV mode may benefit by a switch to AC mode.

- Assist control (AC)
  - Complete control mode (RR and tidal volume)
  - Patient-triggered breaths
  - Pros
    - ARDS/ALI (acute lung injury) usage
  - Cons
    - Hyperinflation (barotrauma), tachypnea complications (alkalosis)
- Synchronized intermittent mandatory ventilation (SIMV)
  - Support mode
  - May be for a set volume or rate (demand-type mode)
  - Pros
    - Patient-triggered work (synchronized)
    - Guaranteed minimum settings (prevents complications)
  - Cons
    - Increase work of breathing

- Pressure support
  - Weaning mode (turn off sedation)
  - Pressure helps breath through the constriction of the ETT
    - Typically 5–10 cm H_2O pressure
  - Pros
    - Patient manages everything but pressure
    - Strengthens respiratory muscles
    - Good for chronically ventilated patients (chronic obstructive pulmonary disease [COPD], deconditioned, rehab)
  - Cons
    - No backup settings
    - Not an effective mode for any patients on higher-than-normal settings (elevated PEEP [positive end-expiratory pressure], higher than 40% FiO_2)
    - Patient may become tired (respiratory failure)
      - Anxiety and restlessness are an early sign of difficulty breathing and hypoxia

Less commonly used modes include a variety of **high-frequency ventilation (HFV)**. Mechanical ventilation never begins with these modes; they are all rare and considered rescue therapies. The general premise of HFV is the prevention of **volutrauma** while maximizing oxygenation. Some of the latter modes are used for surgeries and procedures to minimize thoracic movement.

- High-frequency oscillatory ventilation
  - Very high respiratory rates (above 60/min)
  - Very small tidal volumes
  - Most common high-frequency mode used
  - ALI and ARDS patients
- High-frequency percussive ventilation
  - Severe traumatic brain injury (TBI) patients
    - Issues related to intercranial pressure (ICP)
- High-frequency jet ventilation
- High-frequency positive-pressure ventilation

Ventilator Settings

- Respiratory rate
  - 12–16/minute for standard patients
- Tidal volume
  - 8–10 mL/kg for standard patients
  - 6 mL/kg for ARDS
- Positive end-expiratory pressure (PEEP)
  - 5 cm H_2O standard
  - Aids in expansion of alveoli
    - ARDS
  - Risk for decrease in cardiac output as PEEP increases (intrathoracic pressure)
  - Risk for barotrauma as PEEP increases

- Fraction of inspired oxygen (FiO_2)
  - 40%: minimum before extubation
  - 50%: extubation might be considered
  - 100%: maximum

Patient Care Considerations

- Assess ETT level (at the lip) minimum per shift
- Always have an ambu-bag in the room of a ventilated patient (in case of accidental extubation)
- Rotate ETT position (prevent pressure ulcers on the lip)
- Deep suction when needed, not frequently for no reason
- Prevention of self-extubation (sedation, restraints, teaching, etc.)
- Prevention of ventilator-associated pneumonia (VAP) can be found in the respiratory chapter

At times, a patient may acutely decompensate while on mechanical ventilation. Continuously assess for respiratory distress. Some common reasons are:

- ETT dislodgment or migration
- Pneumothorax
- Pulmonary embolism
- ETT obstruction (mucus plug or frequent biting)

Troubleshooting Ventilators

No matter the potential issue you are presented with from a ventilator, in the moment, the best reaction is to assess the patient first. Start at the patient and move onward to the technology itself. This behavior is good for a wide variety of technology troubleshoots, not just ventilators.

High-Pressure Alarms

Oftentimes the simplest explanation for a high-pressure alarm is the patient waking up or becoming anxious while ventilated. Assess the patient/situation. Increasing sedation is not always the correct intervention.

- Obstruction related
  - Biting/coughing
  - Kinging of ETT
  - Water in tubing circuitry
  - Thick secretions/mucus plug
  - Decreased lung compliance (ARDS)

Low-Pressure Alarms

- Circuit disconnection (tubing fell off of ETT)
- Leaks

> **CCRN Tip**
>
> If the patient continuously fights the ventilator and is desaturating, it is often helpful to disconnect them from the ventilator and bag them (unless high PEEP is required). Breaking of the circuitry should be a last resort, however, given the risk of VAP. If the problem persists, contact the physician about changing ventilator settings or sedation. Never ignore a ventilator alarm.

Weaning to Extubate

Research is very clear that prolonged ventilation is directly related to poor outcomes and mortality. The goal is to extubate as soon as possible, but *safely*. To do this, there is protocol to be closely followed:

- Patient on minimal settings (50% or less FiO_2)
- Initiate spontaneous breathing trial
  - Turn off sedation (patient should be awake)
  - Pressure support mode
- Assess patient vital signs
- Assess ABG
- Weaning parameters performed (typically by respiratory therapy)
  - Vital capacity
  - Negative inspiratory force (NIF): greater than 25 cm H_2O
- Decision to extubate made

Failure Criteria for Breathing Trials
- Tachycardia or tachypnea
- Respiratory distress (accessory muscle usage)
- Hypoxia (SpO_2)
- Changes in cardiac rhythm
- Changes in hemodynamics

Sedation and Neuromuscular Blockade

Adequate sedation for patients in the ICU can be of utmost importance. Adequate sedation allows ventilators to synchronize better, thus ventilating better; however, the primary reason for sedation is certainly to *reduce anxiety and pain*. Be cautious about oversedation, as this affects the ability to extubate within an appropriate amount of time and overall morbidity. The drug dexmedetomidine (Precedex) is becoming popular for this exact reason.

Assessing for Adequate Sedation

The goal of adequate sedation is for a calm yet arousable patient who can follow commands. The reality can oftentimes be different, but that is the goal. There are many scales ranking the sedation of patients, two of the most common are below.

Richmond Agitation Sedation Scale (RASS)
- +4 to +1: levels of agitation
- *0: alert and calm (goal)*
- *–1: drowsy (goal)*
- –2: light sedation
- –3: moderate sedation
- –4 : deep sedation
- –5: unarousable

CCRN Tip

In most cases, as described above, the patient should be arousable. There are circumstances in an ICU where nurses provide moderate sedation using midazolam and fentanyl. The most common situation sedation scales will be utilized on the CCRN exam are in relation to ventilated patients.

Ramsey Scale

- 1: anxious or agitated
- *2: oriented and calm (goal)*
- *3: follows commands (goal)*
- 4: brief response to stimuli
- 5: minimal response to stimuli
- 6: no response to stimuli

Neuromuscular Blockade Agent (NMBA)

Blocking a patient's ability to move their body is no small decision, but there are times it is incredibly useful. When using a paralytic agent, *train-of-four* is used to assess appropriate dosing and titration of the IV medication. *Bispectral index monitoring* is used to assess adequate sedation. Some of the reasons for neuromuscular blockade are as follows:

- Aid in the improvement of ventilation
  - Lung compliance
  - Patient fighting ventilator
- ARDS (very poor ventilation ratio)
- Hypothermia (prevent shivering)

CHAPTER 2

Cardiovascular

The cardiovascular section makes up roughly 21 questions on your CCRN exam, which means that approximately 17% of the exam is devoted to this section alone. Because it reflects such a large portion of a singular topic, it is important to focus more energy on these concepts. You may receive only a few questions on immunology, but the cardiovascular section is a guaranteed certainty. If you have not done so already, remember to read the critical care overview chapter. It outlines hemodynamic concepts and ECG information applied to many cardiovascular issues.

Acute Coronary Syndromes (ACS)

Understanding the different types of ACS is commonplace on the CCRN exam. Are you able to differentiate between the signs and symptoms if presented? What if an ECG is provided for myocardial infarctions (MIs)? What area of the heart is likely being affected by simply looking at an ECG? Master which leads affect which areas of the heart. ACS include unstable angina and myocardial infarctions.

Quick A&P Review

- Main branches
  - Left main coronary artery (LCA)
    - Left anterior descending (LAD)
      - Septum perfusion
      - Anterior wall (left ventricle) perfusion
    - Circumflex
      - Lateral (free) wall (left ventricle) perfusion
  - Right coronary artery (RCA)
    - Right marginal arteries
      - RA and RV perfusion
      - Conduction system perfusion
    - Posterior descending
      - Posterior wall perfusion
- Coronary arteries perfuse during diastole
- Tachyarrhythmias may lead to ischemic issues (decreased coronary perfusion)

The heart uses roughly 70% of the oxygen that flows through the coronary arteries. This number is significantly higher than other areas of the body (25%). It goes to show how reliant the heart is on oxygen flow through the coronaries.

Figure 2-1   Coronary arteries

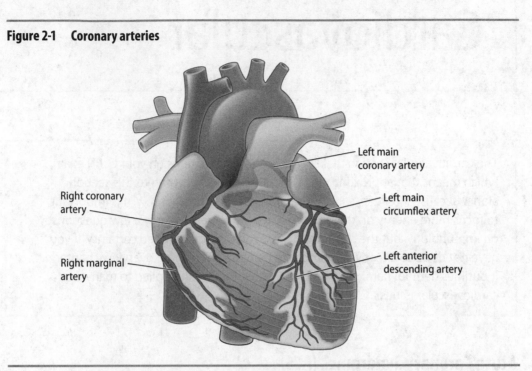

Left main coronary artery

Right coronary artery

Left main circumflex artery

Right marginal artery

Left anterior descending artery

Anatomy Point

It is worth noting that people may have different anatomies. The posterior descending artery may also branch off of the LCA (left dominant circulation). Roughly two-thirds of the time, however, it branches from the RCA (right dominant circulation). The heart is fairly good at creating anastomosis as well to compensate for any fluctuations in blood flow.

ACS

Etiology
- Demographic factors (sex, age, genes)
- Lifestyle factors (smoking, alcohol, diet, sedentary)
- Medical factors (CAD, diabetes, metabolic syndrome, etc.)
- Pharmacological factors (chemotherapy, vasopressin)

Signs and Symptoms
- Stable angina
  - Pain upon activity
- Unstable angina
  - Random (occasionally sustained) onset of chest pain/pressure
  - ST depression or T-wave inversion
  - Negative cardiac markers

CCRN Tip

Atypical presentation: Women, the elderly, and diabetics may not have typical chest pain; flu-like symptoms, jaw pain, and feelings of malaise should not be ignored.

- Non-ST elevation myocardial infarction (NSTEMI)
  - Chest pain
  - Positive cardiac markers (troponin)
  - ST depression and T-wave inversion
- ST elevation myocardial infarction (STEMI)
  - Chest pain
  - Positive cardiac markers (troponin)
  - ST elevation (multiple leads)
  - New-onset left bundle branch block (LBBB)

Diagnostics
- Vital signs, rapid assessment
- EKG
  - **ASAP** (perform *first* within 10 minutes)
  - Large-peaked T waves → onset of injury
  - ST elevation → injury → minutes to hours after
  - T-wave inversion → ischemia → hours after
  - Q waves → infarct → hours to days after

Table 2-1 details ECG changes in MIs. This information is very important; you will encounter it on the CCRN exam!

Table 2-1   ECG Changes in Myocardial Infarctions

INFARCT AREA	LEAD CHANGES	CORONARY ARTERY
Anterior left ventricle	V1, V2, V3, V4	Left anterior descending
Inferior left ventricle	II, III, aVF	Right coronary artery
Lateral (free) left ventricle	V5, V6, I, aVL	Circumflex
Posterior left ventricle	V1, V2	Right coronary artery
Right ventricle	V3R, V4R	Right coronary artery

Note: The "R" in the leads reflects a right-sided ECG. The lead placement is mirrored, same positions on the right side of the chest.

Figure 2-2   ECG infarct areas

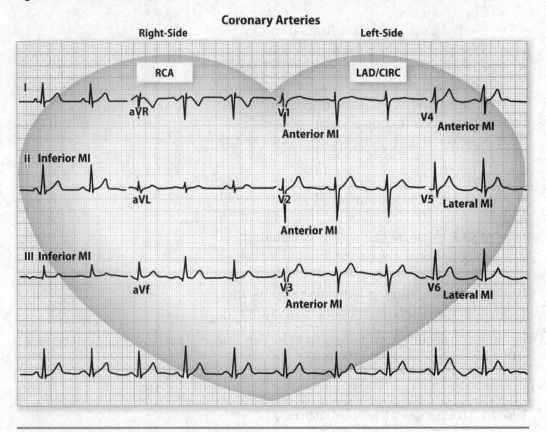

The above figure displays a 12-lead ECG. What you are looking at is an easy-to-use method of interpreting what type of myocardial infarction is occurring and where. By using the image of a heart, you will see, for example, that if an ST elevation was found in leads II and III, an inferior MI is likely. Think of the ECG as a reflection of the heart as a whole. You can even hold a 12-lead ECG up to your own chest to see how the leads fall over the heart. This is also helpful in determining which coronary artery is potentially affected.

Figure 2-2 shows ECG infarct areas. The probability of a question popping up regarding specific leads for specific infarcts is incredibly high. Do NOT ignore this information.

Diagnostics (cont.)

- Labs
  - Cardiac markers, CBC, chem panel, coag panel
  - Troponin is best (1.5 ng/mL or higher)
  - D-dimer if pulmonary embolism is suspected
- Chest x-ray
  - Differential diagnosis (may be something else)

Interventions for NSTEMI
- Pharmacology (heparin, nitroglycerin)
- Reperfusion NOT necessary
- Observation (trend cardiac markers)
- Delayed (12–24 hours) PCI if symptoms persist or worsen

Interventions for STEMI
- Pharmacology
  - If nitroglycerine does not alleviate chest pain, advanced intervention is likely (see below)
- PCI (cardiac catheterization)
  - Door to balloon (90 minutes)
  - **Priority** assessments post-procedure
    - Bleeding (sheath site)
    - Perforation of aorta (radiating back pain and vital sign changes)
    - Neurovascular checks on sheathed extremity
    - Re-occlusion may occur (ST elevation, cardiac markers trending)
- Fibrinolytic therapy
  - Door to drug/needle (30 minutes)
  - **Priority** assessments
    - Reperfusion (abatement of chest pain, normalizing cardiac markers and ECG)
    - Bleeding (neuro, internal)
    - Arrhythmias (VT, VF)
    - Re-occlusion
  - Contraindications (prior brain bleeds, active bleeding, recent major surgery)

Anterior Wall MI
- See **leads** affected (Table 2-1)
- LAD occlusion (most serious MI, worst prognosis)
- Assess for *heart failure*
  - Contraction issues of ventricular wall (poor ejection fraction)
- Assess for second-degree type II heart block or right bundle branch block (RBBB)
- Complication
  - Ventricular septal defect (assess for murmur)

Right Ventricular MI
- See **leads** affected (Table 2-1)
- RCA occlusion
- Signs of right-sided heart failure (JVD, CVP)
- IV fluids and inotropes may be needed
- Hypotension likely if SA node affected

Inferior Wall MI

- See **leads** affected (Table 2-1)
- RCA occlusion
- Assess for arrhythmias (bradyarrhythmias, heart blocks, AV dysfunction)
  - *3rd-degree HB*
- **Papillary muscle rupture** (mitral regurg systolic murmur—listen at **apex**)
  - Large V wave on pulmonary artery occlusion pressure (PAOP)

> **CCRN Tip**
>
> Papillary muscle rupture is potentially fatal. It typically arises secondary to an MI. Rapid-onset cardiogenic shock often appears. Look out for symptoms of further complications of an MI; a murmur is oftentimes the red flag.

Lateral Wall MI

- See **leads** affected (Table 2-1)
- Left circumflex artery

Prinzmetal's Angina

Variant angina, also called Prinzmetal's angina, is often caused by stimulant usage, such as cocaine. The coronary arteries spasm causing chest pain and cardiac changes.

- Transient ST elevation (normalizes quickly, especially with nitroglycerin treatment)
- Negative cardiac markers
- Treat the underlying cause if possible

Pharmacology for ACS

- High-dose aspirin
  - FIRST administration
  - Chew and dissolve
  - Contraindications may exist (current anticoagulation therapy, bleeding disorders, current bleeding, etc.)
- Anticoagulants and antiplatelets
  - Heparin/enoxaparin
  - Clopidogrel, prasugrel, ticagrelor
  - Abciximab, tirofiban, eptifibatide
- Beta blockers
  - Do NOT use in variant angina caused by cocaine
  - Lowers oxygen demand and afterload
  - Metoprolol is good (cardioselective); propranolol is bad (noncardioselective)
- Nitroglycerin
  - Aids in vasodilation and pain relief
  - Decrease preload and heart demand
- Morphine
  - Reduces pain and may aid in vasodilation
  - Inhibit catecholamine release from pain

> **CCRN Tip**
>
> Many people still use the acronym MONA (morphine, oxygen, nitroglycerin, aspirin) to remember early interventions for an MI. While these interventions are still performed, it is important to know that oxygen is no longer provided unless the patient is desaturating. Oxygen may cause decreased coronary blood flow.

Post-Cardiac Injury Syndromes

Damage caused by cardiac events may trigger an autoimmune response, causing inflammation within the heart. This may include inflammation not only of the pericardium but also the myocardium and endocardium. These inflammatory responses may be triggered by a number of events, MI included. This specific response is often called *Dressler syndrome*, named after the researcher who made the connection between MI and pericarditis.

- Post-myocardial infarction syndrome (Dressler syndrome)
- Post-traumatic pericarditis
- Post-pericardiotomy syndrome
- Iatrogenic causes
  - PCI
  - Pacemaker lead insertion
  - Radiofrequency ablation

The general idea is these inflammatory responses may be caused by any cardiac injury, small or large. Treatment generally includes steroids and antibiotics.

Cardiac Procedures/Surgeries

A good way to approach interventions in general is with a sense of least invasive to most invasive. This rule applies to cardiac issues as well. While a patient may require cardiac surgery, it is not the first thought. Can this problem be managed medically? Is there a less invasive way to fix this problem? This requires some knowledge about inclusion and exclusion criteria—something that may come up on the CCRN.

Cardiac Catheterization

While the type of percutaneous coronary intervention performed is the decision of the medical team, one of the common features that arises on the CCRN exam are complications of these procedures, especially evaluating if it worked or not, re-occlusion or failure of a stent being one example. Interventional cardiology as a whole includes a wide array of procedures:

- Coronary stenting (acute failure within **24 hours**)
- Balloon angioplasty (re-occlusion high risk)
- Pacemaker and ICD placement
- Ablation

Post-Procedural Nursing Care

The vast majority of cardiac catheterization procedures go without a hitch, but the job of the nursing staff is to catch potential complications when they do arise. To name a few:

- Stent failure
  - New-onset MI symptoms (ST elevation, chest pain, elevated cardiac markers)
- Sheath-site hematoma
  - Additional compression may be required (bleeding)
  - 15-minute site checks immediately after, then every 30 minutes
- Hematoma formation
  - Intramural dissections may occur due to stent placement or balloon inflation; the walls may "crack" and blood pools in
  - Coronary compression → MI symptoms
  - Rupture → radiating back pain
- Retroperitoneal bleeding
  - Assess for **lower back pain**
  - Most common in femoral sheath access
  - Patient is anticoagulated (high risk)
  - Patient may require fluids and blood products

For any cardiac procedure, **arrhythmias** are a common complication. These patients require telemetry at minimum. Certain topics are more likely to come up on the CCRN exam simply because they occur more frequently in the real-world. Stent **re-occlusion** being one. Stents last, on average, roughly 5 years for healthy patients who heed lifestyle changes, but immediate post-procedural risk is of prime focus.

- Neurovascular checks
  - Distal blood flow (DP and PT pulses) for sheathed extremity
- Renal function
  - Urine output and labs
  - Secondary to occlusion or bleeding → poor perfusion to kidneys (prerenal acute kidney injury [AKI])
- Extremity immobilization
  - Affected extremity → 4 hours

Cardiac Surgery

Open-heart surgery may be required if other interventions do not correct the problem. The CCRN exam does not inquire so much into intraoperative or even preoperative issues and assessments. Rather, the focus is on post-operative complications and what the nurse is required to do following these procedures. Many of the considerations apply to all open-heart surgeries.

Coronary Artery Bypass Grafting (CAB)

- Multi-vessel disease especially left main coronary artery
- Post-op assessments
  - Hemodynamics (correct preload first → albumin and crystalloids)
  - Electrolyte imbalances (potassium, magnesium)
    - Keep potassium above 4.0 mEq/dL
    - Keep magnesium above 2.0 mEq/dL
  - Arrhythmias (atrial fibrillation, tachyarrhythmias, bradyarrhythmias)
  - Hyperglycemia (insulin drip common)
    - Maintain glucose less than 180 mg/dL
  - Paralytic ileus
  - Poor renal perfusion (oliguria)

> **CCRN Tip**
>
> **Atrial kick** accounts for 20–30% of ejection fraction. With blood pressure being potentially sensitive, a change from normal sinus to atrial fibrillation may cause hypotension. A loss of atrial kick is common in tachyarrhythmia when filling time is decreased.

Cardiac Tamponade

Many cardiac surgeries remove the pericardial sac to access the heart. In some cases, the pericardial sac is preserved. The purpose of chest tubes in these surgeries is to remove the blood pooling in the mediastinum and pleural cavities. Regardless, pericardial effusion and **cardiac tamponade** are potential risks of open-heart surgeries. Be aware of any sudden hemodynamic changes, lack of chest tube output, increased jugular venous distention (JVD), and muffled heart sounds. Two red flags to consider are **narrowing pulse pressure** and **pulsus paradoxus** (see Figure 2-3). Urgent pericardiocentesis is required for survivability.

> **CCRN Tip**
>
> Patients who have pulmonary artery catheters will display a diastolic plateau in cardiac tamponade. The CVP, PAD, and PAOP are all within 2 to 3 mmHg of each other.

Figure 2-3   Pulsus paradoxus

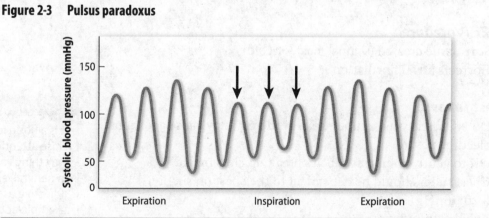

Pericarditis

If the pericardium is preserved or retained, it is possible for pericarditis to complicate recovery. Pericarditis may lead to a constriction of the heart itself and cardiac tamponade. New-onset chest pain with fever and difficulty breathing should be immediately assessed. Post-MI pericarditis is addressed above under the topic ACS; this is Dressler syndrome.

Pericardial friction rubs may be auscultated. The pain associated with pericarditis can often be relieved by leaning forward. If scar tissue forms over time leading to chronic pericarditis, it is likely the pericardial sac will be removed via pericardiectomy.

Valve Replacements
- Biological valve
  - Shorter lifespan
  - Long-term anticoagulation not needed
- Mechanical valve
  - Longer lifespan
  - Long-term anticoagulation required (thrombosis risk)
  - Transcatheter aortic valve replacement (TAVR)
    - Minimally invasive
- Post-op assessments
  - Similar to coronary bypass grafting (CABG)
  - Arrhythmias more common (surgery near SA or AV nodes)
    - Heart blocks
    - Patients typically come out of open-heart surgery with epicardial wires attached to a temporary pacemaker. If required, utilize it.
  - Review pacing in Chapter 1, "Critical Care Overview"
  - Anticoagulation required
    - Single or dual therapy (aspirin, clopidogrel)

MAZE Procedure
- Scar tissue created (scalpel, heat, or cold)
- Corrects atrial fibrillation

Chest Tubes
- Do NOT strip chest tubes unless ordered (may cause additional bleeding)
- OK to gently compress tube to break up clots inside
- Chest tubes should be dependent to the chest on suction (–20 mmHg)
- Avoid clamping
- 100 mL or more per hour → hemorrhage
- Sanguineous drainage normal directly after surgery

CCRN Tip

It is a good idea to pay close attention to the way things are worded in general, especially adjective usage. For the example above with chest tubes, stripping the tubes would be a bad idea, but if the word "gently" or "softly" is used, this makes more sense. Pay attention to word usage. It makes a huge difference!

Figure 2-4   Chest tubes

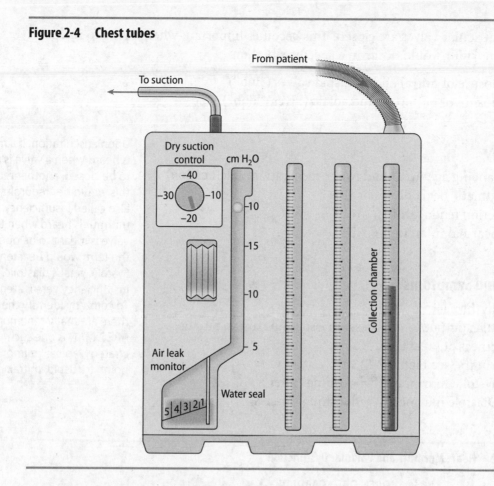

On-Pump/Off-Pump

Cardiac surgery may be performed on-pump or off-pump. When a patient is placed *on-pump*, the heart and lungs are bypassed (cardiopulmonary bypass). When bypass is used, be aware of common effects that it has on the body after surgery:

- Inflammatory response
  - Fever and tachycardia
- Increased capillary permeability (fluid leaks)
  - Edema (possibly pulmonary)
- Anticoagulation and platelet dysfunction
- Delirium (postperfusion syndrome, aka "pumphead")

Valvular Heart Disease

The heart contains four heart valves, semilunar or atrioventricular, each of which could have potential issues of insufficiency or stenosis. How these issues are addressed is dependent on multiple factors, but many go unnoticed until the patient becomes symptomatic. The general function of the valves: semilunar are open during systole, the

> **CCRN Tip**
>
> Use the diaphragm of a stethoscope for S_1 and S_2 auscultation. Use the bell for S_3 and S_4 heart sounds. S_3 is a ventricular gallop directly after S_2. S_4 is an atrial gallop late in diastole (right before S_1).

atrioventricular valves are closed. This becomes important when trying to imagine which murmur would occur in a specific situation.

- S_1: closure of mitral and tricuspid valves ("lub")
- S_2: closure of pulmonic and aortic valves ("dub")

Etiology

- Advancing age (wear and tear, degeneration, calcification)
- Rheumatic heart disease
- Infection (endocarditis)
- Myocardial infarction/CAD

Signs and Symptoms

- Arrhythmias
- Cardiac output/blood pressure issues (dizziness, fatigue, shortness of breath)
- Murmurs (see Figure 2-5)
  - Systolic murmur = "whooshing" after S_1
  - Diastole murmur = "whooshing" after S_2

> **CCRN Tip**
>
> Upon auscultation, if a murmur is heard when a valve is meant to be closed, another term for this would be "regurgitation," also called insufficiency. If the murmur is heard when the valve is meant to be open, the term would be "stenosis." Systolic versus diastolic, insufficiency versus stenosis. To correctly identify the valve there are many mnemonics. APE 2 MAN is one such strategy: apical, pulmonic, erb's point, tricuspid, mitral.

Table 2-2   Heart Murmurs and Valvular Dysfunction

VALVE(S) ISSUE	OPEN OR CLOSED	CARDIAC CYCLE	S&S
Aortic/pulmonic stenosis	Open	Systole	• Aortic: LV dysfunction • Pulmonic: RV dysfunction
Mitral/tricuspid insufficiency	Closed	Systole	• Mitral: LV dysfunction • Tricuspid: RV dysfunction
Aortic/pulmonic insufficiency	Closed	Diastole	• Aortic: LV dysfunction • Pulmonic: RV dysfunction
Mitral/tricuspid stenosis	Open	Diastole	• Mitral: LV dysfunction • Tricuspid: RV dysfunction
Ventricular septal defect	NA	Systole	• Auscultate over left sternal border (5th ICS)
Papillary muscle rupture	NA	Systole	• Auscultate over apex • Potentially inaudible if complete rupture
Aortic valve rupture	NA	NA	• Occurs due to trauma (contusion of heart) • Anterior blunt trauma • Chest pain with ST elevation

Table 2-2 details heart murmurs and corresponding heart dysfunction. It is more common for the CCRN exam to speak about aortic or mitral issues since these tend to be more life-threatening with BP and pulmonary dysfunction.

Figure 2-5   Murmurs

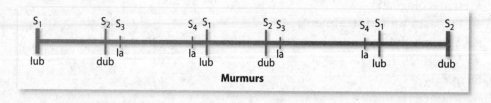

Murmurs

Interventions

How valvular disease is treated depends on the progression of the *disease process* and if the patient is *symptomatic*. A patient will likely have follow-up examinations and be educated on risk factors if the disease is not far along enough for surgery. A stenotic aortic valve forces the left ventricle to work harder. If cardiomyopathy develops, an aortic valve replacement is likely. Echocardiograms are a common diagnostic tool to assess valvular disease progression.

Acute Peripheral Vascular Insufficiency (PVI)

The main word here being "acute." Embolus is typically the main culprit, with the lower extremities most commonly affected.

Etiology

- Peripheral arterial disease (PAD)
- Trauma

Signs and Symptoms

- The 6 P's
  - Pallor
  - Pain
  - Paresthesia
  - Paralysis
  - Pulselessness
  - Poikilothermia
- Ankle–brachial index
  - Not clinically sensitive
  - A ratio of 1.00 to 1.40 is considered normal
  - Stenosis of arteries causes a decrease in the index

Diagnostics

- CT angiography
- Doppler study

> **CCRN Tip**
>
> Neurovascular checks are performed postoperatively to ensure patent vessels. A stent or bypass could potentially fail. Understand the potential risks of anticoagulation in these patients as well as the lab values associated with either warfarin or heparin use.

Interventions

- Pharmacological
  - Heparin (initial treatment)
  - Thrombolytics
  - Vasodilators
- Surgical
  - Endarterectomy
  - Fem-pop bypass
  - Peripheral stents
- Nursing considerations
  - Neurovascular checks
  - Anticoagulation (heparin)
  - Keep affected extremities dependent (increases perfusion)

Carotid Artery Stenosis

An oddball out on the CCRN exam, carotid artery disease may come up.
- Increases the risk of stroke
- Carotid duplex studies
- Endarterectomy performed to improve circulation
  - Prior to procedure the patient should receive anticoagulation (heparin)

Cardiomyopathies

There are quite a few types of cardiomyopathy (see Table 2-3). Luckily, they follow similar symptoms, potentially leading to heart failure. Many cardiomyopathies are asymptomatic until advanced enough to be considered heart failure.

Table 2-3   Types of Cardiomyopathy

Dilated	Hypertrophic
• *Systolic issue*	• *Diastolic issue*
• Most common form	• Thickening of myocardium
• Enlarged heart	• Decreased ventricular filling
• Weakened muscle	• S3/S4 heart sounds
• Mitral valve regurg	• *Sudden cardiac death* risk
Idiopathic	**Restrictive**
• Unknown causes	• *Diastolic issue*
	• Rigidity of walls (noncompliant)

CCRN Tip

You will see as you read on to the heart failure section, a very important piece of information to understand is the difference between a systolic and diastolic dysfunction. The exam often presents questions where being able to differentiate between the two is crucial.

Heart Failure

For the sake of easy learning, this section is split into systolic and diastolic heart failure. This mirrors the common presentation of questions on the CCRN exam. Previous learning on this topic likely separated heart failure into the side affected—right versus left. This foundational knowledge is also required for the exam.

The CCRN exam does not often ask about the classification of heart failure, but it is fairly straightforward. Heart failure is typically classified by patient symptoms followed by more objective observation. The New York Heart Association classifies the severity of patient symptoms with a numbered range 1 through 4 (class 1 = not bad; class 4 = really bad) and objective assessment with a similar lettered range A through D (class A = not bad; class D = really bad). Table 2-4 gives the details of the classification (the lettered classes are not listed in the table but follow the same mentality of bad to worse).

Table 2-4   Classifications of Heart Failure (NYHA)

CLASSIFICATION	SYMPTOMS
Class 1	No limitation on physical activity Ordinary physical activity does not cause symptoms
Class 2	Slight limitation on physical activity Comfortable at rest Ordinary physical activity results in symptoms
Class 3	Marked limitation on physical activity Comfortable at rest Less than ordinary activity results in symptoms
Class 4	Unable to perform physical activity without discomfort Symptoms of heart failure at rest Any physical activity causes increased discomfort

Systolic Heart Failure

Systolic heart failure (SHF) describes problems with the heart's ability to eject blood in a normal manner. As the body attempts to compensate (catecholamine release), the problem may become worse.

Etiology
- Dilated cardiomyopathy
- Coronary artery disease
- Valvular disease

Signs and Symptoms
- Enlarged cardiac silhouette (x-ray): left shift
- Increased BNP
- Low ejection fraction (≤40) showing hypokinesis

- Tachycardia and/or atrial fibrillation (**red flag**: dilated atria)
- Increased end-diastolic pressures
- Pulmonary edema (adventitious lung sounds)
- Advanced decompensation leads to loss of cardiac output and blood pressure

Interventions

- Improve preload, afterload, and contractacility (see Figure 2-6)
- Drugs that prevent compensatory hormones
  - ACE/ARBi: inhibit angiotensin I and II
  - Angiotensin receptor neprilysin inhibitor (ARNI)
    - New class first-line drug (Entresto)
  - Beta blockers: inhibit norepinephrine
  - Aldosterone antagonists: inhibit aldosterone
- Diuretics (loop and potassium sparing)
- Vasodilators
  - Decrease SVR to decrease afterload and improve systolic function
- Positive inotropes (digoxin, milrinone, dobutamine, etc.)
- Do NOT give negative inotropes (will cause further decompensation)
- Prevent constipation (vaso-vagal)

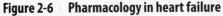

Figure 2-6   Pharmacology in heart failure

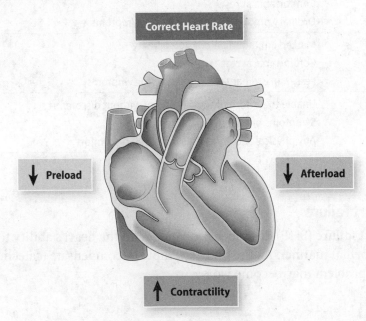

Ejection Fraction Review

- Normal ejection fraction: 50–70%
- Mild dysfunction: 41–49%
- Moderate dysfunction: 30–39%
- Severe dysfunction: <30%

The previous numbers come from the American Heart Association and are also corroborated by The American College of Cardiology. These numbers reflect left ventricle ejection fraction (LVEF).

- Preserved ejection fraction: diastolic heart failure
- Reduced ejection fraction: systolic heart failure

Diastolic Heart Failure

Diastolic heart failure (DHF) describes problems with the filling of heart chambers. If there is not enough space or time for blood to pool, the amount ejected and circulated decreases.

Etiology
- Hypertrophic and restrictive cardiomyopathy
- Hypertension
- Valvular disease

Signs and Symptoms
- Normal heart size on x-ray
- Normal ejection fraction
- Increased BNP
- Increased end-diastolic pressures
- Pulmonary edema
- Hypovolemia causes acute decompensation (decreased fluid on top of decreased filling)

Interventions
- Similar to SHF with the following exceptions
  - Calcium-channel blockers are ok with diastolic heart failure, NOT systolic
  - Do NOT give positive inotropes (will cause further decreased filling time)
    - Includes digoxin

> **CCRN Tip**
>
> Important to note, tachyarrhythmias affect filling problems. If the ventricles already fill poorly, the heart speeds up and the filling time further decreases. This is oftentimes why the initial treatment is to slow down the heart with a beta blocker.

Cardiogenic Shock

As a type of shock, the general description is a severe drop in circulation and blood pressure that is fatal if not corrected. This presents the condition as a medical emergency and action must be taken. Cardiogenic shock is unique in the fact that this drastic loss in blood pressure is caused by failure of the heart and inability of the body to appropriately compensate.

Etiology

- Cardiomyopathies and heart failure
- Dysrhythmias
- Myocardial infarction
- Mechanical dysfunction (valve, papillary muscle, defects)

Signs and Symptoms

- Hemodynamics
  - Decreased CO
  - Hypotension
  - Increased PAOP
  - Increased SVR
- Classic symptoms of shock (cool and clammy skin)
- Pulmonary edema (crackles)
- Acidosis (metabolic and lactic)
  - Assess lactic acid (lactate)

> **CCRN Tip**
>
> By the time a patient is advancing into a progressive stage of cardiogenic shock (see Figure 2-7), if they are not already intubated, it is highly likely they will be. The respiratory compromise will be too much for a patient to compensate on their own.

Figure 2-7   Stages of cardiogenic shock

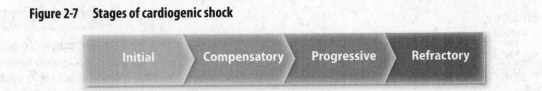

Initial | Compensatory | Progressive | Refractory

Interventions

- Increase inotropic action
  - Dobutamine
  - Dopamine (high dose: 4–10 mcg/kg/min)
- Decrease afterload
- Intra-aortic balloon pump (IABP)
  - Improves coronary perfusion (inflation)
  - Improves afterload (deflation)
  - Triggered by ECG (R-wave) or arterial waveform (dicrotic notch)
- Ventricular assist device (VAD)
  - Bridge-to-transplant
  - Bridge-to-recovery
  - Risk for bleeding and thrombosis
  - Assists with ventricular failure (typically LV)
- ECMO

> **CCRN Tip**
>
> As with most things, the goal is to correct the underlying problem. If cardiogenic shock is secondary to a fixable primary problem such as MI or arrhythmias, those problems become the goal to fix. If the shock is caused by a more advanced or chronic problem, stabilization becomes a priority.

Hypertensive Crisis

While having a drastically elevated blood pressure carries certain risks, a true hypertensive crisis or emergency displays further damage to the body. The true risk of death in a patient with a hypertension (HTN) emergency is acute intracerebral hemorrhage (stroke).

Etiologies

- Aortic dissection
- Acute pulmonary edema
- AKI
- Pheochromocytoma
- MAOI interactions with tyramine
- Eclampsia
- Intracranial hemorrhage

Signs and Symptoms

- Hypertension (180 mmHg systolic or higher)
  - HTN **urgency** → no acute target organ damage
  - HTN **emergency** → target organ damage
- Epistaxis
- Headache

> **CCRN Tip**
>
> Understand basics of pharmacology. For example, nitroprusside causes vasodilation of the arteries and veins affecting both preload and *afterload*.

Interventions

- Nitroprusside (at times nitroglycerin)
  - Cyanide toxicity risk (do not use longer than 24 hours)
    - CNS changes (LOC and mental status)
  - Slow and steady reduction of BP (too quick and perfusion may become an issue)
- Beta blockers (esmolol, labetalol)
- Nicardipine (for AKI or stroke)

Acute Pulmonary Edema

For the ICU nurse, we typically see pulmonary edema to the degree of severe hypoxemia and hypercapnia; patients often require noninvasive ventilation or intubation. Table 2-6 describes the types of pulmonary edema.

Table 2-6   Types of Pulmonary Edema

CARDIOGENIC	NONCARDIOGENIC
• Decompensating heart failure	• ARDS
• Elevated CVP and/or PAWP	• TRALI (blood products)
• Stabilize hemodynamics	• AKI
	• Drowning
	• No CVP of PAWP changes
	• Multiple treatment modalities (correct underlying issue)

Signs and symptoms of pulmonary edema may include adventitious lung sounds (crackles), diminished lung sounds, cough, and frothy sputum. Hemodynamically, the PAWP may rise above 25 mmHg. Oxygenation being the more on-the-nose sign. An x-ray will show interstitial edema.

Aneurysms and Dissection

Aortic aneurysms can be thoracic or abdominal in nature. Be able to differentiate between the two (see Table 2-7).

Table 2-7   Types of Aneurysms

TYPE	SYMPTOMS	TREATMENT
Thoracic (25% occurrence)	• Tearing pain radiating to back and shoulders • Dyspnea	• Surgery most common • Correct exacerbating factors (BP)*
Abdominal (75% occurrence)	• Pulsating mass in abdomen • Abdominal bruit ("whoosh") • Typically asymptomatic unless large	• Monitoring • Correct exacerbating factors (BP)* • If greater than 5 cm, intervention likely

*Beta blockers are a typical first-line drug to alleviate hypertension in a patient with an aneurysm. If the aneurysm remains small, surgery may be avoided. New treatments are less invasive, such as endovascular repairs with a graft.

Aortic Dissection

A dissection requires immediate medical and likely surgical intervention. Without it, the injury would likely be fatal. Most dissections occur in the arch or ascending part of the aorta. Complaints of a tearing or ripping feeling should be taken with a sense of ominous risk.

Aortic Rupture

Rupture may occur due to direct trauma to the aorta or, more commonly, via a ruptured abdominal aneurysm. As with dissections, be aware of any new-onset tearing pain. New retroperitoneal (flank) bruising may also indicate aortic rupture. This emergency has an incredibly high mortality rate; many patients do not make it to the hospital before death.

Structural Heart Defects

Congenital versus acquired? Was the defect present at birth or acquired through wear and tear? That is the main difference between heart defects. Surgical or percutaneous closure of defects are most common, but the choice for intervention typically is decided by patient symptoms and size of the defect.

Congenital Heart Defects

- Atrial septal defect (ASD)
  - Left-to-right shunt
  - Dyspnea
  - Right-sided heart failure

CCRN Tip

Left atrial appendages are oftentimes removed in patients with atrial fibrillation to reduce the risk of embolic stroke.

- Ventricular septal defect (VSD)
  - Left-to-right shunt (most common, can go both ways)
  - Arrhythmias
  - Pulmonary hypertension

Acquired Heart Defects

- Valvular disease

Cardiac Pharmacology

The following tables give a more advanced view of the pharmacology used in the ICU and why. Begin with understanding the types of receptors medications work on (Table 2-8).

Brief A&P Review

This overview is specific to the ICU. This is certainly not all-inclusive. For example, we know dopaminergic receptors are largely involved in the CNS affecting a multitude of disorders. For the purposes of critical care, the following information has been focused.

Table 2-8   Receptors of the Cardiovascular System

RECEPTOR	TISSUES AFFECTED	RESULT
Alpha 1	Arteries, veins	Smooth muscle
Alpha 2	Arteries, veins, CNS	Smooth muscle, sedation
Beta 1	Heart	Heart rate (chronotropy), contractility (inotropy), automaticity (dromotropy)
Beta 2	Arteries, veins, lungs, kidneys	Vasodilation
Dopaminergic	Kidneys	Vasodilation

Sympathetic/Parasympathetic

Sympathetic effects speed up the cardiovascular system, whereas parasympathetic effects slow it down. Many people think of sympathetic effects as the "fight or flight" response, and parasympathetic effects as "rest and digest." Cardiac output rises to increase blood flow and oxygen to the heart, brain, and muscles.

- Catecholamine release (sympathetic): increases body response
- Vagus nerve stimulation (parasympathetic): decreases body response

Hemodynamic Medications

Aside from learning the particulars of alpha versus beta medications, another useful method to learn hemodynamic pharmacology is to ask the following: Do medications affect the **preload**, **afterload**, or **contractility** of the heart? Table 2-9 details cardiac pharmacology and corresponding receptors. You likely have a fair understanding of these medications from using them in the ICU. For the CCRN exam, the expectation is really knowing how they are applied to specific patient scenarios.

Table 2-9   Cardiac Pharmacology and Receptors

Alpha Meds	Beta Meds

• Agonist
  • α_1: norepinephrine, phenylephrine, midodrine
  • α_2: clonidine, dexmedetomidine (Precedex)
• Antagonist (blockers)
  • Not typically seen in ICU
  • Labetalol has beta and alpha effects
	• Agonist
	  • β_1: dobutamine, norepinephrine, isoproterenol (heart transplant)
	  • β_2: rescue inhalers
	• Antagonist (blockers)
	  • β_1: metoprolol

Combined Alpha/Beta Meds	**Dopaminergic Meds**

• Catecholamines
  • Pressors (affect alpha receptors more)
  • Inotropes (affect beta receptors more)
	• Dopamine
	  • Low-dose* (1–2mcg/kg/min)
	  • Medium-dose (3–5mcg/kg/min)
	  • High-dose (>5mcg/kg/min)

Non-adrenergic Meds	

• Milrinone (phosphodiesterase inhibitor)
  • Positive inotrope
  • Pulmonary artery vasodilator	

* A renal dose of dopamine does increase renal perfusion and diuresis; however, there is little evidence that this increases survival rates in the ICU. Regardless, it is still used for this purpose.

Review Questions

Questions 1–3 refer to the following case.

A 56-year-old patient was admitted to the CVSICU 2 hours ago post-CAB. During the first hour, chest tube output was 75 mL. This past hour, chest tube output was 10 mL and BP consistently 100/75. BP has trended down the last 15 minutes despite inotropic titration of drips and a single albumin bolus. Patient currently remains sedated and intubated.

BP: 85/72 MAP: 76	HR: 120 Sinus tachycardia	R :24
SpO$_2$: 93% on 40% FiO$_2$ Intubated	T: 98.5°F (37°C)	Pain: 0/10 Sedated
CO: 2.7 L/min	CVP: 15 mmHg	PAP: 17/9 mmHg
PCWP: 15 mmHg		

Assessment

- Current arterial waveform pattern

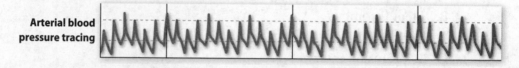

Arterial blood pressure tracing

- Positive JVD
- Clear lung sounds
- Abdomen soft and nontender
- Urine output = 35 mL for last hour

1. Based on the following vitals, hemodynamics, and brief assessment, what is the likely explanation for this continued hypotension?

   A. Acute pulmonary edema

   B. Left ventricular dysfunction due to graft failure

   C. Hypotension due to tachycardia

   D. Cardiac tamponade

2. Which of the following signs and symptoms would support the above diagnosis?

   A. Bounding peripheral pulses

   B. Equalization of filling pressures

   C. ST elevation

   D. Low-grade temp

3. The nurse recognizes that the above patient will likely require what?

   A. Emergency surgery

   B. Pleuracentesis

   C. Removal of the chest tubes

   D. Nitric oxide

Questions 4–6 refer to the following case.

Three hours after a PCI with stent placement was performed, the patient complains of chest pain. They are visibly diaphoretic and anxious. EKG was performed and shows ST elevations. Current vital signs are as follows.

BP: 155/80 MAP: 105	HR: 110 Sinus Tachycardia	R: 20
SpO$_2$: 94% on 2L NC	T: 98.6°F (37°C)	Pain: 5/10

4. Which complication does the nurse recognize?

   A. Retroperitoneal bleeding

   B. Stent thrombus

   C. Pericarditis

   D. Reperfusion injury

5. The nurse would understand which of the following is priority?

   A. Administer a beta blocker IV

   B. Increase oxygen, improving perfusion

   C. Have the patient lean forward to alleviate pain

   D. Obtain a crash cart, expect a code

6. The patient requires which intervention at this point?

   A. Coronary bypass surgery

   B. Repeat PCI with thrombectomy or angioplasty

   C. Emergent chest x-ray

   D. Fluid bolus and IV heparin

7. A patient is brought to the ER via ambulance due to complaints of chest pain. A bar owner called the ambulance after witnessing the collapse of the patient. Friends state the patient may have been using cocaine. Which of the following medications is contraindicated in this situation?

   A. Nitroglycerin (NTG) sublingual

   B. Metoprolol IV

   C. Aspirin chewable

   D. Morphine IV

8. Variant (Prinzmetal's) angina is often attributed to ingestion of stimulants like cocaine or nicotine. Which statement below is correct regarding this unique type of angina.

   A. Chest pain subsides after NTG administration, troponin trends downward
   B. NTG administration does not correct problem, PCI is needed
   C. ST elevation and chest pain subsides with NTG administration
   D. ST elevation and cardiac marker elevation takes 2–3 days to recover

9. A patient is admitted to the CCU due to a workup for aortic stenosis. Which of the following signs and symptoms are related to early-stage aortic stenosis?

   A. LV dysfunction, bradycardia, shortness of breath
   B. LV dysfunction, chest pain, ST elevation, dizziness upon activity
   C. Systolic murmur at right upper sternal border, dizziness upon activity, increased left-sided filling pressures
   D. Systolic murmur at left sternal border 4th intercostal space, heart palpitations, and tachycardia

10. In reference to the murmur associated with aortic stenosis. When would you hear the murmur?

    A. After S_1 during systole, semilunar valves are open
    B. After S_2 during diastole, semilunar valves are closed
    C. During regurgitation of blood through the aortic valve
    D. During systole, AV valves are open

11. The patient in question 8 and 9 is curious about the advantages and disadvantages of a mechanical valve versus a biological valve. Which of the following statements is true regarding these types of valves?

    A. Biological valves have longer lifespans, short-term anticoagulation needed
    B. Mechanical valves have longer lifespans, long-term anticoagulation not needed
    C. Biological valves have shorter lifespans, long-term anticoagulation not needed
    D. Mechanical valves have shorter lifespans, long-term anticoagulation needed

12. A 56-year-old patient with diabetes, hypertension, and hyperlipidemia is admitted for symptoms of peripheral arterial disease (PAD). The distal area of the left extremity is cool to the touch with absent palpable pulses. The left dorsalis pedis pulse is faintly heard with Doppler. Right lower extremity pulses are +2. The physician decides to perform a fem-pop bypass on the left lower extremity. Which of the following is most important in providing post-operative care?

    A. Keep the affected extremity elevated increasing perfusion
    B. Hold anticoagulation due to risk of bleeding
    C. Administer antiplatelet medications like aspirin
    D. Recognize an ankle–brachial index of 0.5 is normal

13. During rounding of a patient in the ICU post-STEMI, the morning EKG shows QT prolongation. Which of the following medications should be considered for discontinuation?

    A. Haloperidol
    B. Furosemide
    C. Metoprolol
    D. Clopidogrel

14. The patient in question 13 converts into torsades de pointes, the patient remains hemodynamically stable. Torsades is confirmed via emergent ECG. What treatment plan may help correct the underlying issue?

    A. Immediate transcutaneous pacing
    B. Aggressive diuresis
    C. Administer magnesium sulfate
    D. Administer amiodarone

15. A 35-year-old patient with Marfan's syndrome has been admitted to the SICU due to an enlarged abdominal aortic aneurysm. The aneurysm is larger than 5 cm in diameter and will likely require intervention. The nurse understands that which of the following represents appropriate immediate post-op care?

    A. BP management, assess for tearing pain radiating to the neck and arms
    B. Assess urine output, administer antihypertensives as ordered
    C. Vomiting is common, administer antiemetics, continue to monitor
    D. Administer antibiotics prophylactically

16. A 70-year-old patient with class 4 systolic heart failure is admitted to the CCU for close monitoring of an acute exacerbation. Current ejection fraction shows 30%. What clinical findings would confirm the presence of an acute exacerbation in this case?

    A. PAOP of 19, cough with frothy sputum, tachycardia
    B. PAOP of 12, lung sounds clear, shortness of breath
    C. CVP of 12, dependent edema, elevated JVD
    D. Normal PA pressures, PaO_2 of 70%, chest pain

17. A 78-year-old patient with a history of hypertension, obesity, diabetes, and CAD was admitted to the ICU yesterday for treatment of hypertensive crisis, BP 210/105 with signs of AKI (creatinine 2.2). The family states he has been confused lately and may not have taken his medication. The patient has been receiving a nitroprusside drip and morphine for pain. Which of the following answers reflects an improvement in condition?

    A. BP 143/85, increase in urine output, improvement in azotemia
    B. BP 115/70, decrease in thiocyanate levels, decrease in pain
    C. BP 140/90, creatinine 2.0, urine output 250 mL for shift (12 hours)
    D. BP 125/80, HR 115, glucose 75

18. The patient in question 17 has been showing improvement on the nitroprusside. Which of the following signs and symptoms should the nurse be acutely aware of?

    A. Bradycardia, hypotension, seizure activity
    B. Metabolic alkalosis, confusion, tachycardia
    C. Respiratory acidosis, tachypnea, hypotension
    D. Metabolic acidosis, confusion, change in level of consciousness

19. A 72-year-old female patient was observed unconscious in a store when 911 was called. Paramedics arrived on the scene and obtained immediate vitals—BP 88/60, HR 125, RR 28, SpO_2 86%. Oxygen was started with improvement. Upon arrival to the ER, vitals have slightly improved and the patient is now awake complaining of chest pain. An ECG is ordered immediately showing ST elevation in leads V2, V3, V4. Which statement about this STEMI is correct?

    A. Anterior wall MI, monitor for heart failure
    B. Posterior wall MI, monitor for second-degree heart block
    C. Inferior wall MI, monitor for right ventricular failure
    D. Anterior wall MI, monitor for papillary muscle rupture

20. The patient in question 19 was given aspirin chewable and continued oxygen. The nurse was in the room when the monitor now reveals the following rhythm and hemodynamics.

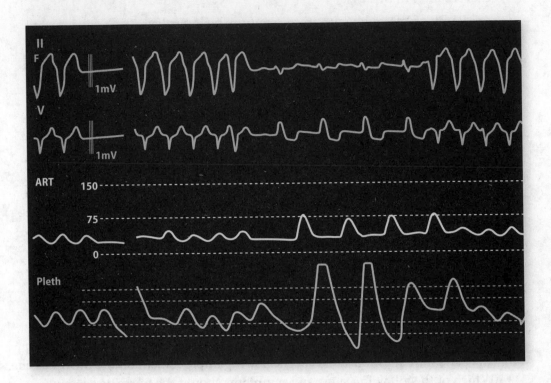

What order of interventions would be the most appropriate for the nurse to perform?

A. Normal saline bolus, administer atropine, perform ECG

B. Increase oxygen, fluid bolus, perform ECG, administer amiodarone

C. Increase oxygen, prepare for immediate intubation,

D. Zero transducers: abnormal waveforms

Answer Key

Question 1

Answer: D

Rationale: Cardiac tamponade after an open-heart surgery is certainly rare, but not unheard of. When they open and salvage the pericardial sac, blood may pool post-op and lead to pericardial effusion and cardiac tamponade. Eventually the tamponade is so great that cardiogenic shock begins. The narrowing pulse pressure (85/72), low cardiac output and BP, equalizing filling pressures (CVP, PAP, PAOP), JVD, and pulsus paradoxus shown on the A-line waveform all suggest cardiac tamponade. The other big thing of note is the drastic reduction of chest tube output in a short period of time. We do want to see a reduction in output over the course of the patient's recovery; however, the first post-op hours are crucial as to avoid buildup.

Pulmonary edema is not likely here since the lungs are clear. An x-ray would be able to differentiate between this, potentially showing infiltrates (edema) versus enlarged cardiac silhouette (tamponade). An echocardiogram is also typically used as confirmation of tamponade.

Some of these symptoms match left ventricular dysfunction, which, technically speaking, cardiac tamponade includes; however, it is not due to graft failure. Similar to stent failure, if a graft fails, reemerging symptoms of an MI would occur. Since the patient is sedated and pain cannot be readily assessed, a primary go-to would be assessing the ECG and rule out ST elevations along with a troponin draw. The full clinical picture here suggests tamponade not graft failure.

This patient is hypotensive, but they are not hypotensive due to tachycardia. The tachycardia, in fact, is likely one of the things stabilizing the BP as the body attempts to compensate.

Question 2

Answer: B

Rationale: The above rationalization for question 1 explains the majority of this question's signs and symptoms. Muffled heart tones along with increased JVD and hypotension is sometimes called *Beck's triad*. In addition, ST elevation and a low-grade temp would be indicative of pericarditis, not cardiac tamponade.

Question 3

Answer: A

Rationale: Emergency surgery is most likely in this case. Since the sternum was cracked only hours ago, the surgeon will likely take the patient back to the OR to correct. If the sternum was intact, pericardiocentesis or a pericardial window is also an option.

Pleurocentesis is for a pleural effusion, not a pericardial effusion. Removing the chest tubes is the last thing you want to do. We *want* the blood or fluid to come out that is causing the tamponade. Nitric oxide is occasionally used in pulmonary edema.

Question 4

Answer: B

Rationale: Stent thrombosis most commonly occurs acutely (<24 hours post-PCI) and mimics signs and symptoms of a typical MI (chest pain, ST elevations). The actions that follow are also similar to an MI; make sure to contact the HCP if symptoms of re-occlusion occur.

Retroperitoneal bleeding is noticeable via the classic low back pain. Depending on the severity of the bleeding, the patient may become hypotensive and require fluids and/or blood products. A patient with pericarditis could have chest pain and ST elevations; however, the temperature of this patient is normal. Reperfusion may cause arrhythmias, mostly due to the "stunning" of the myocardium. At times, reperfusion injury can be fatal, hence the goal of reestablishing blood flow as soon as possible.

Question 5

Answer: A

Rationale: As explained in the previous question, stent occlusion will match symptoms and interventions of a typical MI. Therefore, administering a beta blocker is the best option here; remember cardioselective is best (metoprolol, not propranolol). The beta blocker will take the stress off the heart by lowering the heart rate and likely improving the blood pressure.

The pulse ox is adequate here at 94%; do not administer oxygen unless it is needed. Leaning forward may help alleviate pain in a patient with pericarditis. Current signs and symptoms of this patient do not warrant an expecting code—at least not yet. If the patient was experiencing frequent runs of V-tach or advancing heart blocks, it may be a good idea to keep a crash close at hand.

Question 6

Answer: B

Rationale: If a patient post-PCI is having symptoms of another MI, stent occlusion should be the first rule-out. It is also the most likely complication given the clinical picture here. The patient will require a thrombectomy or angioplasty.

The question does not state which coronary artery is affected, but surgery at this point is a jump. If all noninvasive measures do not correct the problem, at that point a surgeon may be consulted. Two large inclusion criteria for CAB is left main disease and/or triple vessel disease. An x-ray would not be needed here, all symptoms point to re-occlusion. The patient does not appear hypovolemic with a BP of 155/80. A fibrinolytic or thrombolytic may be used; heparin does not break up clots and is not a thrombolytic. That is tPA (alteplase). As a side note, it is not uncommon for the CCRN to test your knowledge about contraindications to the use of tPA, such as a prior hemorrhagic stroke.

Question 7

Answer: B

Rationale: Beta blockers are contraindicated if the ACS is caused by stimulants such as cocaine. The medication may inhibit vasodilation. The vasospasms are treated with nitroglycerin, with pain typically subsiding afterward. A first-line medication for ACS is aspirin. While it won't effectively prevent or fix the problem, it may be given and oftentimes is if the practitioners were unaware of the prior cocaine use. Pain relief may also aid in vasodilation; therefore, morphine is not contraindicated and remains a common medication for ACS.

Question 8

Answer: C

Rationale: Prinzmetal's angina, also called "variant" angina, is treated with nitroglycerin (NTG). Once administered, the chest pain and ST elevations normalize. The medication isosorbide dinitrate may also be seen on the CCRN. Remember it is a "nitrate," a vasodilator.

Troponins are not elevated in Prinzmetal's. PCI is not needed in Prinzmetal's unless medical management does not work. It may be utilized as a diagnostic tool in search of vasospastic activity in the coronaries. The ST elevations with Prinzmetal's are transient, returning to normal upon treatment.

Question 9

Answer: C

Rationale: A systolic murmur in the right upper sternal border coincides with aortic stenosis. Remember the "APE 2 MAN" strategy on auscultation locations of valves. The dizziness is due to left ventricular dysfunction leading to reduced cardiac output and hypotension.

The patient would be tachycardia, not bradycardic. ST elevations and chest pain could be seen if the aortic stenosis is so severe it is not inhibiting blood flow into the coronaries. This would be advanced, however, not early stage. A murmur in the left fourth intercostal is indicative of a problem with the tricuspid valve (sternal border) or mitral valve if it was more mid-clavicular.

Question 10

Answer: A

Rationale: The semilunar valves are open during systole; the AV valves are closed. This would include aortic stenosis as in this question, or a pulmonic stenosis. A murmur after S_2 would be diastolic in nature; the semilunar valves are closed. Regurgitation of blood through the aortic valve is describing insufficiency during diastole, not stenosis.

Question 11

Answer: C

Rationale: Biological valves are more common in younger patients, mostly because long-term anticoagulation and taking of meds is not needed, as opposed to mechanical valves, where anticoagulation is absolutely necessary to prevent thrombosis. Biological valves do not last as long as mechanical valves.

Question 12

Answer: C

Rationale: Like many diseases of the vascular system, stabilizing perfusion is the goal. Preventing occlusion with antiplatelets (aspirin, clopidogrel) and/or anticoagulants (heparin, warfarin) is mainstay administration. Dual-therapy treatments are becoming more and more common.

   The affected extremity should be lower (dependent) than the heart to increase perfusion. Elevation will decrease blood flow. Holding anticoagulation will increase the risk of a failed surgery and occlusion of the new bypass. An ankle–brachial index below 1 is abnormal and would warrant investigation.

Question 13

Answer: A

Rationale: Antipsychotics like haloperidol may lead to QT prolongation. Other drugs like amiodarone and other antiarrhythmics—specifically, the IA Class (procainamide, quinidine)—have been known to prolong the QT. Loop diuretics (furosemide) could eventually lead to QT prolongation, but that would be related to the loss of potassium (hypokalemia), not the drug itself. The other medications, metoprolol and clopidogrel, are not known to cause QT prolongation. If the patient has been consistently bradycardic, metoprolol may be discontinued to allow the interval to speed up.

Question 14

Answer: C

Rationale: Magnesium sulfate has been proven to be effective in torsades and is the first-line therapy to correct it. Transcutaneous pacing may be advisable if other interventions do not work. Because this patient is currently hemodynamically stable, there is some time to correct the underlying problem. Diuresis would likely make the problem worse since electrolyte imbalances have been known to cause torsades. If the patient was severely hyperkalemic, remember that insulin with D50 would be a primary intervention. Antiarrhythmics, especially IA Class and amiodarone, will prolong the QT further worsening the problem here.

Question 15

Answer: B

Rationale: Managing post-operative blood pressure is of utmost importance. Antihypertensives should be administered as ordered and as often as needed. Common medications include hydralazine IV PRN, beta blockers IV PRN, or if

HTN persists, a drip of nicardipine or nitroglycerin. The surgeon often orders a specific range for blood pressure; the nurse titrates to the desired effect. Assessing the urine output is also important so any prerenal AKI can be quickly corrected. This may be due to a lack of blood flow to the kidneys during surgery or potentially (albeit more rarely) a graft that is blocking the renal arteries.

A tearing pain radiating to the neck and arms is more in line with thoracic aortic dissection, not an abdominal aneurysm. Vomiting is not common; it may be a symptom of a complication with the aneurysm. Antiemetics would want to be administered to prevent vomiting that may increase blood pressure. Antibiotics are given prophylactically before or during the surgical repair, not after. This is oftentimes the case with many cardiovascular surgeries. Prophylactic antibiotics will also be used in patients with grafts before any dental procedures.

Question 16

Answer: A

Rationale: Severe LV dysfunction as indicated here by the ejection fraction can lead to a number of signs and symptoms. Elevated pulmonary pressures including a wedge (occlusive) pressure is in line with left-sided failure as the fluid backs up into the lungs. This also leads to pulmonary edema (frothy sputum). Reflex tachycardia here is the body attempting to compensate for the low cardiac output.

Lung sounds would not be clear. Crackles would exist in pulmonary edema caused by severe LV dysfunction. **Remember that an answer has to be 100% correct to be correct on the CCRN exam.** This patient may be short of breath due to low cardiac output, but the rest of the complete answer is wrong. Elevated CVP with dependent edema and JVD is indicative of right-sided heart failure. The ejection fraction here implies left. Myocardium may become ischemic (chest pain) if the cardiac output is low causing decreased perfusion to the coronaries, however, pulmonary pressures again would not be normal.

Question 17

Answer: A

Rationale: The goal of blood pressure treatment in an HTN crisis is not to drastically reduce the BP, but a slow and steady downturn away from the dangerously elevated BP. Too quick of a reduction of BP may send the patient into a pseudo-shock-like state. The improvement in urine output and azotemia also displays correction of the kidney damage.

BP 115/70 is too far too quick. Thiocyanate levels would be monitored if cyanide poisoning was suspected. There are no signs and symptoms in this question that point to poisoning. A creatinine of 2.0 and urine output of 250 mL over 12 hours still shows kidney damage. Improvement would be a correction of these issues. A HR of 115 also displays that the body continues to compensate. The patient may be a diabetic, but the problem here was not glucose related.

Question 18

Answer: D

Rationale: Cyanide poisoning is a possibility with the use of nitroprusside. Patients experiencing any change in mental status or level of consciousness should be immediately assessed for poisoning. Metabolic acidosis without any underlying cause is another red flag. The thiocyanate levels of this patient will be monitored to evaluate correction.

Question 19

Answer: A

Rationale: Leads V2, V3, and V4 indicate an anterior wall MI. The risk of heart failure is great in these patients due to ventricular damage. Make sure to study ACS MIs and the leads displayed. This will certainly come up on the CCRN exam.

Question 20

Answer: B

Rationale: ABCs. First and foremost, correct the hypoxia and blood pressure issues. This is done by increasing the oxygen and increasing preload via bolus. An ECG is performed to confirm the rhythm. The monitor here is showing likely runs of V-tach. In theory, this could also potentially be a code situation if the V-tach simply continues. There is no way of knowing here and the answers do not point to a code.

The patient may be intubated if increasing the oxygen and other interventions do not work to correct the hypoxia. The patient is not bradycardic here, atropine is not needed. The full hemodynamic picture does not lead to suspicion of the technology itself. If only one waveform was off, that may warrant a zeroing of transducers.

CHAPTER 3

Respiratory

The respiratory section makes up roughly 19 questions on your CCRN exam, so approximately 15% of the exam is devoted to this topic. Respiratory is the second-largest area on the CCRN exam. Certain things in this chapter are a MUST KNOW. Arterial blood gas (ABG) tests will absolutely be on the CCRN exam. This chapter may give brief A&P reviews before certain diseases, but it is wise to ask yourself if you truly understand the underlying pathophysiology or not. It is better to really grasp the info than regurgitate memorized information. Review mechanical ventilation and respiratory monitoring devices in Chapter 1.

Oxygen and Oxygenation Concepts

While Chapter 1 runs through some of the monitoring tools utilized for oxygen, let's discuss some basics regarding this all-important molecule for the human body. Hemoglobin carries 98% of oxygen, with the remaining dissolved in the blood itself.

- SpO_2: oxygen saturation of hemoglobin detected by pulse ox
- SaO_2: oxygen saturation of hemoglobin from arterial blood
- PaO_2: oxygen pressure/dissolved in arterial blood
- SvO_2: oxygen saturation in the pulmonary artery (mixed venous)

SpO_2 is undoubtedly the most common method of immediately assessing oxygen status. While useful, understand this number may be deceiving depending on underlying pathology (anemia, carbon monoxide poisoning).

SaO_2 is the saturation form of PaO_2. They are essentially the same number presented in alternate formats. Saturation is in the form of a percentage, whereas a partial pressure is in the form of mmHg. These numbers do tend to correlate; however, different diseases may manipulate the numbers. This is called the *oxyhemoglobin dissociation curve* (see Figure 3-1).

CCRN Tip

Temperature makes for an easy explanation of this curve. An increase in temperature allows chemical reactions to move more easily, aka oxygen leaving hemoglobin. This is taking it back to chemistry, but remember these reactions are easier with heat/energy.

Left Shift

- Oxygen clings to hemoglobin
- Alkalosis
- Hypothermia
- Carbon monoxide poisoning
- Decreased 2,3-diphosphoglycerate (DPG)
  - Many PRBC transfusions

Right Shift

- Oxygen unloads of hemoglobin
- Acidosis
- Hyperthermia
- Increased 2,3-DPG
  - Decreased hemoglobin (anemia)

Figure 3-1   Oxyhemoglobin dissociation curve

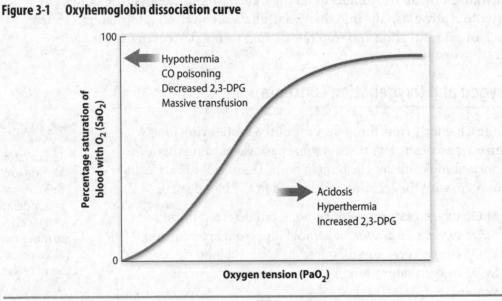

Understanding the concept of the oxyhemoglobin dissociation curve is important for the exam. (See Figure 3-1.) It is likely to come up in a question requiring you to apply your knowledge using the concept and showing why a curve or oxygen problem may react a certain way in a disease.

The affinity of oxygen to hemoglobin by acidity of blood and carbon dioxide is called the *Bohr effect*. It is represented in this curve. As you likely know, an increase in carbon dioxide worsens acidity. This enables oxygen to leave hemoglobin more readily, and vise versa.

Carbon Monoxide Poisoning

Remember that the SpO_2 will give deceiving results here. It may show a saturation of 95%, but pulse ox is for hemoglobin saturation, not necessarily just oxygen. In this case, carbon monoxide has locked onto hemoglobin over oxygen and carbon dioxide.

Signs and Symptoms
- Dull headache
- Changes in mental status or LOC
- Tissue hypoxia → organ failure → death

Interventions
- 100% FiO_2
- Trend carboxyhemoglobin numbers (3% or less is normal)

Lactic Acidosis

When organs are no longer being perfused with the amount of oxygen required for cellular metabolism, anaerobic respiration will begin and lactic acid will build up. Drawing a lactic acid (lactate) is standard on assessing overall stability, or severity of decline, in the patient. Most ABGs include a lactate level.

Many causes exist as to why a cell may not be able to use oxygen: septic shock, carbon monoxide (CO) poisoning, hypovolemia, lung disease, etc. All of these lead to the same problem with cellular metabolism and the body's inability to create energy (ATP).

ABG Interpretation

You likely have a fair amount of experience and practice with ABG draws and how to interpret the results. That is a good thing because the CCRN will absolutely test you on it. This is a staple and a requirement of a trained critical care nurse. Everything listed below is a must know.

Normal ABG Values
- pH: 7.35–7.45
- $PaCO_2$: 35–45 mmHg
- HCO_3: 22–26 mmol/kg
- PaO_2: 80–100 mmHg

$PaCO_2$: respiratory (quick changes)
HCO_3: metabolic (slow changes)

A normal anion gap is 5–15 mEq/L. This number may come up in certain diseases such as DKA.

> **CCRN Tip**
>
> Smokers generally have a slightly elevated carbon monoxide level (10%). In carbon monoxide poisoning, we also look for the carboxyhemoglobin level to drop below 10% while on 100% oxygen. That is an indication of improvement.

> **CCRN Tip**
>
> Hydrogen ions (H^+) build up as the pH decreases, leading to acidosis. There is an inverted relationship with hydrogen ions and $PaCO_2$; when one increases, the other decreases, and vice versa.

Table 3-1   Acid–Base Imbalances

ACID–BASE IMBALANCE	CAUSES	SIGNS AND SYMPTOMS	TREATMENT
Respiratory acidosis	Respiratory depression (bradypnea), diaphragm paralysis, decreased gas exchange	LOC changes, dysrhythmias, hypoxia, hypercapnia	Increase RR, improve LOC, suctioning, bronchodilators, diuretics
Respiratory alkalosis	Pain, fear, hypermetabolic states, CNS stimulation	Headache, dizziness, paresthesias	Treat underlying cause
Metabolic acidosis	Increased production of acids, impaired renal function, loss of bicarb (diarrhea), toxic ingestion (salicylates)	Abnormal anion gap (DKA), dysrhythmias, tachypnea (compensation)	Treat underlying cause, administer bicarb
Metabolic alkalosis	Loss of gastric acid (vomiting or NG suctioning), diuretics, steroids, hypovolemia, hypokalemia	Electrolyte imbalances, dysrhythmias, CNS changes, bradypnea (compensation)	Acetazolamide, chloride replacement, potassium replacement

Fully compensated: normal pH
Partially compensated: pH remains abnormal

> **CCRN Tip**
>
> Evaluate a partially or fully compensated ABG. Understand how to interpret these results. If the primary problem is respiratory in nature, the body compensates metabolically. If the primary problem is metabolic in nature, the body compensates respiratorily. Think of DKA: the patient is exhibiting Kussmaul breathing in an attempt to breathe off acid in the form of CO_2.

Acute Pulmonary Embolism (PE)

Dead space refers to the anatomical or alveolar space where gas exchange does not occur. To a degree, this is normal in all of us. In a PE, however, dead space is drastically increased and ventilation suffers. This is called alveolar dead space. The alveoli affected are not perfused and no gas exchange occurs. Oddly enough, many PEs go undiagnosed and are oftentimes confused for other things.

Deep vein thrombosis (DVT) is the number one cause of pulmonary embolism. Understand the main risk factors for DVT and how they are prevented. (See Table 3-2.)

> **CCRN Tip**
>
> *Virchow's triad* is an easy way to remember DVT risk. It includes hypercoagulability, stasis, and endothelial injury.

Table 3-2   DVT Risk Factors and Prevention

RISK FACTOR	PREVENTION
• Fractures, surgery, trauma • Prolonged bed rest, sitting • Oral contraceptives, pregnancy, hormone replacement • Obesity, age	• SCDs, compression stockings, ambulation, range of motion • Heparin (low-molecular weight or unfractionated) • Weight loss • Adequate hydration

Etiology

- Venous DVT (Doppler scan)
- Fat emboli
    - Long bones (femur), especially in open fractures (compound)
    - Pelvis
- Less common (air, tumor, septic)

Signs and Symptoms

- Dyspnea and tachypnea with *hypoxemia*
- Cough with or without hemoptysis
- Chest pain (pleuritic)
- V/Q mismatch
- S_3 and/or S_4
- Increased pulmonary artery pressure
    - May lead to R-sided heart failure
- Cardiac arrest (if clot large enough)
- *Petechiae (fat emboli)—especially on the thorax*
- PEA or sudden shock (massive PE)

Diagnostics

- CT pulmonary angiography (primary and "gold standard")
- Ventilation (V)/perfusion (Q) scan
- Positive D-dimer
- ABG
    - Respiratory alkalosis (minor PE)
    - Respiratory acidosis (massive PE)
- MRI

Interventions

- Oxygen therapy (NIV if needed)
- *Push fluids*
- Heparin and warfarin
- Fondaparinux
- Fibrinolytic therapy (advanced PE)

V/Q Scan

Know this! The normal V/Q ratio is 0.8 or 4 L of ventilation/min for every 5 L of perfusion/min. This normal V/Q ratio should exist for a patient on room air (21% FiO_2). A V/Q mismatch occurs when ventilation or perfusion is affected. For a PE, perfusion is the problem. In pneumonia, covered later in this chapter, ventilation is the problem. (See Figure 3-2.)

A *shunt* occurs when a V/Q mismatch is severe, such as in ARDS. Blood is passing through the lungs but not becoming oxygenated. One indicator of a shunt via oxygenation is called an "alveolar–arterial gradient." This gradient shows if gas exchange is occurring and to what degree. If a shunt is severe, the gradient will be worse. A normal alveolar–arterial gradient is less than 10 mmHg.

Figure 3-2   Ventilation/profusion

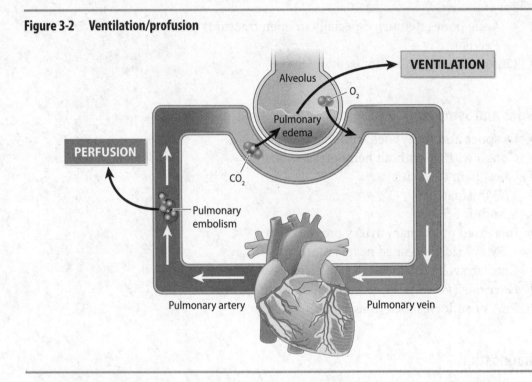

Acute Respiratory Distress Syndrome (ARDS)

A dangerous syndrome, ARDS is a multifactorial complication that brings patients into the ICU if not developed in the ICU directly. Pathophysiologically, the entire syndrome is due to a large inflammatory response that causes damage to the cells in the lungs (see Figure 3-3). Increased membrane permeability leads to edema. Decreased surfactant leads to decreased lung compliance (static and dynamic) and increased work of breathing. Eventually, if ARDS progresses, the result is shunting, serious *refractory hypoxemia,* and potential multiple system organ failure.

Figure 3-3   Pathophysiological changes in ARDS

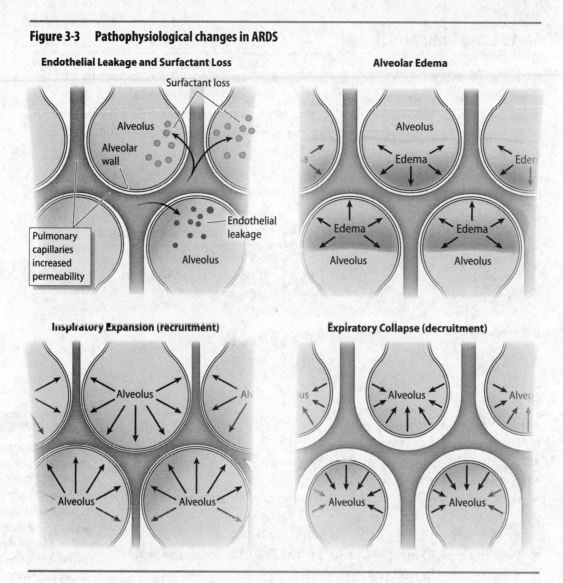

- **Refractory hypoxemia**: *hallmark sign*, a state of emergency where the body no longer responds to increases in oxygen. PEEP must be added to increase alveolar ventilation. Refractory hypoxemia is one of the requirements to make a diagnosis of ARDS. By increasing the PEEP, FiO_2 may be decreased if the patient tolerates.

- **Lung compliance**: the measurement of the lungs' ability to expand. It is measured by the change in volume and change in pleural pressure. Dynamic compliance is affected by the movement of air (asthma), whereas static compliance is affected by volume (lungs). Surfactant increases compliance by decreasing surface pressure. Compliance is also affected by positioning; supine is bad. *Decreased compliance → increased work of breathing.*

Acute Lung Injury (ALI)

A precursor to ARDS, ALI is similar in pathophysiology and risk factors to ARDS (see Table 3-3). The difference between the two is in the P/F ratio. The cut-off value for the P/F ratio is 200 mmHg. ALI is a less severe form of ARDS and is considered at a P/F ratio between 201 and 300 mmHg. A ratio below 200 mmHg signifies ARDS.

Table 3-3   Etiology of ARDS/ALI

PRIMARY/DIRECT	SECONDARY/INDIRECT
Pneumonia (most common)	Shock (any etiology)
Aspiration	• Septic most common
• Decreased LOC	*Blood transfusion (TRALI)*
Inhalation injury	Burns
• Smoke inhalation	DIC
Drowning	
Chest trauma	

Signs and Symptoms

- Dyspnea and tachypnea
- Hypoxemia (PaO_2 <60 mmHg on room air)
- Hypercapnia ($PaCO_2$ >50 mmHg)
  - Respiratory alkalosis (first due to hyperventilation until fatigue)
  - Respiratory acidosis (later sign on ABG)
- PaO_2/FiO_2 ≤200 mmHg (the higher the FiO_2, the lower the ratio)
  - ≤200 mmHg ARDS
  - 201–300 mmHg = ALI
  - 300–400 mmHg = normal ratio
- Crackles upon auscultation (*noncardiogenic* pulmonary edema)
  - PAWP <18 mmHg
- Diffuse bilateral infiltrates on chest x-ray

Pulmonary Interventions

- Mechanical ventilation with 100% FiO_2 (if needed)
- Increased PEEP: 12 cm H_2O or more (expand alveoli)
  - May cause hypotension
- Plateau pressure 30 cm H_2O or less (avoid barotrauma)
- Tidal volume 6 mL/kg
- Prone positioning

CCRN Tip

When assessing monitoring devices, allow for a clinical picture you are typically not used to seeing. The numbers will not be perfect. Below are some expected ranges when monitoring a patient in ARDS:

- SpO_2: 88–95%
- Arterial pH: 7.30–7.45
- PaO_2: 55–80 mmHg

At times, *permissible* hypercapnia leading to a pH of 7.20 can be expected in a patient.

Supportive Treatment

- Conservative fluid management
  - Follow lower central pressures (CVP)
- Manage cardiac output
  - Vasoactive/inotropic medications
- DVT prophylaxis
  - Low-molecular-weight heparin (enoxaparin)
- Stress ulcer prophylaxis
  - PPI, H_2 antagonist, sucralfate
- Nutritional needs
  - Enteral is best (protein a plus)
- **Steroids no longer routinely used**

Acute Respiratory Failure (ARF)

When there is a failure of oxygen passing from the lungs to the blood, a state of respiratory failure exists. Acute failure is fast in onset; chronic slower in onset. There are many types of acute respiratory failure, but by following the primary cause, it can be more easily understood (see Table 3-4).

Table 3-4   Types and Etiologies of Acute Respiratory Failure (ARF)

HYPOXEMIC	HYPERCAPNIC	BOTH
Pneumonia	Respiratory depression	ARDS
Pulmonary edema	COPD	COPD
Cystic fibrosis	Spinal cord injury	Asthma
No hypercapnia	Diaphragm weakness	
$PaO_2 < 60\ mmHg$	Brain stem issues	
Most common in ICU	*With hypoxia*	
	$PaCO_2 > 50\ mmHg$	
	pH <7.35	

Signs and Symptoms

- SpO_2 <88% on RA
- Tachypnea and dyspnea (hypoxemic ARF)
- Cyanosis (very low oxygen)
- Arrhythmias
- Changes in LOC and mental status

CCRN Tip

In hypercapnic respiratory failure, an increase in lung dead space and/or decreased minute ventilation (hypoventilation) often contribute to the problem.

Interventions

The primary goal of treatment is to increase the oxygen delivery to the lungs and aiding in the removal of carbon dioxide. Once the patient is stabilized, focus on treating the underlying condition.

- Oxygen supplementation
  - Nasal cannula, NIV (CPAP or BiPAP), mechanical ventilation
    - CPAP (in): hypoxic ARF
    - BiPAP (in and out) : hypoxic and hypercapnic
  - Do not over-oxygenate
- Pharmacology
  - Nebulizer treatments (bronchodilators)
  - Steroids
  - Antibiotics, diuretics (as needed)
- Nursing care
  - Turning patient (maximize V/Q areas of lungs)
  - Incentive spirometry (if possible)
  - Suctioning as needed

> **CCRN Tip**
>
> Be careful when assessing the need for NIV versus mechanical ventilation. There are times when the patient really should be intubated to preserve either the airway or ventilation. Intubation may also occur if the patient is simply too sick, affecting not only the pulmonary system but also cardiovascular (arrhythmias, hypotension, etc.), among other body systems.

Pneumonia

Pneumonia is fairly common in the ICU. The infection oftentimes leads to advancing respiratory failure. Therefore, prompt treatment of pneumonia is crucial. Pneumonia remains a leading cause of death for patients in the ICU. The most common pathogen causing inflammation of the alveolar space (pneumonia) is bacteria, followed by viral and fungal infections (see Table 3-5). Flu vaccines and pneumococcal vaccines (over 65 y.o.) are used as preventive measures.

> **CCRN Tip**
>
> Pay attention to the story of the patient. A culture takes time to return, but a story can point to the type of causative pathogen the patient may have. A hospital-acquired pneumonia is typically caused by *Staphylococcus aureus,* whereas a community-acquired pneumonia is typically caused by *Streptococcus pneumoniae.*

Table 3-5 Etiologies/Risk Factors of Pneumonia

MEDICAL	DEMOGRAPHIC/LIFESTYLE	COMMON PATHOGENS
Respiratory disease	Age	**Bacterium**
• COPD, asthma	• Infants	*Streptococcus pneumoniae*
• Cystic fibrosis	• Elderly	• Most common
Heart disease	Smoking	• Pneumococcal
Atelectasis	Sedentary	*Klebsiella pneumoniae*
• Post-op risk	Poor nutrition	*Staphylococcus aureus*
LOC issues	Poor hygiene	*Legionella pneumophila*
• Decreased cough	Occupation	
• Aspiration	Recent travel	**Viral**
Immunocompromised	Contact with animals	*Haemophilus influenzae*
• AIDS		Respiratory syncytial virus
• Chemotherapy		
• Transplants		**Fungal**
Ventilator/tracheostomy		*Pneumocystis jirovecii*
Recent cold or flu		• Most common in immunosuppressed (AIDS)

Signs and Symptoms

- Tachypnea, dyspnea, accessory muscle use
- Productive cough—purulent sputum
- Chest pain upon breathing and/or cough
- P/F ratio ≤250
- Lobar infiltrates (chest x-ray) and diminished breath sounds
- Confusion (elderly)
- Lab values
    - WBC (does not have to be increased)
    - C-reactive protein—increased

Interventions

There are a number of potential treatments for pneumonia, but remember to reasonably address the infection based on presentation. Least invasive interventions are always performed first.

- Bad lung up, good lung down
- Administer FiO_2 as needed
- Suction as needed
- Respiratory therapy
    - Chest physiotherapy (postural drainage)
    - Assist cough (do not suppress)
- Antibiotics
    - Draw culture and sensitivity before antibiotics
    - Empirical therapy (treatment using knowledge of local pathogens and patterns)
- Corticosteroids (community-acquired)
- Pleural fluid culture
- Bronchoscopy and/or mechanical ventilation (if necessary)

Complications

- Respiratory failure
- Septic shock
- Pleural effusion and/or **empyema**
- Renal failure

Empyema

A new addition to the 2020 CCRN blueprint, a collection of purulent material in the pleural cavity defines an empyema. It may develop from pneumonia (most common) or by thoracic surgery or trauma. Initial chest x-ray, ultrasound, and CT scan assist in the diagnosis of any effusion. Once a thoracentesis is performed, the fluid will be sent off for testing to determine the bacterium present in the empyema. Be careful not to contaminate cultured fluid of any kind (use blood culture tubes if possible). Antibiotics will follow to treat the infection along with, most commonly, a tube drainage from the pleural cavity. If the problem cannot be solved by a chest tube, video-assisted thoracotomy (VAT) or open thoracotomy is warranted.

Ventilator-Associated Pneumonia (VAP)

VAP increases the length of stay and mortality in the hospital. Many preventive measures are well established and commonly part of a bundle. The obvious and easy way to prevent VAP is to minimize unnecessary intubations.

- Elevate head of bed (HOB) (30 degrees or more)
- Oral care q4hr (minimum) w/ CHD
- Maintain ETT cuff pressure
- Administer PPIs as ordered
- Continuous subglottic suctioning
- Monitor nasogastric (NG) tube feedings/confirm placement with x-ray
- Do not break circuitry (unless absolutely necessary)
- Coordinate care with respiratory therapy
- Sedation vacations

Air Leak Syndromes (ALS)

An air leak syndrome is essentially respiratory distress due to the movement of air into places it does not belong, typically from alveoli bursting. There are some conditions like subcutaneous emphysema that do not affect respiratory status; however, for the sake of this section, all topics are related to respiratory distress. Motor vehicle accidents remain one of the leading causes of traumatic pneumothorax.

Pneumothorax

There are many ways pneumothorax may be classified. One common method is based on the etiologies in Table 3-6. They can be further classified based on the types of injuries (simple vs. tension, open vs. closed). A tension pneumothorax describes any time the collapse causes a mediastinal shift and cardiovascular compromise.

> **CCRN Tip**
>
> Blunt trauma may also cause a pneumopericardium, a collection of air in the pericardial sac. It may lead to cardiac tamponade.

Table 3-6   Types of Pneumothorax

SPONTANEOUS	TRAUMATIC	IATROGENIC
Occur without any trigger or event Primary • No known lung disease Secondary • Known lung disease	Open • Sucking wound (stab or penetrating) • Fractured ribs • Flail chest Closed • Intact rib cage • Blunt injury • Falls	Needle aspiration Barotrauma • Ventilators Central line placement • Subclavian most common Surgical

Tension Pneumothorax

A medical emergency, tension pneumothorax can compress major arteries and veins, causing cardiovascular collapse along with the obvious respiratory complications. This is also one of the big differences to recognize between a tension pneumothorax and a "normal" pneumothorax. Is the patient exhibiting signs of cardiovascular problems? Is the problem sudden and drastic?

- Tachycardia
- Hypotension
- Reduced venous return (distended neck veins)
- Tracheal deviation **away** from collapse

Signs and Symptoms

How a pneumothorax looks can be very different depending on the type and severity. Some collapses are relatively minor and the patient remains asymptomatic. If the pneumothorax is large, hypoxemia can certainly be expected.

- Tachypnea, dyspnea
- ABG: respiratory acidosis
- Absent or diminished breath sounds
- Tracheal deviation
    - Ipsilateral (spontaneous pneumothorax)
    - Contralateral (tension pneumothorax)
- Ipsilateral pleuritic chest pain
- Reduced chest expansion

Interventions

See table 3-7 for Pneumothorax treatments.

Table 3-7   Treatments for Pneumothorax

SIMPLE	OPEN	TENSION
• High-Fowler's • Supplemental oxygen (nasal cannula 4–6L) • Follow-up chest x-ray • Tube thoracostomy (chest tube) placement if larger	• Occlusive dressing • Tube thoracostomy • Monitor for tension pneumothorax • Monitor for bleeding	• *Emergency* tube thoracostomy • Needle aspiration (if necessary)

CCRN Tip

Chest tube placement is preferred over needle aspiration (thoracentesis). The goal of both, however, is to restore the negative pressure of the pleural cavity. Chest tube placement will also take precedence over other advanced interventions like intubating the patient.

Hemothorax

Common in a majority of open traumatic pneumothoraces, a hemothorax is a collection of blood in the pleural cavity. It may also occur due to a closed (blunt) trauma to the chest wall. Once confirmed, if the amount of blood is large, chest tube placement is likely. Monitor for continued signs of bleeding. This condition may lead to shock.

Aspiration

Any foreign substance that is inhaled into the lungs would be considered an aspiration. Contents are typically aspirated through the oral route or by stomach contents falling into the airways. The severity of the resulting disease is dependent on the nature and amount of the contents aspirated (bacterial, stomach contents, etc.). The disease is also often classified based on the acute or chronic nature of the aspirations.

- **Aspiration pneumonia**: typically caused by bacterial inhalation from the oral or nasal pharynx
- **Chemical pneumonitis**: typically caused by the aspiration of stomach contents causing inflammation due to the acidity

Etiology

- Esophageal issues
  - Elderly (common)
  - Dysphagia
  - GERD

- Impaired swallowing (dysphagia)
- Decreased level of consciousness
  - Alcohol and drugs
  - Anesthesia
- Neurological conditions
  - Stroke and seizures
  - Multiple sclerosis
  - Parkinson's
- Artificial airways
  - Endotracheal tube
  - Tracheostomy
- NG tube feeding
- Prolonged supine position

Signs and Symptoms

- Hyperthermia or hypothermia
- Tachypnea and tachycardia
- Hypoxemia with acute respiratory distress
- Crackles/rales
- Decreased breath sounds
- Hypotension (septic shock)

Interventions

How aspiration is treated depends on the type of aspirate. Antibiotics, corticosteroids, and immunomodulating medications may be used in certain situations; you do not need to know when. Go back to basics, culture then administer if needed. Be especially aware of potential complications and the nursing considerations detailed in Table 3-8.

> **CCRN Tip**
>
> Diagnostic tools like an x-ray are helpful in displaying the severity of an aspiration. Most cases affect the **right lung** rather than the left due to a more vertical position of the right main bronchus. Position of the patient may also change the likely location of an aspirate, but, on average, the right side is the most common.

Table 3-8   Treatments for Aspiration

COMPLICATIONS	NURSING CARE
ARDS: intubation and ventilation **Septic shock**: vasopressors	• Patient position → Fowler's, right side to clear • Suctioning as needed • FiO_2 **Preventive** • HOB elevated • Oral hygiene • Swallow evaluations • PPI (if intubated)

Foreign Body Aspiration

Choking is the term generally used when a foreign body is inhaled and occludes the airways causing acute respiratory distress. If less invasive measures to remove the foreign object fail, a bronchoscopy may be performed in an attempt to immediately restore a patent airway. If bronchoscopy fails, a thoracotomy may be necessary.

Chronic Obstructive Pulmonary Disease (COPD)

While a chronic issue, COPD like many diseases, may be complicated by an acute exacerbation. Often called acute on chronic, these types of exacerbations may land people in the ICU due to advancing respiratory distress. COPD in general, is characterized as a combination of emphysema and chronic bronchitis.

COPD Basics

- SpO_2: 88–92%
- Chronic acidosis (may be compensated)
- Barrel chest (larger antero-posterior diameter)
- Decreased peak expiratory flow (PEF)

Etiology/Triggers of Acute Exacerbation

An acute event occurs when inflammation overpowers body mechanisms to protect the airway. This leads to tissue damage and decreased lung function.
- Respiratory infections (most common)
  - Bacterial, viral, atypical
- Environmental pollution

Signs and Symptoms
- Dyspnea and wheezing
- Increased cough and sputum production
- Decrease in forced expiratory volume (FEV_1)
- Respiratory distress
  - Worsening acidosis and hypoxemia
- V/Q mismatch

Interventions

COPD is nonreversible. With an acute exacerbation, the immediate goal is to improve respiratory function and stabilize the patient. Remember that a COPD patient already has decreased function, so the expected outcomes of treatment will not be perfect. Noninvasive ventilation has been shown to be incredibly effective in COPD patients with acute exacerbations. Early intervention may prevent a worsening condition and avoid intubation and mechanical ventilation.

CCRN Tip

Understanding the class of medications is oftentimes important on the CCRN exam. Names of medications may not always be provided for easy recognition—albuterol being a good example for COPD. Short-acting rescue inhalers are common for both COPD and asthma; the class being *"beta₂ agonist."*

- Oxygen
  - SpO_2: 90% or higher
  - PaO_2: 60% or higher
- Bronchodilators (inhaled, not oral)
  - Short-acting (albuterol, ipratropium)
  - Long-acting (salmeterol)

Steroids and antibiotics may be added to treatment protocols depending on causes and severity. Consider the adverse effects of steroids if they are used (hyperglycemia). Other considerations may include nutritional goals, management of secretion, and monitoring hemodynamics.

Asthma

The largest differentiation between asthma and COPD is the fact that respiratory compromise of asthma can be reversed with treatment. Pathophysiological changes to the lungs in a COPD patient are already permanent. Signs and symptoms along with treatment of asthma are similar to COPD(see Table 3-9). One potentially fatal acute exacerbation of asthma is status asthmaticus.

Status Asthmaticus/Acute Severe Asthma

A medical emergency, status asthmaticus can be fatal and requires immediate treatment. The largest treatment problem is the issue of no response to traditional bronchodilator therapy. Similar to COPD exacerbations, the most common causes of status asthmaticus are upper respiratory infections. Patients who have been intubated previously for near-fatal exacerbations of asthma remain the highest risk for death.

- **Stage 1:** Respiratory alkalosis, normal PaO_2
- **Stage 2:** Respiratory alkalosis, decreased PaO_2
- **Stage 3:** Normal pH, decreased PaO_2
- **Stage 4:** Respiratory acidosis, decreased (severe) PaO_2

> **CCRN Tip**
>
> Initial treatment in the ER should increase PEFR and FEV_1 by 70% or more of what would be expected. Anything less warrants a hospital admission. An ICU admission would be warranted for even worse pulmonary function numbers (less than 50%), in addition to arrhythmias, cardiac or respiratory collapse, and mental status or level of consciousness changes.

Table 3-9   Signs and Symptoms of Status Asthmaticus

GENERAL	SEVERE
Tripod position (leaning forward)	Accessory muscle use
Tachypnea	Pulsus paradoxus
Dyspnea	Decreased to absent breath sounds
Tachycardia	Respiratory acidosis
Wheezing	V/Q mismatch (air trapping)
Decreased peak flow (PEFR) or FEV_1	Hypoxemia → lactic acidosis
Mental status changes	PEFR or FEV_1 → 50% or more reduction

Interventions
- Bronchodilators, anticholinergics, steroids
- Therapeutic gases
  - Oxygen is typically low dose unless the exacerbation is severe
  - Heliox, a combination of helium and oxygen, aids in reduced work of breathing
- Noninvasive ventilation for up to 24 hours
- Intubation as indicated below

Clinical Indicators to Intubate
- Cardiopulmonary arrest
- Decreasing LOC (obtunded or coma)
- Increasing accessory muscle use
- Absent lung sounds/absent speech

Sedation/Paralytics/Ventilator Settings
When caring for an intubated patient with status asthmaticus, it is important to choose sedatives carefully. The primary concern being ventilator synchrony. Some sedatives may also complicate the respiratory status with histamine release and/or bronchoconstriction. Paralytics are generally avoided due to the possibility of myopathy; however, if desynchrony continues, at times they are added with caution.

Ventilator Considerations
- Monitor PEEP carefully
- Increase exhalation time → low respiratory rate
- Reduce tidal volume → prevent auto-PEEP
- Monitor peak pressures (suction as needed)

Pulmonary Fibrosis

Injury to the lungs is followed by inflammation. Normally the body regulates these processes, but in fibrosis, overactivation by irritants may cause a remodeling of the overall lung structure. This may lead to fibrosis, lesions, and, eventually, respiratory compromise.

Etiology
- *Injury → inflammation → tissue repair*
- Continuous irritants
  - Allergens (allergic airway inflammation)
  - Toxic chemicals
  - Radiation (thoracic)
- Idiopathic fibrosis (unknown cause)
- Cystic fibrosis/cystic lung disease

Signs and Symptoms

- "Honeycomb" appearance on radiography
- Decreased oxygen diffusion → hypoxemia
- Often eventually fatal

Interventions

- Treat underlying conditions (remove allergens, etc.)
- Lung transplantation
- Palliative care

Pulmonary Hypertension

The normal systolic blood pressure of the pulmonary arteries tends to range between 15 and 30 mmHg; however, when discussing pulmonary hypertension the *average or mean* is used. Echocardiogram may be used to assess a ballpark pressure, but direct right-sided catheterization is needed to diagnose. In the ICU, pulmonary artery (Swan-Ganz) catheters are used for continuous monitoring of pulmonary pressures.

> **CCRN Tip**
>
> When assessing measurements of pressures, remember that the patient should be at rest and at end expiration. PAWP/PAOP may be normal or decreased in PH (<15mmHg)

Etiology

There are many potential causes of pulmonary hypertension (PH). The most common is left-sided heart disease. Pulmonary embolism and COPD are other causes you may see in the ICU.

Signs and Symptoms

- PAP (mean): 25 mmHg at rest or higher
- Earliest symptom → dyspnea on exertion
- Left-sided heart failure symptoms (SOB, fatigue)
- Right-sided heart failure symptoms (JVD, edema)
    - Angina (demand ischemia)
    - Hepatomegaly
- Pulmonic valve murmur (left 2nd IC)

Remember to take into account diagnostic tools. A BNP may be elevated due to heart failure (>180 is particularly worrisome). A chest x-ray may show hypertrophy of the ventricles and dilated pulmonary vessels. Pulmonary function tests may be ordered along with standard ECG. If a PE is suspected, a V/Q scan may be ordered. The entire clinical picture is often complicated; follow the trail of symptoms.

Interventions

- Dilatory medications
  - Phosphodiesterase-5 inhibitors (sildenafil)
  - Prostacyclin/epoprostanol, iloprost (inhaled preferred, also IV)
- Nitric oxide (if intubated, cautious use)
- Treat symptoms and underlying factors

Thoracic Surgery

Many thoracic surgeries and procedures have been covered above in this chapter. Utilize the information regarding the types of surgeries and proceedures in Table 3-10 to gauge overall understanding of individual topics. The CCRN is more likely to discuss post-operative care of these patients as well as the reasons that landed them in the OR.

Table 3-10   Types of Thoracic Surgery/Procedures

MINOR	ADVANCED
Bronchoscopy	Open thoracotomy
Video-assisted thoracoscopic (VAT)	Lobectomy
• Wedge resection	Pneumonectomy
Tracheostomy	Pleurectomy
	Lung transplantation

Aside from common post-operative care like preventing DVT and infections, most thoracic surgery patients come out of surgery with a chest tube. Understand the following nursing considerations in the management of a chest tube:

- Assess for signs of re-collapse (pneumothorax)
- Avoid kinking of tubing; keep the system below insertion site
- Never strip tubing without orders (massage gently, not "strip")
- Do not clamp the chest tube (especially in pneumothorax patients)
  - Expect bubbling—an improvement is decreased bubbling
- Manage pain
- Manage accidental tube dislodgement

Thoracic Trauma

Due to the anatomical area and the vital organs that are held there, thoracic trauma oftentimes has increased morbidity and mortality. Because of this, thoracic trauma makes up a large percentage of trauma-related deaths. Be cognizant of potential cardiac and pulmonary compromise. A FAST exam—focused assessment with sonography for trauma—is performed to isolate potential bodily damage commonly in addition to x-ray/CT. Whether surgery is required is determined by the severity and type of injury. Many traumas require only observation until the body heals on its own.

- **Blunt trauma** (most common): motor vehicle accidents and falls
- **Penetrating trauma**: gunshots and stabbings

Fractured Ribs

- Risk for contusions, pneumonia, delayed hemothorax
- Risk for pneumothorax
- Flail chest
  - Multiple fractures in multiple places
  - Contusions lead to pulmonary compromise

Lung Contusion

- Bruising of the lung (capillaries and alveolar burst)
- Chest pain, hemoptysis (severe)
- Risk for pulmonary edema → hypoxia
- Risk for ARDS

Tracheal Perforation

- Rare but life-threatening
- Dyspnea and respiratory distress
- Subcutaneous emphysema
- Hemoptysis (severe)
- Stridor

Pulmonary Pharmacology

Many of the issues discussed in this chapter involve medications that affect a multitude of systems. For our purposes here, specific pulmonary meds commonly used in the ICU are discussed— those that affect the respiratory system directly via airways. Pharmacology is added here as a brief refresher. More detail is provided in individual disease areas. Some CCRN questions simply state the class, such as "administer a bronchodilator," but it is possible for a specific drug name to come up.

Bronchodilator Therapy

Patients with compromise of the airway frequently receive bronchodilator therapy. Table 3-11 details the types of bronchodilator therapy. These medications are also commonly used along with pulmonary function tests to assess effectiveness. The same thought process is applied in the ICU with the use of

CCRN Tip

You may be familiar with theophylline. It is typically used more as an add-on therapy if the therapies outlined in Table 3-11 do not correct the problem. The drug itself (theophylline) is a fairly weak bronchodilator; many studies do not show effectiveness in its addition to treatment.

these medications. If the patient is intubated, monitor the ventilator along with the patient for signs of improvement.

Table 3-11 Types of Bronchodilator Therapy

CLASS	MEDICATION NAMES	RESULT
Inhaled β_2-agonists	Short acting (SABA): albuterol Long acting (LABA): salmeterol	Smooth muscle relaxation Bronchodilation
Inhaled corticosteroids*	Beclomethasone Budesonide Fluticasone	Inhibit inflammatory response
Anticholinergics**	Ipratropium bromide Tiotropium bromide	Inhibits bronchoconstriction and secretions through parasympathetic inhibition

*Be aware of side effects
**More common in COPD

Review Questions

1. A recent ABG for a patient with an exacerbation of COPD is as follows:

    $pH = 7.25$
    $CO_2 = 58$ mmHg
    $HCO_3 = 28$ mEq/L
    $PaO_2 = 65$ mmHg

    After increasing the oxygen to 4L via the nasal cannula, which intervention would the nurse perform next?

    A. Suction the patient using the in-line catheter
    B. Call the respiratory therapist and MD for emergency intubation
    C. Administer bicarbonate
    D. Administer a bronchodilator

2. A patient was recently admitted to the ICU due to status asthmaticus. They were recently placed on CPAP with 21% FiO_2. Upon rounding, the patient appears to be in respiratory distress. Which intervention is appropriate at this time?

    A. Obtain a stat ABG
    B. Administer salmeterol
    C. Consider switching to BiPAP
    D. Increase the pressure for NIV

3. Which of the following symptoms would be expected with a patient in ARDS?

    A. PAWP >18 cm H_2O
    B. Increased wheezing
    C. Alveolar–arterial gradient = 8 mmHg
    D. Refractory hypoxemia

4. A patient with right-sided pneumonia, crackles, and a productive cough is currently intubated and ventilated. A high-pressure alarm is triggered. Which of the following actions would be most appropriate for the nurse at this time?

    A. Increase the oxygen flow, bag using an ambu-bag if necessary
    B. Assess lung sounds, suction as needed
    C. Administer a bronchodilator
    D. Place a bite guard around the endotracheal tube

5. After hyperoxygenation and suctioning, the current pulse ox of the patient in question 4 remains 88%. Which of the following interventions is most appropriate for this patient to improve oxygenation?

   A. Prepare for a bronchoscopy

   B. Place the patient on the left side

   C. Administer PRBCs

   D. Increase the FiO_2

6. All of the following are used for reducing ventilator-associated pneumonia EXCEPT for which intervention?

   A. Administration of pantoprazole

   B. Swap out ventilator circuitry when liquid is present

   C. Q2hr oral care

   D. Maintain HOB 30 degrees

7. A gunshot victim has just arrived at the trauma bay in the ED. Immediate vital signs show hypoxia and tachycardia. Diminished lung sounds exist on the left side with tracheal deviation to the right. What complication is likely occurring in this patient?

   A. Pleuritis

   B. Hemothorax

   C. Tension pneumothorax

   D. Tracheal perforation

8. A patient was recently admitted due to a suicide attempt. Symptoms include nausea, confusion, and headache. Carbon monoxide poisoning is suspected. He is lethargic but follows commands. Which of the following interventions is most important at this time?

   A. Maintain 100% FiO_2

   B. Keep HOB elevated to 90 degrees

   C. Maintain a SpO_2 above 93%

   D. Achieve a carboxyhemoglobin level of 30% or lower

9. A hypothermic patient was recently admitted to the ICU. An ABG was drawn due to evident hypoxia. Analysis of the ABG shows respiratory acidosis. What is the best explanation for the oxygen use in this patient at this time?

   A. Oxygen will hold stronger to hemoglobin due to acidosis

   B. Oxygen is readily picked up by tissues and cells due to acidosis

   C. Oxygen is easily released to tissues due to hypothermia

   D. Oxygen is easily released to tissues due to hyperthermia

10. A trauma patient was recently admitted to the ICU after an open reduction of the femur. An hour later the patient complains of shortness of breath. Focused assessment shows slight crackles at the bases of the lungs but otherwise clear and a petechial rash on the upper chest and neck. Which complication is likely happening here?

    A. Post-operative pneumonia

    B. Atelectasis

    C. Fat embolism

    D. Pleural effusion

11. A patient on a BiPAP for acute respiratory failure is severely obtunded and hypoxemic. Which of the following interventions is likely for this patient at this stage?

    A. Intubation and mechanical ventilation

    B. Increasing the NIV pressures

    C. Prone positioning

    D. Repeat an ABG

Questions 12 and 13 refer to the following case.

While assessing a sedated ventilated patient, the end-tidal CO_2 is noted at 55 mmHg. Further assessment of an ABG is shown below. The patient was admitted and intubated earlier this morning due to an overdose of benzodiazepines.

pH = 7.28
CO_2 = 50
HCO_3 = 24
PaO_2 = 85%

12. Based on the current condition of the patient, which priority action is likely?

    A. Increase the FiO_2

    B. Increase the respiratory rate

    C. Decrease the tidal volume

    D. Increase the sedation

13. The physician orders a chest x-ray on a recovering stroke patient. The x-ray displays bilateral infiltrates. Which condition is the patient likely suffering from?

    A. Atelectasis

    B. Tension pneumothorax

    C. Aspiration pneumonia

    D. ARDS

14. Treatment of the likely condition of the patient in question 13 would include which priority intervention?

    A. Respiratory hygiene
    B. Bronchoscopy
    C. Positioning with the bad lung up
    D. Intubate for deep suctioning

15. Which of the following reasons necessitates mechanical ventilation?

    A. Increasing need for FiO_2
    B. Protection of the airway
    C. Patient has difficulty clearing secretions
    D. Current respiratory rate of 8 BPM

16. Positive end-expiratory pressure is often used for patients with refractory hypoxemia. When using PEEP, which complications may arise?

    A. V/Q mismatch and hypoxemia
    B. Bradycardia and barotrauma
    C. Hypertension and bradycardia
    D. Hypotension and barotrauma

17. An elderly female was recently admitted to the ICU complaining of severe dyspnea. A smoker for many years, the patient states she has lost weight this past year and cannot perform household tasks without becoming tired. The physician has diagnosed her with emphysema and ordered nasal cannula oxygen. All of the following are assessment findings for emphysema EXCEPT:

    A. Hyperresonance on percussion of lung fields
    B. Decreased breath sounds
    C. Decreased forced inspiratory volume (FIV_1)
    D. Complaints of productive cough

18. If an intubated and mechanically ventilated patient develops increased plateau pressures, what is the best explanation for the current problem?

    A. The ventilator has to work harder to deliver air into the patient (pushes harder)
    B. The ventilator has high pressures during no air movement in the circuitry
    C. The ventilator senses an increase of pressure during exhalation
    D. The ventilator senses lung compliance as adequate and normal

19. A 70-year-old male is being admitted to the ICU following a house fire that burned large portions of his body. The physicians are concerned about smoke inhalation and intubate the patient to protect the airway. The following day the patient develops bilateral crackles, tachypnea, and hypoxemia. Which findings would suggest ARDS?

   A. PaO_2/FiO_2 ratio = 250 mmHg, Hypercapnia, PAWP = 20 mmHg
   B. PaO_2/FiO_2 ratio = 300 mmHg, Infiltrates on x-ray, hypoxemia
   C. PaO_2/FiO_2 ratio = 180 mmHg, Hypercapnia, PAWP = 15 mmHg
   D. PaO_2/FiO_2 ratio = 150 mmHg, Hypoxemia, PAWP = 22 mmHg

20. The current ABG is pH 7.50, $PaCO_2$ 50, HCO_3 36. Given the results of this ABG, what may be a potential etiology? Is the ABG compensated?

   A. Severe pain: full compensation
   B. Electrolyte imbalances: partial compensation
   C. Hyperkalemia: no compensation
   D. Decreased gas exchange: partial compensation

Answer Key

Question 1

Answer: D

Rationale: A good way to approach treatment or intervention questions like this one is to approach it with a "least invasive to most" mentality. Will this patient potentially be intubated? Of course, but it is not the first thing we would do. By administering a bronchodilator, we are attempting to correct the underlying problem with a COPD exacerbation: inflammation. This ABG shows respiratory acidosis with hypoxemia. By increasing the oxygen, our goal is to correct the hypoxemia first. This question is asking what comes next.

The bicarb of 28 shows partial compensation. Administering additional bicarbonate in this situation will not fix the underlying problem. If the question stated a patient coughing with thick secretions and crackles, suctioning would make more sense in this situation. As stated earlier, this patient may end up intubated, but it is not an appropriate intervention at this time to call the physician for emergency intubation. If a bronchodilator fixes the problem and the patient stabilizes, the nurse has fixed the current issue.

Question 2

Answer: A

Rationale: Nursing process continues to follow all of us in practice and examinations. The CCRN is no different. ADPIE can certainly be used in these situations. Without a proper assessment, it is hard to know which intervention may benefit the patient fully. Obtaining an ABG will show if the patient is truly having an oxygenation or ventilation problem. Many circumstances are not what they seem. It is not uncommon for patients on CPAP or BiPAP to lack a good seal on the mask.

With this thought in mind, the other answers here could be potential interventions, but not until the problem is fully understood. A logical next step would be to administer a bronchodilator given the diagnosis of status asthmaticus. This could be albuterol, salmeterol, tiotropium, etc. A switch to BiPAP, increase in CPAP pressure, or intubation would be down-the-line interventions if no other interventions work. Remember *least invasive to most*.

Question 3

Answer: D

Rationale: One of the hallmark signs of ARDS is refractory hypoxemia. There will be no improvement, with an increase in FiO_2 often requiring 100%. PAWP is < 18 mmHg in ARDS. A higher wedge pressure would be indicative of something else, like left-sided heart failure. A normal alveolar–arterial gradient is < 10 mmHg. When the gradient increases above normal, shunting is likely. Less common is the inability of oxygen to diffuse into the blood. Increased wheezing may sound good given the association with respiratory disorders, but it is more associated with airway resistance issues (COPD, asthma).

Question 4

Answer: B

Rationale: As mentioned in an earlier question, the nursing process remains every bit as important in critical care as in other specialty areas. Why is there a high-pressure alarm in this patient? We do not know yet; the nurse must assess. Given the diagnosis of pneumonia with a productive cough, it is likely this patient is having difficulty clearing their own secretions. It is important to note the wording here "suction as needed." It is no longer good practice to suction without an assessment that warrants it. The lining of the trachea may be damaged by obsessive suctioning. The patient may begin showing signs of injury like blood-tinged sputum.

It is also entirely possible the patient is not adequately sedated and is biting the ETT, but we would not know without assessing first. Placing a bite guard will not help a high-pressure alarm if the alarm is not due to patient biting. A high-pressure alarm is not related to current patient oxygenation. It is a ventilation issue; the machine recognizing higher-than-normal pressures in the circuitry. If an assessment shows wheezing or adventitious lung sounds, a bronchodilator makes sense. Again though, we would not know until assessing.

Question 5

Answer: B

Rationale: "Bad lung up" is the saying. This is a right-sided pneumonia; position the patient on the left side. There is also a component of the understanding "least invasive to most" here. The FiO_2 may be increased, however other interventions should be performed first to avoid the patient needing more oxygen. Less is more in this sense as long as the ABG is stable. A bronchoscopy may be performed down the line if the secretions are too thick to suction out or the consolidation grows. It is not the primary intervention here. Administering PRBCs may increase oxygenation in a patient, if they're anemic—this question provides no information about the patient being anemic, and therefore the answer is moot.

Question 6

Answer: B

Rationale: Ventilator circuitry should only be broken as an absolute last resort. Not only does it open the patient up to infection, it also causes a loss of PEEP. If the patient condition requires PEEP for improvement, this loss of pressure can further exacerbate problems. Administering a PPI such as pantoprazole is important in preventing VAP. By decreasing the amount of any potential reflux, risk of VAP is reduced. Frequent oral care reduces the bacterial flora in the mouth. A minimum of Q4hr oral is required. The more frequent, the better. Any elevation of the head of the bed is important in VAP reduction: 30 degrees may be considered the minimum, but if the patient can tolerate higher, the higher the better.

Question 7

Answer: C

Rationale: Gunshot wounds to the chest may result in a number of complications given the sensitive territory of organs. This patient is showing signs of tension pneumothorax with the diminished lung sounds and tracheal deviation. Pleuritis or pleurisy, an inflammation of the pleural lining, causes chest pain. Hemothorax may be caused by trauma and become a medical emergency; however, tracheal deviation is not found. Tracheal perforation is rare and presents with difficulty breathing and potential changes to the voice.

Question 8

Answer: A

Rationale: Carbon monoxide poisoning is potentially life-threatening. The tissues may not receive adequate amounts of oxygen due to hemoglobin carrying carbon monoxide. Placing the patient on 100% FiO_2 is an immediate and vital intervention to stabilize oxygenation levels. High oxygen is maintained until the carboxyhemoglobin level trends downward, the goal being less than 10%. Elevating the head of the bed may aid the patient in breathing, but it will not affect the physiological change to the hemoglobin. A pulse ox will show a false positive in carbon monoxide poisoning cases; the number cannot be trusted. The benchmark for improvement is 10%, not 30%, in relation to carboxyhemoglobin. Remember that smokers do tend to have a slightly elevated number.

Question 9

Answer: B

Rationale: Understanding the oxygen dissociation curve is important. This involves the factors that may affect a right or left shift in affinity to hemoglobin by oxygen. In this patient, they are acidotic, causing a right shift and an easier release of oxygen from hemoglobin to tissues. The other answers are not a correct understanding of oxygen affinity in this patient.

Of note, hyperthermia (answer 4) does also cause a right shift and an easier release of oxygen, so this answer is medically correct. It does not, however, define the patient in this question. This patient is hypothermic, not hyperthermic.

Question 10

Answer: C

Rationale: A big red flag in this story is the petechial rash on the thorax. The patient is also at risk for embolism given the fracture of a long bone (femur). Differentiating between a normal embolism or a fat embolism lies in the petechial rash. Shortness of breath and crackles at the bases of the lungs could be a number of things; the petechial rash points to fat embolism.

Pay close attention to the timing of things. This patient was recently admitted to the ICU. Post-op pneumonia does not develop in a matter of hours. The same rule would apply to pleural effusion or atelectasis, a precursor to pneumonia.

Question 11

Answer: A

Rationale: BiPAP and NIV are typically utilized as a last resort before intubation and mechanical ventilation. This patient is severely obtunded and unable to protect their airway. The poor oxygenation will likely lead to death if imminent action is not taken.

NIV pressures are fairly predetermined based off of patient body size. They may be changed by physician recommendation, not by nursing judgment. As stated above, this patient is no longer a good candidate for NIV given they're severely obtunded. Prone positioning is utilized on occasion in ARDS, not this. Repeating an ABG at this stage will not assist in the problem. The clinical presentation appears grim. Immediate intervention is required. The question also says the patient is hypoxemic; a follow-up ABG is redundant.

Question 12

Answer: B

Rationale: Ventilator settings are moved to stabilize the patient and an ABG. This patient displays respiratory acidosis. To correct this the respiratory rate can be increased or the tidal volume. Oftentimes, respiratory rate is the first to change. Increasing tidal volume can cause barotrauma.

The FiO_2 does not need to be increased. A PaO_2 is adequate. Decreasing the tidal volume would worsen the acidosis. This question says nothing of the patient fighting the vent or potentially contributing to the acidosis on the ABG. There is no reason to increase the sedation at this time.

Question 13

Answer: C

Rationale: There is not an overwhelming amount of information in this question to go off of. This may be seen on the CCRN exam as well. The ability to extrapolate conclusions from incomplete data is crucial in these types of exams. The thing we do know is this is a recovering stroke patient. Dysphagia is a very common problem in this patient population. Impaired swallowing often leads to aspiration pneumonia.

ARDS is also a condition where bilateral infiltrates may be seen; however, there is no story in this question to fit the bill. Aspiration is much more likely. Atelectasis would display diminished lung sounds or space on the x-ray, but not infiltrates. A tension pneumothorax has different signs and symptoms. The x-ray would show a mediastinal shift.

Question 14

Answer: A

Rationale: Aspiration patients require strict respiratory hygiene and depending on their ability to swallow, potential changes to the diet or temporary NPO order. There is no reason to intubate this patient. Deep suctioning is not a reason to intubate a patient although it may be a benefit on the side. This patient has bilateral infiltrates, there is no "bad" lung to put up. Both lungs at this moment are bad. Bronchoscopy may be performed down the line if the infiltrates become much worse. Remember *least invasive to most*.

Question 15

Answer: B

Rationale: Intubation with mechanical ventilation is considered a final resort if at all possible. There are many medical emergencies that require immediate intubation, loss of airway being one. For whatever reason, an inability to protect the airway is considered an emergent need for intubation. This could be due to drug overdose, smoke inhalation, or something more expected like anesthesia and surgery.

Remember that 100% FiO_2 can be given without intubation. A nonrebreather mask, for example, has the ability to deliver 100% FiO_2. While it certainly is somewhat easier to suction a patient with an in-line catheter through an ETT, this is not a reason for intubation either. A patient may be deep suctioned with a normal rubber catheter while awake (nasally or orally). A patient with a respiratory rate of 8 BPM does not necessarily warrant intubation. More information would be needed, like a pulse ox and an ABG. There are many ways to stimulate a patient and increase the RR.

Question 16

Answer: D

Rationale: An increase in intrathoracic pressure decreases the preload back to the heart. This will cause reduced cardiac output and hypotension. The increase in pressure may also cause damage to the lungs (barotrauma). Pressure does not affect ventilation or perfusion of the alveoli. Pressure also does not affect oxygenation. With a reduced cardiac output, the patient would likely become tachycardic, not bradycardic.

Question 17

Answer: C

Rationale: Patients with emphysema have difficulty with exhalation, NOT inhalation. There would be a decreased expiratory volume (FEV_1) in this patient, not inspiratory. All of the other answers are potential symptoms of emphysema.

Question 18

Answer: B

Rationale: A plateau pressure is measured when there is no air movement in the circuitry. Poor lung compliance may increase plateau pressures. Inhalation or exhalation periods do not describe a plateau pressure.

Question 19

Answer: C

Rationale: The PaO_2/FiO_2 ratio indicative of ARDS is less than 200 mmHg. The rest of this is memorization of the signs and symptoms of ARDS: hypercapnia and a wedge pressure below 18 mmHg. Infiltrates and hypoxemia are also often seen in ARDS patients. Remember the answer has to be 100% correct or it is not correct at all. There is no partial credit.

Question 20

Answer: B

Rationale: This ABG shows metabolic alkalosis with partial compensation. Study ABGs until you are able to find the conclusion of ABGs perfectly. This WILL be on the CCRN exam. The only answer in the list that may lead to metabolic alkalosis is electrolyte imbalances. Severe pain would lead to hyperventilation and respiratory alkalosis. Hyperkalemia would not be the direct cause of an acid–base imbalance, but rather a sign of the underlying problem, such as kidney failure. Decreased gas exchange or V/Q would lead to respiratory acidosis as CO_2 retention increases.

CHAPTER 4

Endocrine

The endocrine section makes up roughly five questions on your CCRN exam, so about 4% of the exam is devoted to this topic. Endocrine is a relatively small area on the CCRN exam, but there are a handful of key points to learn and master.

Acute Hypoglycemia

Mild hypoglycemia can affect anyone, but it is much more common in diabetics given the treatment regimens and the complex nature of glucose regulation. Severe hypoglycemia—glycemic emergency—almost exclusively affects diabetics and requires immediate treatment. Remember, there is a difference between Type 1 and Type 2 diabetes mellitus (DM). Type 1 DM has a higher risk of complications due to regular insulin administration. The brain requires glucose to function, and worsening states of hypoglycemia can lead to coma and death. (See Table 4-1.)

Table 4-1   Levels of Hypoglycemia Severity

LEVEL 1 MILD HYPOGLYCEMIA	LEVEL 2 MODERATE HYPOGLYCEMIA	LEVEL 3 SEVERE HYPOGLYCEMIA
• Glucose level < 80 mg/dL • Early signs	• Glucose level < 54 mg/dL	• Glucose level < 40 mg/dL • Late signs • Severe cognitive impairment

Etiology

- Insulin and oral antidiabetic agents
- Increased metabolic requirements
  - Exercise
- Changes in food intake
- Excessive alcohol intake in a diabetic

Signs and Symptoms

- Early signs → sympathetic stimulation
  - Tachycardia
  - Cold and clammy or diaphoretic
  - Headache
  - Anxiety or irritability
- Late signs → brain lacks glucose
  - Confusion
  - Slurred speech
  - Double vision
  - Seizures and convulsions (severe)
  - Loss of consciousness (severe)

CCRN Tip

Be cautious in diabetic patients also taking a beta blocker like metoprolol. Tachycardia is an early sign of hypoglycemia and will be masked with the use of these medications. Be cautious in patients with diabetic autonomic neuropathy as well.

Interventions

- Simple sugars (juice, glucose tablets, honey, candy, etc.)
- Dextrose
  - Crystalloids IV drip (5% or 10%)
  - 50% IV bolus
- Glucagon IM or IV

Diabetic Ketoacidosis (DKA) and Hyperglycemic Hyperosmolar Nonketotic Syndrome (HHNK)

Both DKA and HHNK are medical emergencies that may emerge in a diabetic patient. DKA is the more commonly hospitalized problem of the two. These emergencies are often discussed together because both are hyperglycemic in nature, and both are in relation to diabetics. Learn about the differences between them in the following section.

DKA

Etiology

- Uncontrolled Type 1 DM
  - Lack of insulin disables cells' ability to absorb glucose
  - Body utilizes fatty acids for energy → ketone production
- Infection (pneumonia, flu)
- Dehydration (6L loss of total body water)
- Fast onset

Signs and Symptoms

- Glucose: >250 mg/dL
- Metabolic acidosis on ABG
- Anion gap: >12
- Urinalysis
  - Positive: ketones
  - Positive: glucose

- Polyuria, polydipsia, polyphagia
- Acetone (fruity) breath
- Kussmaul breathing → compensation, breathe off carbon dioxide

Interventions
- Crystalloid treatment (**PRIORITY**)
  - 0.9% or 0.45% saline (assess natremic status)
  - Dextrose (when glucose reaches 250 mg/dL)
- Insulin treatment (secondary priority)
  - Assess serum potassium → replace if necessary
  - Drip to begin
  - SubQ (when anion gap is closed and acidosis resolved)
- Monitor potassium levels
  - Acidosis causes an increase in serum potassium
  - Insulin causes a decrease in serum potassium
    - Replace if necessary
- NPO order

HHNK

HHNK is now commonly called hyperosmolar hyperglycemic state (HHS).

Etiology
- Dehydration (9 L loss of total body water)
- More prevalent in elderly and Type 2 DM
- Slow onset

Signs and Symptoms
- Glucose: >600 mg/dL
- Osmolality: >320 mOsm/kg
- Hot and dry (dehydrated)
  - Elevated specific gravity
- Polyuria, polydipsia, polyphagia

Interventions
- Crystalloid treatment (**PRIORITY**)
  - 0.9% or 0.45% saline
  - Dextrose (when glucose reaches 300 mg/dL)
- Insulin treatment (secondary priority)
  - Drip to begin
  - SubQ
- NPO status

CCRN Tip

Slow and steady decreases are required for DKA and HHS. Too fast a decrease of glucose and/or sodium may lead to cerebral edema. A 50–100 mg/dL/hr for glucose reduction is key. There is also a risk of overshooting the mark creating *hypoglycemia and hypokalemia.*

Diabetes Insipidus (DI) and Syndrome of Inappropriate Secretion of Antidiuretic Hormone (SIADH)

Often referred to as a "master gland," the pituitary gland oversees a number of endocrinologic processes. For the purpose of this section, we are focusing on the water/salt concentration regulation of the pituitary gland. Antidiuretic hormone (ADH) is produced in the posterior pituitary with an end influence on the kidneys. Monitoring serum and urine osmolality allows for assessment of the kidneys' ability to concentrate urine and what amount of spillover may be occurring.

An interesting side note for learning: alcohol suppresses ADH, causing people to urinate more upon drinking. This is why patients coming into the hospital for alcohol-related injuries are typically dehydrated.

Serum Osmolality (275–295 mOsm/kg)

- Affected by sodium, BUN, and glucose. An increase in all these leads to an increase in osmolality. Back to basics: *water follows concentration*, osmosis. Where do we see these problems?
  - Sodium → DI and SIADH
  - BUN → acute kidney injuries
  - Glucose → DKA and HHS
- Hyperosmolar: >295 mOsm/kg
  - Concentrated blood → lab values go up (typically)
  - Hematocrit is a common lab value that trends with osmolality, but only if the hemoglobin is stable (no anemia or polycythemia)
- Hypo-osmolar: <275 mOsm/kg
  - Diluted blood → lab values go down (typically)

Urine Osmolality vs. Specific Gravity

These two values correlate quite well when the sample of urine is clean. Much of the time, specific gravity is utilized to estimate osmolality and overall fluid volume status. Osmolality is a much more accurate predictor, however. Do not confuse the two—the values are inverted and can be easily mistaken. (See Table 4-2.)

Table 4-2   Urine Osmolality vs. Urine Specific Gravity

URINE OSMOLALITY	URINE SPECIFIC GRAVITY
• 500–850 mOsm/kg • Increase → concentrated • Decrease → diluted	• 1.010–1.030 • Increase → dehydrated • Decrease → normovolemic or fluid overload

CCRN Tip

Specific gravity may be confusing in the setting of DI and SIADH because they do not follow traditional reasoning. While an increased specific gravity tends to imply dehydration in the patient, urine in a DI patient is dilute, whereas urine in a SIADH patient is concentrated. This is due to the condition itself.

Diabetes Insipidus (DI)

DI is characterized by decreased secretion of ADH.

Etiology

- Head injury (surgery or trauma)
- Tumor
- Hypoxic brain injury

Signs and Symptoms

- Increased serum osmolality (>295)
- Extreme polyuria (greater than 3 L/day)
  - Oftentimes greater than 6 L (calculate 24-hour urine output)
  - Dilute urine (low specific gravity)
- Monitor electrolytes
  - Hypernatremia
- Polydipsia, nocturia

Interventions

- Fluid replacement (often liter for liter)
- DDAVP
  - PO, intranasally, subQ, or IV
- Desmopressin, vasopressin
- Monitor electrolytes, especially sodium

> **CCRN Tip**
>
> Severe changes in fluid volume and sodium can lead to seizures and death. Any neurological changes in the patient should be regarded as potentially life-threatening. Keep this in mind during treatment as well. Rapid increases or decreases are dangerous.

Syndrome of Inappropriate Secretion of Antidiuretic Hormone (SIADH)

SIADH is characterized by increased levels of ADH.

Etiology

- CNS issues
  - Stroke, infection, trauma
- Malignancies
  - Small cell lung cancer (oat cell carcinoma)
- Pneumonia (viral, bacterial, tuberculosis)
- Medications
  - Carbamazepine, phenytoin

Signs and Symptoms

- Dilutional hyponatremia (nausea, malaise)
  - Vomiting (**RED FLAG**) → seizure activity
- Oliguria
- Decreased serum osmolality (<275)

Interventions

- Treat the underlying condition
- Fluid restriction w/ oral salt tabs or hypertonic saline (if necessary)
- Vasopressin antagonists (tolvaptan)—rare use (hepato/nephrotoxic)

Adrenal Insufficiency and Crisis

Most cases of adrenal insufficiency, also called Addison's disease, are relatively minor and often go undiagnosed. In critical care, the leading concern is the life-threatening nature of adrenal crisis and imminent shock states. Serum cortisol, ACTH, and chemistry panels should be assessed early to rule out adrenal crisis.

Etiology

- Iatrogenic (caused by treatments → glucocorticoids)
  - Lack of appropriate titration
- Autoimmune damage
- Adrenal stress or hemorrhage, infections, cancer

Signs and Symptoms

- Salt cravings
- Hyponatremia, hyperkalemia
- Hypotension → shock
- Skin pigmentation/poor skin turgor

Interventions

- Glucocorticoid/mineralocorticoid replacement (hydrocortisone, dexamethasone)
- Treat underlying infection if necessary
- Manage hemodynamic instability
- Dextrose administration for hypoglycemia

Hyperthyroidism vs. Hypothyroidism

It is not uncommon for critically ill patients to have some abnormalities with thyroid hormone levels. It is also associated with longer ventilator times and hospital stays if left untreated. The pathophysiology for these secondary hypothyroidism or hyperthyroidism states are not very well known and are not covered on the CCRN exam. It is, however, important to distinguish **primary** hypothyroidism or hyperthyroidism that brings a patient into the ICU. (See Table 4-3.)

CCRN Tip

The relationship between T3/T4 and TSH/TRH is inverted. A decrease in TSH/TRH will result in an increase in T3/T4. Be aware of this when analyzing the correlation.

Table 4-3   Comparisons of Hypothyroidism and Hyperthyroidism

	HYPOTHYROIDISM	HYPERTHYROIDISM
Etiologies	Decreased T3 and T4 Increased TSH Hashimoto's thyroiditis Iodine deficiency Infection (may trigger myxedema)	Increased T3 and T4 Decreased TSH Graves' disease Exogenous hormone (levothyroxine)
Clinical emergency	*Myxedema coma*	*Thyroid storm/crisis*
Signs and symptoms	Fatigue, malaise, weight gain Cold intolerance Stupor, coma Respiratory depression Bradycardia Hypotension Swelling of face, tongue	Agitation, weight loss Heat intolerance Hyperthermia Hypotension Dysrhythmias Respiratory compromise Delirium/psychosis
Interventions	Intubation and mechanical ventilation if necessary T3/T4 administration Slow central rewarming Isotonic fluid resuscitation Steroids	NIV or intubation with mechanical ventilation if necessary Beta blockers Methimazole Propylthiouracil Stabilize hemodynamics Body cooling Plasmapheresis

Review Questions

1. A patient diagnosed with a brain tumor was recently admitted to the ICU due to suspected diabetes insipidus. The previous hour urine output totaled 500 mL. The physician has ordered lactated Ringer's fluid replacement and desmopressin. Which of the following lab values would indicate improvement of the condition?

   A. Serum sodium 151 mEq/L

   B. Serum osmolality 270 mOsm/kg

   C. Serum potassium 4.0 mEq/L

   D. Serum osmolality 290 mOsm/kg

2. Aside from polyuria for the patient in question 1, what other findings would the nurse recognize as likely diabetes insipidus?

   A. Urine specific gravity 1.002

   B. Serum osmolality 265 mOsm/kg

   C. Serum sodium 121 mEq/L

   D. BP 135/70, HR 90

3. A patient with a history of small cell lung cancer was recently brought to the ED due to excessive vomiting. Current labs include Na^+ 115 mEq/L, urine output 20 mL/hr, and a serum osmolality of 255 mOsm/kg. Which of the following would be the most important for the nurse to do first?

   A. Administer hypertonic saline 100 mL/hr IV

   B. Assess for tremors, seizure activity

   C. Administer furosemide 40 mg IV

   D. Assess deep tendon reflexes

4. A 78-year-old female with Type 2 diabetes was admitted from a nursing home due to continued high fingerstick glucose checks with worsening confusion. The most recent glucose taken was 650 mg/dL. Which of the following would indicate a diagnosis of HHS instead of DKA?

   A. Osmolality 330 mOsm/kg, glucose 650 mg/dL

   B. Osmolality 260 mOsm/kg, polyuria

   C. Osmolality 275 mOsm/kg, serum pH 7.20

   D. Osmolality 330 mOsm/kg, tachypnea

5. The patient in question 4 was started on normal saline and an insulin drip in the ICU. Current labs show glucose 290 mg/dL, serum osmolality 300 mOsm/kg, BP 110/80 mmHg, HR 95. Which of the following interventions is appropriate at this time?

   A. Assess for glucosuria
   B. Stop the insulin drip
   C. Decrease normal saline infusion to 25 mL/hr
   D. Dextrose IV continuous

6. A hospitalized patient with diabetes and hypertension has been prescribed metoprolol by the physician. What would the nurse emphasize in the teaching to this patient at discharge?

   A. Call the physician if bradycardic
   B. Understand signs and symptoms of hypoglycemia
   C. Increase glycemic food intake
   D. Hold metoprolol if hypoglycemic

7. Which of the following symptoms may the patient in question 6 expect if hypoglycemic?

   A. Changes in vision
   B. Tachycardia
   C. Fever and diaphoresis
   D. Oliguria

8. A patient remains intubated in the ICU post-op day 2 from a complicated thoracotomy. The patient is currently sedated with tube feedings at 50 mL/hr. Morning labs showed abnormal sodium at 150 mg/dL. The physician decides to add-on a serum osmolality to lab work; the result is 320 mOsm/kg. Which of the following interventions is indicated at this time?

   A. Decrease rate on tube feedings
   B. Decrease rate on normal saline drip
   C. Add free water flushes to tube feedings
   D. Begin hypotonic infusion

9. Serum osmolality is affected by a multitude of factors. In which of the following would the nurse expect to see increases to the serum osmolality?

   A. SIADH
   B. Alzheimer's patient with excessive water intake
   C. Decreased BUN (urea)
   D. Dehydration in a elderly diabetic patient

10. An 18-year-old patient was recently admitted after being witnessed collapsing outdoors on a hot day. Upon admission their skin is cold and clammy to the touch. The patient remains obtunded and unable to answer questions. A classmate is bedside and states she believes the patient to be diabetic. Which of the following findings would the nurse expect?

    A. Glucose 45, HR 50, urine specific gravity 1.010

    B. Glucose 600, HR 140, acetone breath

    C. Glucose 60, BP 160/80, polyuria

    D. Glucose 45, HR 130, BP 90/60

Answer Key

Question 1

Answer: D

Rationale: The normal range for serum osmolality is 275–295 mOsm/kg. Patients experiencing diabetes insipidus have a hyperosmolar state >295 mOsm/kg. If the treatment is working, a corrected osmolality is expected on the higher end of normal. A normal sodium between 135 and 145 mEq/L would indicate improvement of DI. The potassium of 4.0 mEq/L is a normal number, but this is not the main concern for DI.

Question 2

Answer: A

Rationale: Questions like this that ask you to list signs and symptoms of diseases are relatively common on the CCRN exam. For diabetes insipidus, a diluted urine is expected; this is shown in a specific gravity of 1.002. Nocturia along with polyuria and polydipsia are also expected in DI. Serum osmolality and sodium would be elevated in DI, not reduced. With a patient voiding excessive amounts of fluid, it can be expected the patient may be hypovolemic with a low blood pressure and reflex tachycardia.

Question 3

Answer: B

Rationale: The patient is showing signs and symptoms of SIADH. The excessive vomiting is especially worrisome, as it is an indication of dilutional hyponatremia. The biggest risk at this moment is seizure activity that may lead to death if left unmanaged. The nurse should assess seizure activity first, then move on to treatments. A hypertonic solution may be used, but 100 mL/hr is excessive. Remember that the goal of sodium movement is incremental improvements. Changes that are too quick are dangerous. A diuretic is used at times in SIADH, but it is not the immediate priority. Deep tendon reflex changes are often seen with changes in serum magnesium, not sodium levels.

Question 4

Answer: A

Rationale: A diagnosis of HHS over DKA can be seen first by serum osmolality. HHS is a hyperosmolar disorder; DKA is not. The elevated osmolality above 320 mOsm/kg displays HHS. Glucose is typically much higher in HHS than DKA as well, typically above 600 mg/dL. Polyuria can be a symptom of both HHS and DKA. HHS is not an acidic state like DKA. Deep tachypneic breathing (Kussmaul) is seen in DKA, not HHS.

Question 5

Answer: D

Rationale: The treatment for this patient has been working. There has been improvement in both glucose and serum osmolality. At this time, it is appropriate to add dextrose to the crystalloid treatment. When the glucose falls below 300 mg/dL, it is time to add dextrose. The insulin drip will be decreased by protocol but is not discontinued until the osmolality issues have been resolved and mental status has improved. The hydration via normal saline will also continue until osmolality has resolved. Assessing glycosuria is not needed, the diagnosis of HHS already exists.

Question 6

Answer: B

Rationale: Extra care must be given to diabetic patients prescribed beta blockers like metoprolol. Tachycardia is an early sign of hypoglycemia; with a beta blocker, the medication will mask this symptom and the patient may not be aware they are hypoglycemic. It is important for the patient to understand the full picture of what hypoglycemia may look like for them. Unless the patient is experiencing other problems, bradycardia does not warrant calling the physician for this patient. Increasing foods high in sugar is not a good idea for any diabetic patient. It may assist this patient from avoiding hypoglycemia, but they will likely experience hyperglycemia and unregulated diabetes due to the drastic dietary change. Patients do not choose to hold meds on their own accord; changes to scheduled medications require a higher scope of practice.

Question 7

Answer: A

Rationale: Diabetic patients who take metoprolol should be taught the signs and symptoms of hypoglycemia they may expect. Later signs of hypoglycemia are often the *first* signs these patients experience. Vision changes and other CNS issues (slurred speech, confusion) may be seen. While diaphoresis is considered an early sign of hypoglycemia, something this patient may not experience due to the beta blocker, a fever with diaphoresis is more aligned with HHS. Oliguria is not a symptom of hypoglycemia.

Question 8

Answer: C

Rationale: This patient is showing possible signs of dehydration or at the least hypernatremia with hyperosmolality. Sodium changes should be done slowly. By adding free water flushes to the tube feeding, the patient will receive more fluid enterally. This is also considered a less invasive measure than other options like a hypotonic infusion. Decreasing the tube feeding or a current isotonic infusion would make the problem worse. This patient needs more fluid, not less.

Question 9

Answer: D

Rationale: Dehydration may come about for many reasons: vomiting, diarrhea, sweating, burns. Decrease in overall body fluid causes an increase in the concentration of fluids (osmolality). It is especially important for the elderly to receive enough fluid intake. A dehydrated elderly diabetic patient has increased risk of developing HHS if not corrected early enough. SIADH, excessive fluid intake, and a decreased BUN would cause a decrease in serum osmolality, not increase. Remember that the main particles of osmolality include sodium, BUN, and glucose.

Question 10

Answer: D

Rationale: The story and symptoms most closely match hypoglycemia with likely dehydration given the hot day. Hot weather may also precipitate hypoglycemia due to increased body metabolism. The heart rate will be increased with other symptoms of dehydration (increased urine specific gravity, increased serum osmolality, decreased blood pressure). Acetone breath is seen in DKA. Polyuria is seen in hyperglycemia.

CHAPTER 5

Gastrointestinal

The gastrointestinal section makes up roughly eight questions on your CCRN exam, so 6% of the exam is devoted to this topic. The majority of the concepts listed in this chapter you are likely familiar with from previous studies and/or clinical application. A fair number of these issues are common. As is with all critical care knowledge, a strong foundation in anatomy and physiology helps overall understanding. Revisit the basics on anatomy if you feel weak in this area. General assessment points are also included in this chapter.

Abdominal Physical Assessment Review

Given the multiple organs and large body area covered by the GI system, a brief review of physical assessment is helpful. The following points are not all-inclusive, but rather focus on the top CCRN exam questions that may appear.

Abdominal Pain

Pain is the most common manifestation associated with GI issues. Focus on the location of the pain (see Figure 5-1), the intensity, duration, and any radiating. Based upon the pain findings along with symptoms (diarrhea, nausea, vomiting, melena, jaundice, etc.), a more thorough train of thought is formed.

Figure 5-1   Abdominal Assessment Locations

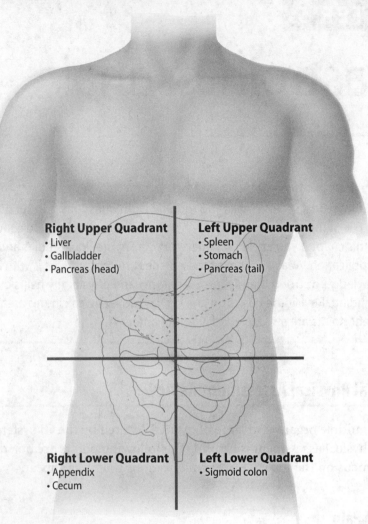

Right Upper Quadrant
- Liver
- Gallbladder
- Pancreas (head)

Left Upper Quadrant
- Spleen
- Stomach
- Pancreas (tail)

Right Lower Quadrant
- Appendix
- Cecum

Left Lower Quadrant
- Sigmoid colon

Abdominal Compartment Syndrome (ACS)

You may be quite familiar with the term *compartment syndrome* in relation to an extremity and the medical emergency involving potential loss of limb. The same idea applies to abdominal compartment syndrome. The increase in abdominal pressure may lead to ischemia of the bowels and abdominal organs. If blood flow is not reestablished, infarctions and permanent damage may occur, leading to organ dysfunction and failure. The syndrome is fatal if not corrected. (See Table 5-1.)

CCRN Tip

Abdominal perfusion pressure (APP) is similar to MAP. Both numbers should ultimately be above 60 mmHg to demonstrate adequate perfusion.

Table 5-1   Etiology: Primary vs. Secondary

PRIMARY ACS	SECONDARY ACS
Abdominal blunt or penetrating trauma	Significant fluid shifts
Hemorrhage	• Ascites
Abdominal aortic aneurysm (AAA) rupture	• Burns
Intestinal obstruction	• Large volume fluid resuscitation
Retroperitoneal bleeding	Intra-abdominal sepsis (peritonitis)

Signs and Symptoms

The most common method of assessing ACS is through bladder pressures. Make sure the patient is lying flat and the transducer is placed at the **symphysis pubis**. Measure at the end of breath expiration if possible.

- Intra-abdominal hypertension (IAH): >12 mmHg (typically via bladder pressures—foley cath)
  - Severe IAH: >20 mmHg
- Distended or tense abdomen (hemorrhage, fluid)
  - *Cullen's sign* → ecchymosis around umbilicus
  - *Grey Turner's sign* → ecchymosis of flank (retroperitoneal)
  - *Kehr's sign* → left shoulder pain (ruptured spleen)
- Secondary organ problems
  - Cardiac: decreased cardiac output, increased CVP
  - Pulmonary: increased peak airway pressures, decreased ventilation
  - Renal: oliguria (decreased renal perfusion)

Interventions

The primary goal is to reduce IAH and prevent the progression to ACS. Once ACS is reached and/or symptoms of organ dysfunction exist, the treatment modalities become more aggressive.

- Intra-abdominal hypertension (IAP 12–19 mmHg)
  - Decrease abdominal pressure (positioning, remove constrictive devices or clothing)
  - NG tube to low-intermittent suction and rectal tube placement (decompression)
  - Move the bowels if possible (induce defecation → enema, medications)
  - Manage pain, keep the patient comfortable
  - Drain abdominal fluid → needle aspiration
  - Neuromuscular blockade in vented patients (if necessary)
- Abdominal compartment syndrome (IAP >20 mmHg)
  - Emergency laparotomy
    - Temporary closure/open fascia → wound vac or zipper

Acute Gastrointestinal Hemorrhage

GI bleeding is potentially life-threatening depending on the severity of the hemorrhage. Upper bleeds occur roughly twice as often as lower bleeds. Lower GI bleeds oftentimes resolve spontaneously without intervention; upper GI bleeds have higher mortality rates (upward of 10%). Table 5-2 distinguishes between upper and lower GI bleeds. Any hemodynamic instability and/or active bleeding prompts an ICU admission.

Table 5-2   Upper vs. Lower GI Hemorrhage

UPPER GI BLEED	LOWER GI BLEED
Etiologies Peptic ulcers (50%) • H. pylori • NSAID use Esophageal varices (higher mortality) • Liver cirrhosis Mallory-Weiss tears Malignancy	**Etiologies** Colonic bleeding • Diverticulosis (30%) • Internal hemorrhoids • Ischemic Inflammatory bowel disease (IBD) Malignancy
Signs and Symptoms Hematemesis • Bright red (most serious) • Coffee-ground (less serious) Melena (black tarry)	**Signs and Symptoms** Hematochezia (red, maroon stool)
SEVERE BLEED Signs and Symptoms Hypotension/dizziness Severe dysrhythmias/palpitations Cold and clammy LOC/mental status changes	

Interventions
EGD (<12 hours)
Proton pump inhibitors
 • Esomeprazole, pantoprazole
Peptic ulcers
 • Epinephrine submucosal injection
 • Clips
Esophageal varices
 • Octreotide (vasoactive)
 • Vasopressin
 • Band ligation
 • Sengstaken-Blakemore tube
   • Tamponade bleeding
   • Cut balloon if respiratory distress develops
 • TIPS surgery (last resort)
	Interventions
	Colonoscopy/sigmoidoscopy (<24 hours)
	Mesenteric angiography
	Diverticulosis
	 • Epinephrine submucosal injections
	 • Clips
	Colonic surgical resection is now much less common

Common Interventions for BOTH Fluid resuscitation (isotonic solutions) Transfusions NPO status Oxygen and vasopressors (if necessary)	

CCRN Tip

In cases of severe bleeding, endoscopy would be performed immediately.

> **CCRN Tip**
>
> For patients on medications that predispose excessive bleeding—warfarin, heparin, clopidogrel, NSAIDS, etc.—blood products may be required to correct the underlying problem and/or reversal agents. Review blood products, if necessary, in Chapter 8, "Hematology/Immunology." It is important to know in what cases they may be used (e.g., platelets in thrombocytopenia <50,000).

Endoscopy Procedures

Endoscopy may include EGD, colonoscopy, sigmoidoscopy, and ERCP, among others. Less invasive methods such as wireless capsules are also becoming more popular. Common pre-, intra-, and post-procedural information potentially tested by the CCRN exam include the following:

Pre-procedural
- Upper scope: NPO 6 hours before
- Lower scope: NPO 12 hours before
    - Colonoscopy: bowel prep (polyethylene glycol)
    - Sigmoidoscopy: fleet enemas
- Legal basics (consent, time-out)
- Antibiotic prophylaxis (high-risk patients)

Intra-procedural
- Monitor vitals
- Moderate sedation (midazolam, fentanyl)
- Pathological findings (photo documentation)

Post-procedural
- Monitor for complications
    - Perforation (tachycardia, radiating pain, fever)
    - Bleeding (vomiting blood, blood in stool)
    - ABC issues (chest pain, dyspnea)
- PACU recovery protocols
- Discharge planning

Bowel Infarction

A loss of blood flow to the bowels may lead to ischemia and infarction. If left untreated, the inflammatory process leads to necrosis and potential emergencies like perforation, sepsis, and death. The terminology can get a bit jumbled, but the general consensus among gastroenterologists is the acute or chronic nature of the disease and the ability for a patient to move from one type to another type. (See Table 5-3.)

As with most things, the acute problem is more serious and life-threatening. For the purpose of the CCRN exam, focus on the acute, life-threatening issues; chronic issues are deliberately left short.

Anatomy

- Superior mesenteric artery (SMA): main blood supply to small bowel
- Celiac artery system (pancreaticoduodenal arteries): collateral blood flow to small bowel
- Inferior mesenteric artery (IMA): collateral blood flow

Infarction Types

- Acute mesenteric ischemia (AMI): may lead to intestinal infarction
- Chronic mesenteric ischemia (CMI): also called intestinal angina
- Colonic ischemia (CI): common ischemic-inflammatory process

Etiology

- Vessel occlusions
  - Arterial occlusion by emboli (most common [50%])
  - Thrombus occlusions (stenosis, small vessels, venous)
- Multi-vascular disease
  - Atherosclerosis (highest risk)
  - HTN, diabetes, coronary artery disease
- Major surgery and trauma

> **CCRN Tip**
>
> Acute embolism of the mesenteric arteries is typically the most obvious form of the disease with a blanket of symptoms. A common phrase used is "pain out of proportion," meaning unrelenting excruciating pain unrelieved by meds.

Table 5-3   Signs and Symptoms: Acute vs. Chronic

ACUTE MESENTERIC ISCHEMIA	CHRONIC MESENTERIC ISCHEMIA
Triad • Pain out of proportion (see CCRN Tip) • Fever • Hemoccult-positive stools Nausea, vomiting, diarrhea Peritonitis (red flag → ominous) Intestinal dilation → abdominal distention Gangrenous Monitor for ABC changes; may indicate emergency	Nongangrenous Intestinal angina

Interventions

- Early CT angiography
- Fluids (first) → increase visceral perfusion
- Nasogastric decompression
- Antibiotics and heparin

- Continuous monitoring
  - Electrolytes
  - Lactate levels
  - Acidosis
- Early revascularization → angioplasty and/or stenting
- Emergency laparotomy → resection of necrotic tissue (if emergency)

Bowel Obstruction

Any blockage or failure to move contents forward in the GI tract may be considered a form of obstruction. There are many names and types of obstruction; a review of important ones follows in Table 5-4.. Small bowel obstructions are more common than large bowel obstructions.

Table 5-4   Types of Obstruction

FUNCTIONAL OBSTRUCTION	MECHANICAL OBSTRUCTION
Due to nerve dysfunction	Barrier causing obstruction **Volvulus**: twisting around mesentery **Intussusception**: scoping of bowel

Etiology

- Small bowel obstruction (SBO)
  - Adhesions (most common): scar tissue forming between bowel loops and organs or the abdominal wall
  - External hernia
  - Crohn's disease
  - Neoplasm: metastatic disease
- Large bowel obstruction (LBO)
  - Colorectal cancer (most common)
  - Inflammatory bowel diseases (diverticulitis)
  - Twisting or scoping of the bowel (intussusception, volvulus)

Signs and Symptoms

- Diagnostics
  - KUB → dilated bowels
  - CT scan → partial versus complete obstruction
  - Colonoscopy → large bowel suspected
- Abdominal pain → typically dull and generalized
- Bowel sounds
  - High-pitched → small bowel
  - Low-pitched → large bowel
- Nausea, vomiting, diarrhea
- Electrolyte imbalances (monitor potassium)

Interventions

- Conservative (primary) treatment plan
  - Intravenous fluid therapy
  - Correct electrolyte imbalances
  - NG tube to suction → decompression (prevent aspiration from vomiting)
  - Feedings depend on location of ileus
- Aggressive treatment plan
  - Complete obstruction → laparotomy
  - Strangulation, perforation, gangrene → laparotomy

Bowel Perforation

A known complication of bowel obstruction, a perforation is a medical emergency and will result in death if not immediately treated. There are other causes of perforation such as trauma or invasive procedures; the result is the same: the system (GI tract) is no longer closed. (See Table 5.5.)

Table 5-5   Bowel Perforation

SIGNS AND SYMPTOMS	INTERVENTIONS
Peritonitis	Stabilize hemodynamics
• Rigid, board-like abdomen	Broad-spectrum antibiotics
Pain	NPO and NG tube to suction (decompression)
• Gradual or sudden	Laparoscopic or open laparotomy
• Guarding	• Direct repair and infection control
Sepsis	
• Hyperthermia	
• Tachycardia	
• Tachypnea	
• Loss of BP (shock)	

Hepatic Failure

The full clinical picture for liver failure is rather large simply because of the multitude of functions by the liver itself. For this reason, it may be wise to take a step back and analyze the essential functions of the liver itself.

Etiology

- Acute liver failure
  - Drug-induced liver injury (DILI; most common) → acetaminophen
  - Viral hepatitis (less common)
    - Hepatitis B
  - Ischemic hepatitis (poor perfusion due to shock states)

- Chronic liver failure
  - Alcohol abuse and hepatitis C
  - May lead to cirrhosis (scar tissue → fibrosis)

Signs and Symptoms

- Nausea, vomiting, fatigue, malaise
- RUQ pain (inflammation)
- Ascites (fluid-wave test)
- See table 5-6 for lab value changes in liver failure

CCRN Tip

Fulminant hepatitis is a rare but life-threatening complication of acute viral hepatitis and acetaminophen/paracetamol use. The liver parenchyma experiences enormous **necrosis** with a resulting shrinking of the liver itself. It is often **not palpable** at this stage. The assessment and interventions for fulminant hepatitis is in line with expected liver failure.

The most obvious difference affecting fulminant hepatitis is the **RAPID** onset and fast progression of the disease. Without liver transplantation, death is likely.

Table 5-6   Serum Changes and Implications

INCREASED LAB VALUES	
Ammonia (NH_3) → hepatic encephalopathy	Glucose → hypoglycemia
Transaminitis (AST, ALT)	Albumin (protein) → ascites
Bilirubin → jaundice (icterus)	**Pancytopenia**
PT, PTT → bleeding risk	WBC → infection risk
Creatinine, BUN (azotemia) → renal compromise	RBC → anemia
• Hepatorenal syndrome	Platelets → bleeding risk

Interventions

The following is a generalized approach to liver failure, including interventions for hepatic encephalopathy and portal hypertension.

- N-acetylcysteine → acetaminophen overdose
- Antivirals → viral hepatitis
- Monitor all potential serum lab abnormalities
- Monitor for metabolic acidosis
- Dextrose infusion (prevent hypoglycemia)
  - Add saline to make the solution isotonic
  - Lactated Ringer's is avoided due to lactate being metabolized in the liver
- Prevent cerebral edema (ICP)
  - Semi-Fowler's: midline head position
  - Mannitol administration
  - Hyperventilation
- Nutritional requirements (enteral or parenteral)
- Correct coagulopathy **if active bleeding** exists
- Liver transplant

Hepatic Encephalopathy (HE)

Hepatic encephalopathy, sometimes called hepatic coma, is caused by an increase of ammonia in the blood. It is reversible if the underlying liver disease is corrected. There are also some temporizing treatments given in the meantime. There are four stages of HE. Stage one being the beginning, showing minor changes in mental status such as confusion. As the stages advance to stage four, eventually the patient moves into a coma with no response to stimuli.

Signs and Symptoms

- Confusion → stupor → coma
- Asterixis (hand flapping)
- ICP-related issues
- Fetor hepaticus (musty breath)

Interventions

- Lactulose (oral or enema)
- Neomycin (reduces ammonia forming bacteria in GI tract)
- Avoid Lactated Ringer's
- **Avoid hypokalemia**
- Avoid renal failure and GI bleeding (precipitates encephalopathy)

Portal Hypertension

One of the many potential complications involving liver failure, specifically cirrhosis, is portal hypertension. The increase of pressure in the portal system (see Figure 5-2) above 5 mmHg may suggest portal hypertension. Collateral circulation is created to compensate for this increase in intrahepatic pressure:

- Esophageal varices → hematemesis
- Ascites → risk for bacterial peritonitis
- Caput medusae (periumbilical abdominal veins)
- Spider nevi

> **CCRN Tip**
>
> Esophageal/gastric varices are covered in more detail under GI bleeding. Refer to that section for immediate interventions.

Figure 5-2   Portal system

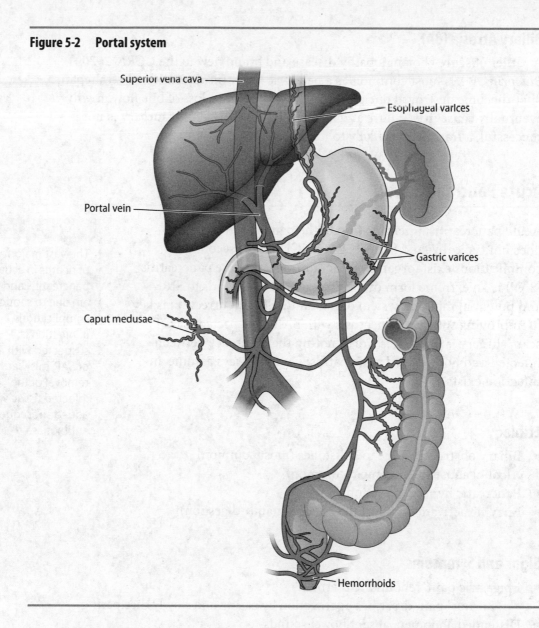

Superior vena cava

Esophageal varices

Portal vein

Gastric varices

Caput medusae

Hemorrhoids

Transjugular intrahepatic porto-systemic shunt (TIPS) has become an effective procedure to reduce the overall pressure in the portal system. It is considered when high mortality complications like esophageal varices, pulmonary compromise, and/or renal compromise are recurrent. Refractory ascites is also an indication for the procedure. Post-procedural complications include the following:

- Hemodynamic compromise
- Sepsis
- Hepatic encephalopathy
- Thrombosis and/or stent occlusion

Biliary Atresia (BA)

A rather obscure cholangiopathy disease and brand new to the *CCRN 2020 Blueprint*, BA is most common as a pediatric issue. Intrahepatic or extrahepatic ducts become destroyed due to fibrosclerosis causing a loss of bile flow. It will eventually cause liver failure and death without treatment. If surgery is not successful, a transplant is likely to follow.

Acute Pancreatitis (AP)

Acute pancreatitis, inflammation of the pancreas, in general does not typically land patients in the ICU unless secondary complications exist (organ dysfunction). Severe acute pancreatitis (SAP) is an extreme form of the disease that often leads to SIRS and potential multiple system organ failure. Early correction is key to improving survival. If necrosis with SAP is suspected via CT scan, surgery is likely. It is worth noting the difference between infected and noninfected pancreatitis. Do not always assume an infection exists.

> **CCRN Tip**
>
> The vast majority of deaths in acute pancreatitis and SAP are due to septic complications. If infection is suspected with AP or SAP, this warrants removal of the infected tissue with added subsequent antibiotics.

Etiology

- Biliary obstruction due to gallstones (most common)
- Alcohol abuse (second most common)
- Pancreatic hyperstimulation
- Enzyme activation within the pancreas (auto-digestion)

Signs and Symptoms

- Epigastric pain, rebound tenderness
  - "Boring" pain describes aggravation by eating and slowly dissipating
- Distended abdomen, absent bowel sounds
- Nausea and vomiting
- Laboratory changes
  - Increased serum amylase and lipase
  - Increased serum glucose
  - **Decreased serum calcium (Trousseau's** and **Chvostek's sign)**
- ERCP or MRCP if biliary causes suspected
- Infection triad if suspected
  - Elevated WBC
  - Fever
  - Pain

Interventions

- Systemic support (fluid resuscitation, oxygen support, nutrition support, correct electrolyte imbalances, manage glucose levels)
  - Assess for secondary complications
  - Pulmonary complications (effusions, atelectasis, ARDS)
- Restrict pancreatitis inflammation and necrosis
  - Antibiotics → if severe
  - Protease inhibitors (octreotide) → reduce pancreatic exocrine release
- Enteral and/or parenteral therapy
  - Enteral → jejunal route
  - Bowel rest → TPN
- Conservative surgery (organ debridement) → SAP
  - Drainage catheters (irrigation and drainage)

Malnutrition and Malabsorption

Most patients in the ICU have some degree of malnutrition upon admission, especially the elderly. Prompt assessment is important to minimize delay and the risk of complications regardless of the admitting diagnosis. Many of the earlier conditions discussed in this chapter further increase this risk of malnutrition due to malabsorption.

A brief reminder of types of malabsorption based on the area of the bowel follows. If large portions of the small intestine are removed, the general resulting malabsorption is termed "short-gut syndrome." In the end, consideration must be made not just for macromolecules like protein, fats, or carbs, but also vitamins and minerals.

- **Small bowel (duodenum/jejunum):** nutrients, minerals, vitamins, lactose intolerance
- **Small bowel (ileum):** bile salts, vitamin B12
- **Large bowel:** water

Table 5-7 outlines the signs and symptoms of malabsorption.

Table 5-7   Malabsorption Signs and Symptoms

PHYSICAL SYMPTOMS	LAB CHANGES
Weight loss/emaciation	**Anemias**
Abdominal pain/cramping	Vitamin B12 (cobalamin)
• Chronic diarrhea	Vitamin B9 (folate)
• Steatorrhea (fatty stools)	Iron (ferritin)
Glossitis (sore tongue)	**Deficiencies**
Cheilosis (dry scaly mucous membranes)	Vitamin A (beta-carotene) → night blindness
	Vitamin D → hypocalcemia and bone issues
	Vitamin K → bleeding issues (petechiae)

Interventions

Most treatments for digestive disorders involve limiting the insulting problem, an example being minimizing fats for a patient not producing enough bile or without a gallbladder. Medications may also be used to treat certain symptoms: for diarrhea, loperamide; for GERD, PPIs. In addition to dietary changes, some patients may not be able to make these changes on their own, prompting enteral or parenteral nutrition.

Enteral Nutrition

Enteral feeding is preferred over parenteral. Oral intake preserves the function of the gut and minimizes the loss of gut flora that aid in digestion. In an ICU patient, feedings should begin regardless of bowel sounds, flatulence, or the passing of stool. Begin at a low feeding rate and slowly increase to goal. The most concerning complication of tube feedings is pulmonary compromise.

- Preventing aspiration
  - Confirm NG tube placement (pH of aspirate, x-ray)
  - Semi-Fowler's position or higher
  - Monitor tube position via length at nares
  - Residuals q4hr
- Feeding intolerance
  - Diarrhea, vomiting
  - Stomach distention

> **CCRN Tip**
>
> Anytime there is concern about aspiration or NG tube placement, enteral feedings should be stopped. Added note: Residuals are no longer a basis for discontinuing a feeding unless very large in size (500 mL or more). Typically, a prokinetic agent like metoclopramide is prescribed before a feeding is stopped altogether.

Parenteral Nutrition

If enteral feedings are not possible, parenteral nutrition may begin with a few general rules. If a patient is unable to achieve at least 60% of the necessary caloric intake after 7 to 10 days, parenteral nutrition is indicated.

- Complications
  - Infection (central venous catheter → CLABSI)
  - Hyperglycemia (TPN contains dextrose)
  - Liver dysfunction

> **CCRN Tip**
>
> If a patient will feasibly be able to begin enteral intake within the 7-day period albeit not at this exact moment, parenteral nutrition is *not* indicated. The risks outweigh the benefits.

GI Surgeries

There are a number of GI surgeries that may be performed on patients for a multitude of reasons. Table 5-8 showcases specific surgeries listed on the CCRN blueprint. As with most surgeries, bleeding and pulmonary complications are fairly common. For this purpose, the complications listed below are specific to that type of surgery.

Table 5-8   Types of GI Surgeries

SURGERY	INDICATIONS	COMPLICATIONS

Whipple (pancreaticoduodenectomy)	Pancreatic ductal adenocarcinoma
	Cystic neoplasm
	Ampullary lesions
	Chronic pancreatitis
		Pancreatic fistula
		Delayed gastric emptying
		  • Rule out obstruction
		Dietary concerns
		  • Low fat, small meals, soft solids
		Anastomotic leak
		  • Assess drain output
		Hyperglycemia

Esophagectomy	Esophageal cancer	Anastomotic leak
		Laryngeal nerve damage
		  • Hoarseness of voice
		Stenosis with dysphagia
		  • Dilation to fix

Bowel resections	Colorectal malignancy	Anastomotic leak
		  • Antibiotics
		  • Washout
		Left ureter damage
		Infection (wound, UTI)

Bariatric
Gastrectomy
Gastric bypass
Gastric balloon
Gastric sleeve
	Weight loss	Anastomotic leak
		Hypoglycemia (due to dumping syndrome)
		Malabsorption
		  • Protein
		  • Vitamins (B12, folate)
		  • Calcium
		  • Iron
		Gallstones (high risk)
		Wound

Anastomotic Leak

Anastomotic leak is a repeating theme in the above surgeries. It is a devastating complication that drastically increases a patient's morbidity and mortality. The below symptoms may show in a patient with a potential leak. Typical onset of symptoms is 3 days post-operative.

- Persistent tachycardia (>120 BPM)
- Fever
- Abdominal pain
- Dyspnea

Review Questions

1. A patient was recently admitted with diffuse abdominal pain, decreased bowel sounds, and a fever of 100.5°F. Upon palpation, a section of the bowel feels hard to the touch. Three hours later, the patient complains of severe 10/10 abdominal pain. Auscultation reveals absent bowel sounds and a rigid abdomen to the touch. What is the immediate intervention at this time?

    A. Prepare for open laparotomy

    B. Increase IV fluids and prepare for colonoscopy

    C. Insert an NG tube and place to suction

    D. Administer metoclopramide STAT

2. Which of the following is NOT a known complication of mesenteric ischemia?

    A. Increasing lactate levels

    B. Necrosis of bowel tissue

    C. Perforation with peritonitis

    D. Metabolic alkalosis

Questions 3–5 refer to the following case.

A patient was recently brought into the trauma unit after a fall from a three-story building. The patient was immediately intubated and an indwelling catheter was placed. During quick assessment, the nurse notes bruising bilaterally to the flank and a rigid distended abdomen.

3. What finding would cause the most concern at this time?

    A. Bladder pressure of 20 mmHg

    B. Abdominal perfusion pressure of 60 mmHg

    C. BP 110/70, HR 110 BPM

    D. Oliguria over the past hour

4. All of the following reflect common complications of intra-abdominal hypertension EXCEPT for:

    A. Increased CVP

    B. Diminished lung sounds

    C. Decreased urine output

    D. Hemorrhagic pancreatitis

5. When assessing the trauma patient above, which of the following reflects the correct protocol for obtaining and analyzing a bladder pressure?

   A. Place the transducer at the phlebostatic axis

   B. Bladder pressures above 20 mmHg reflect a nonpathological abdomen

   C. Place the patient in a supine position, take readings in the same position

   D. Understand a direct measurement may be taken by placing a needle into the bladder

6. A patient is recovering in the PACU after a complicated upper endoscopy. The patient now complains of upper back pain. Current vitals include a BP of 110/80, HR of 120, and a low-grade fever. What is the most accurate concern for this patient at this time?

   A. Reaction to the anesthesia

   B. Perforation of the esophagus

   C. Myocardial infarction

   D. Internal abdominal bleeding

7. A patient was recently admitted with a diagnosis of a small bowel obstruction. KUB displays dilated bowel loops. The patient complains of discomfort but not pain. Which of the following interventions would be appropriate at this time?

   A. Parenteral nutrition therapy

   B. Colonoscopy

   C. Closely monitor electrolytes

   D. Prepare for open laparotomy

8. A patient with chronic liver failure has required repeated paracentesis procedures to remove the excess fluid in his abdomen. He arrives at the hospital in respiratory distress and is placed on 2 L nasal cannula. What is the best explanation for why this patient is having difficulty breathing?

   A. Fluid diffusion causing pericardial effusions

   B. Fluid causing increased pressure against the diaphragm

   C. Increased peak pressures due to fluid in the abdomen

   D. Diminished lung sounds caused by atelectasis

9. A patient recently had gastric bypass one month ago. Understanding the post-op recovery for this patient, which of the following statements if made by the patient displays accurate understanding?

   A. Increasing vitamin K intake will help prevent potential bleeding

   B. Decrease intake of proteins to help prevent gallstone complications

   C. It is important to drink plenty of water during mealtime

   D. A sore tongue may be a sign of vitamin B6 deficiency

10. A critically ill patient has been intubated in the ICU for 5 days and the medical team is beginning discussions about nutrition. Because of the nature of the patient's disease and injuries, parenteral nutrition is the most appropriate. The patient has now been on TPN for 12 hours. Which of the following may be a complication of the TPN?

   A. 1500 mL urine output over a 12-hour shift
   B. Peripheral IV thrombophlebitis
   C. Serum glucose 65 mg/dL
   D. Decreased liver enzymes

Answer Key

Question 1

Answer: A

Rationale: This question is describing bowel obstruction with a subsequent emergency of bowel perforation shown by the absent bowel sounds and severe pain. A rigid abdomen now implies peritonitis, a very serious infection that can lead to sepsis. The most important intervention at this time is emergency surgery. The perforation needs to be repaired and the infected abdomen washed out. Without prompt correction, the patient will develop sepsis which may quickly lead to death. IV fluids, administering metoclopramide, and placing an NG tube to suction are all interventions for bowel obstruction. The problem here has advanced beyond that to the complication of bowel perforation.

Question 2

Answer: D

Rationale: Presentation of mesenteric ischemia (MI) includes metabolic acidosis, not alkalosis. An increased anion gap may also be found. An increase in lactate levels can be assumed anytime tissues are not receiving enough oxygen to function; a switch to anaerobic respiration. Without adequate perfusion, the bowel will eventually become gangrenous and necrotic. Bowel perforation leading to peritonitis is a known complication of MI.

Question 3

Answer: A

Rationale: A bladder pressure of 20 mmHg or higher indicates the emergency abdominal compartment syndrome (ACS). A pressure between 12 and 19 mmHg indicates intra-abdominal hypertension. The pressure does not need to reach 20 mmHg to witness organ dysfunction, however. An abdominal perfusion pressure of 60 mmHg or greater indicates adequate perfusion. Remember that the number mimics a MAP, 60 or greater is good. A blood pressure of 110/70 and a HR of 110 may display some sort of dysfunction: however, it is not at the point of emergency such as the bladder pressure. Oliguria is likely the second most important thing out of these four answers. It shows renal dysfunction and the secondary organ problem. The bladder pressure, however, is the underlying problem and would be considered the most important. If we correct the ACS emergency, renal perfusion will increase.

Question 4

Answer: D

Rationale: Hemorrhagic pancreatitis is NOT one of the common complications of intra-abdominal hypertension. Secondary organ complications may include cardiac, renal, or pulmonary systems. An increased CVP can be seen in cardiac complications, diminished lung sounds in pulmonary complications, and oliguria in renal complications.

Question 5

Answer: C

Rationale: It is important when taking bladder pressures to have the patient be in the same position for every reading. If possible, the patient should be supine. The reading is taken at the symphysis pubis, NOT the phlebostatic axis like an arterial transducer. Bladder pressures above 20 mmHg are indicative of a pathological abdomen. A needle may indeed be used to take a direct measurement, but it is not placed inside of the bladder; it is placed inside the peritoneum.

Question 6

Answer: B

Rationale: Radiating back pain is a "red flag" symptom for many emergencies. In this case, a perforation of the esophagus is a complication, albeit rare, for an upper endoscopy. Thoracic aortic aneurysm rupture, dissection, or arterial perforation post-cardiac catheterization also often show this radiating back pain symptom. The vital signs and fever are also indicative of perforation with potential blood loss.

The anesthesia commonly used for an upper endoscopy includes midazolam and fentanyl. If a patient were to have a reaction, it would likely include some sort of skin abnormalities and/or respiratory distress. There are different types of hypersensitivity, but an allergic reaction would manifest differently than what we have in this question. These symptoms could potentially be in line with a myocardial infarction, but the backstory with the endoscopy and a potential complication of that procedure is NOT an MI. There may be internal bleeding in this patient, but it would not be in the abdomen.

Question 7

Answer: C

Rationale: Some of the standard early interventions for bowel obstruction include IV fluid hydration, placing an NG tube to suction, AND monitoring electrolytes. Enteral nutrition may begin if deemed appropriate for the location of obstruction, but not parenteral. TPN is typically reserved for patients who we do not expect to be able to take enteral intake within the 7-window. A colonoscopy is appropriate if the large bowel is involved, not the small bowel. An open laparotomy is the likely intervention if perforation or emergency is suspected. This patient is not there yet; no pain is reported.

Question 8

Answer: B

Rationale: When the amount of fluid in the peritoneum becomes large, it may cause dyspnea due to the pressure exerted on the diaphragm. Patients typically find relief after the fluid is removed via paracentesis. While liver failure leads to changes in oncotic pressure and may cause pericardial effusions, this question is specifically talking about ascites and respiratory distress. If anything, a pleural effusion would make more sense than pericardial. A peak pressure increases due to conditions like asthma or COPD. A constriction or obstruction of the airways leads to increased peak pressures. Atelectasis certainly leads to decreased breath sounds; however, this is not the best explanation for this patient's dyspnea.

Question 9

Answer: A

Rationale: Vitamin K plays an important role in the clotting cascade. If you reference the hematology chapter (Chapter 8), you will see some important points regarding the cascade as a whole. This also makes sense in the context of coumadin and why we use vitamin K as a reversal agent. To prevent gallstones, the patient is instructed to reduce fat and cholesterol. Drinking water during mealtime may lead to dumping syndrome. Patients are instructed to eat small frequent meals and drink water in between meals. A sore tongue is a potential symptom of pernicious anemia caused by vitamin B12 or cyanocobalamin, not vitamin B6 (pyridoxine).

Question 10

Answer: A

Rationale: The most common complications of TPN use is infection and hyperglycemia like we see here. Polyuria as displayed in answer "A" indicates hyperglycemia. Remember that normal fluid intake for most people and patients is 2–3 L/day. Output greater than 2.5–3 L for a 24-hour period is suggestive of polyuria and warrants investigation. TPN is not administered peripherally. Infection is a risk, but it would be seen through a central line. Hypoglycemia or hyperglycemia are potential risks of TPN usage; a serum glucose of 65 mg/dL is considered normal. Liver failure is a potential complication of long-term TPN usage, so liver enzymes would be elevated (transaminitis), not decreased.

CHAPTER 6

Renal

The renal section makes up roughly eight questions on your CCRN exam, so approximately 6% of the exam is devoted to this topic. With roughly 1 million nephrons per kidney, the renal system as a whole is fairly complex, with many processes affecting the workings inside the kidneys and as a systemic system. Remember to review lab values in the Chapter 1 and previous anatomy and physiology of the kidneys if required. A brief review of important points common in renal critical care follow.

Renal Assessment Review

One crucial job of the kidneys is to remove nitrogenous waste from the body. A decrease in glomerular filtration rate (GFR) will decrease the filtration of these waste products (blood urea *nitrogen* [BUN], creatinine). The result is azotemia, an increase in creatinine and BUN. In addition to GFR, creatinine, and BUN, alternate assessment tools include urinalysis, creatinine clearance tests, bladder scanners, among others. See Table 6-1 for a brief overview.

> **CCRN Tip**
>
> If a patient is spilling protein into the urine, assess serum albumin as well. Protein spillage is indicative of kidney damage.

Table 6-1   Types of Renal Assessment Tools

BLOOD (SERUM)	URINE	DIAGNOSTICS
Creatinine • Renal issues (AKI, CKD) • Non-renal issues (rhabdo, burns) BUN GFR • GFR decreases as *creatinine* increases • 120 mL/min • Decreases in NSAID and ACEi/ARB usage	Urine output • 1.5 L/day (minimum) Urinalysis • Specific gravity • Proteinuria (30–300 mg/day) • Casts • WBC, RBC, glucose, pH 24-hour creatinine clearance • Measures GFR best • Ratio of urine creatinine to serum creatinine Culture/sensitivity • UTI assessment	Ultrasound • Rule out obstructions and post-renal AKI causes Bladder scanner • Urine retention (*suprapubic fullness*) CT imaging • Visualize obstruction

Urine Specific Gravity

Urine specific gravity is the comparison of urine density to the density of water. While specific gravity may be used to estimate osmolality, it is not a very good indicator.

- Well hydrated: <1.010
- Minimal dehydration: 1.010–1.020
- Significant dehydration: 1.021–1.030
- Serious dehydration: >1.030

Fixed Specific Gravity

Certain medical conditions, medications, and factors cause a "fixed specific gravity" that does not fluctuate based on fluid volume status (osmolality). This may be confusing due to the opposite expected shift in specific gravity. It can be helpful to think of the disorders as the spillage of bad urine, whether it is poorly concentrated or not for pathological reasons. In DI, the kidneys do not adequately concentrate urine causing the decreased specific gravity even though we would expect an increased specific gravity due to likely dehydration. Luckily, these conditions are few and far between. (See Table 6-2.)

Table 6-2 Conditions Causing "Fixed" Specific Gravity

"FIXED" INCREASE IN SPECIFIC GRAVITY	"FIXED" DECREASED IN SPECIFIC GRAVITY
SIADH Diabetes mellitus (DM): glycosuria	Diabetes insipidus (1.008) AKI Glomerulonephritis/pyelonephritis Diuretics

Renin Aldosterone Angiotensin System (RAAS)

RAAS regulates blood pressure and SVR through a series of hormones where the system obtains its namesake (see Figure 6-1). Sodium reabsorption, water regulation, and vascular tone are managed by RAAS. RAAS manages more long-term end marks, whereas the baroreceptor reflex deals with acute changes. Many medications, such as ACEi, work by decreasing the effects of RAAS and lowering the blood pressure.

Figure 6-1   Renin aldosterone angiotensin system (RAAS)

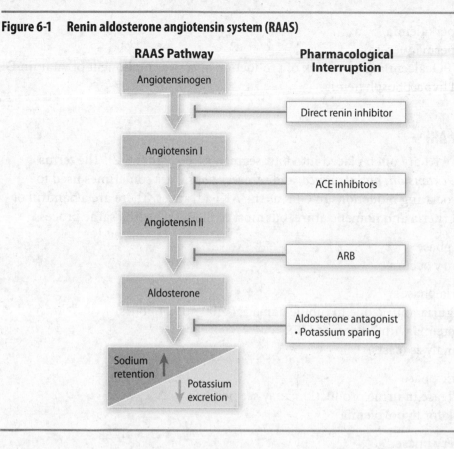

Acute Kidney Injury (AKI)/Acute Renal Failure (ARF)

AKI is typically reversible if assessed and corrected early. It is also relatively common in the ICU with some studies showing up to 65% of the critically ill developing some degree of AKI. There are three common types of kidney injury (the newer term over ARF): prerenal, intrarenal, and post-renal AKI. Be aware that it is possible for a person to have an acute issue on top of chronic kidney disease (superimposed).

Glomerular filtration is pushed by afferent and efferent pressures through the arterioles on either side of the glomerulus. Regardless of the insulting factor, changes in these pressures lead to AKI.

Follow trends from baseline. While all three types of AKI have different etiologies, there are common signs and symptoms seen in all.

- Reduced GFR
- Increased creatinine and BUN
- Oliguria (<30 mL/hr)
- Fluid overload
- Electrolyte imbalances
  - Hypernatremia

CCRN Tip

Creatinine is a much better indicator of renal status than BUN. BUN is affected by shock and hypovolemia, not just renal function. A BUN–creatinine ratio is sometimes used to differentiate between prerenal and intrarenal AKI. Divide BUN by creatinine.

- Prerenal AKI: 20–40:1
- Intrarenal AKI: <20:1

- Hyperkalemia
- Hypermagnesemia
- HYPOcalcemia (due to lack of production of active component of vitamin D and hyperphosphatemia)

Phases of AKI

Phases of AKI are often placed into four segments (see Figure 6-2). The terms *initiation*, *extension*, *maintenance*, and *recovery phases* are sometimes used to reflect associating reductions in GFR as the AKI advances. There are a handful of different criteria and nomenclature, but most of them reflect the same process.

1. Onset phase
   - Injury occurs

2. Oliguria phase
   - Oliguria/anuria due to tubule damage (<400 mL/24 hours)
   - Azotemia with decreased GFR
   - Urinalysis (casts)

3. Diuretic phase
   - Increase in urine production; may see polyuria
   - Risk for hypovolemia

4. Recovery phase
   - GFR increases

Figure 6-2   Phases of AKI

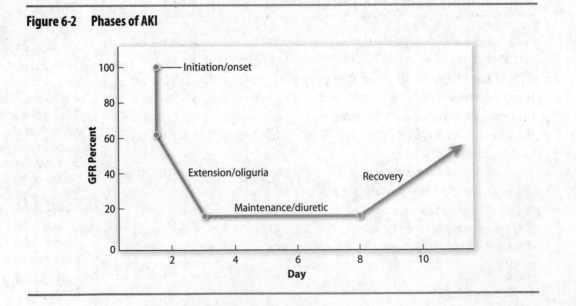

RIFLE/KDIGO Criteria

Most hospitals utilize a RIFLE criteria or KDIGO tool, KDIGO being the newer option. Understand the factors that go into these methods of distinguishing severity of dysfunction. The RIFLE criteria are displayed in Table 6-3; however, both tools mimic similar considerations. Understand those. KDIGO is covered in more detail under CKD.

The CCRN exam will not ask you to specifically call out a lab value per stage. Ballpark memorization is easier and more helpful.

Table 6-3   RIFLE Criteria for Renal Failure

STAGE	SERUM CREATININE	URINE OUTPUT
Risk	Increased creatinine by 1.25 baseline	UO < 0.5 mL/kg/h × 6 hours
Injury	Increased creatinine by 2.0 baseline	UO < 0.5 mL/kg/h × 12 hours
Failure	Increased creatinine by 3.0 baseline or Serum creatinine greater than 4 mg/dL	UO < 0.5 mL/kg/h × 24 hours or UO = 0 (anuria) × 12 hours
Loss	Persistent AKI = complete loss of renal function greater than 4 weeks	
ESRD	End-stage renal disease	

Prerenal AKI

Etiologies

- Reduced perfusion to the kidneys
  - Hypovolemia (hemorrhage, severe burns, GI losses)
  - Decreased cardiac output (cardiogenic shock, acute coronary syndrome)
  - Systemic vasodilation (septic shock, anaphylaxis, anesthesia)
  - Renal vasoconstriction (NSAIDS, iodinated contrast)
  - Efferent arteriole vasodilation (ACE inhibitors, ARBs)

Interventions

- Fluid challenge: if the AKI improves after a fluid challenge, the insult was prerenal in nature
- Correct renal perfusion depending on insulting factor (see Table 6-4)

Table 6-4   Interventions for Prerenal AKI Types

Correct volume if depleted • IV fluid therapy	Correct cardiac function if low • Optimize preload and afterload • Improve ejection fraction/CO
Correct systemic vasodilation if causative • Utilize vasopressors • Treat anaphylaxis	Correct renal vasodilation or vasoconstriction • Hold insulting medications (NSAIDS, ACE, ARBs)

Intrarenal AKI

Etiologies

Two of the most common pathways to intrarenal AKI are listed next. Alternate terms often used for some of these examples are nephrotoxic versus ischemic.

- Acute tubular necrosis (ATN)
  - Most common type of AKI
  - **Ischemic**
    - Prolonged renal ischemia causing ischemia and cell death
  - **Nephrotoxic**
    - Medication induced (vancomycin, aminoglycosides)
    - Contrast-induced nephropathy (see CCRN Tip below)
    - **Rhabdomyolysis—myoglobin** (covered in Chapter 9)
    - Hemolytic diseases—hemoglobin
- Acute interstitial nephritis
  - Antibiotic induced (penicillins)
  - Infections of the kidney (post-streptococcal glomerulonephritis)
  - Autoimmune conditions (systemic lupus erythematosus [SLE], Goodpasture syndrome)
- Vascular damage
  - Malignant hypertension

Contrast-Induced Nephropathy

Due to an increase of diagnostic procedures utilizing contrast medium, it is important to assess high-risk patients beforehand. Monitor any changes in renal function carefully.

High-Risk Patients

- Chronic kidney disease (most common)
- Current underlying nephropathy (diabetes, hypertension, heart failure)
- Advanced age (elderly)

Treatment for Contrast Patients

The *best way* to treat contrast-induced nephropathy is to prevent it before it happens.

- IV fluid therapy with NS (before and after)
  - 1 mL/kg/hr for 6–12 hours before the procedure
  - Continue hydration after the procedure
- Assess current renal function and presence of diabetes
  - Hold insulting medications when appropriate (metformin, etc.)
- Minimize contrast dose as applicable
- Consider an alternate diagnostic scan if possible
- Diuretics
- Dialysis (more common in diabetics)

> **CCRN Tip**
>
> Bicarb is no longer routinely used as a preventive treatment. Studies show no consistent benefit. The exam may mention it, however. Acetylcysteine is another treatment that shows no benefit in prevention of nephropathy.

Interventions

- Acute tubular necrosis is very slow to heal (weeks to months)
- Diuretics (furosemide; cornerstone) during oliguric phase (correct fluid overload and sodium imbalances); high doses may be necessary
- **Correct hyperkalemia immediately** (fatal in AKI)
  - Insulin with IV dextrose
  - Potassium-binding resins (polystyrene sulfonates)
  - Calcium gluconate (protect myocardium)
  - Diuretics
  - Dialysis (last resort)
- Renally adjusted medication dosages
- Nutritional considerations
  - Reduce intake of potassium and phosphorus
  - Administer renal diet (protein is still required → kidney-friendly protein)
- Dialysis (last resort); covered later in the chapter in the section "Chronic Kidney Disease (CKD)"

> **CCRN Tip**
>
> If the condition causing intrarenal AKI is interstitial nephritis, the patient may benefit from steroids. Be cautious of the risk of infection. Most AKI and renal patients have some degree of *immunosuppression* at baseline.

Post-renal AKI

Etiologies

- More common in older patients
- Obstruction in urine outflow (obstructive uropathy)
  - Nephrolithiasis (kidney stones)
  - BPH
  - Urinary retention (neurogenic, etc.)
- Increases in tubular pressure decreases GFR

Interventions

- May lead to intrarenal AKI
- Correct underlying issue
  - Kidney stones → calcium antagonists, lithotripsy
  - BPH → TURP
  - Urinary retention → prazosin, anticholinergics, straight cath
- Indwelling bladder catheter
  - Coude catheter → maneuver around obstruction
  - Suprapubic if necessary
- Ureteral stents/nephrostomy tubes
- Cystoscopy

Chronic Kidney Disease (CKD)

The benchmark definition of CKD exists when the glomerular filtration rate (GFR) drops below 60 mL/min for a period longer than 3 months (chronic). From this point of 60 mL/min or less, CKD is defined into stages, eventually leading to end-stage renal disease (ESRD).

Kidney Disease Improving Global Outcomes (KDIGO)

KDIGO establishes and updates practice guidelines for the treatment of CKD. This includes GFR and albuminuria. Do not memorize the individual areas between stages, simply the progression.

Etiologies
- Diabetes mellitus 2 (most common)
- Hypertension
- AKI progression to CKD
- Advanced age (>65)

Signs and Symptoms
- Early stages (1–3)
  - Asymptomatic typically
- Late stages (4–5)
  - Oliguria/proteinuria
  - Fluid overload (generalized edema, pulmonary edema)
  - Electrolyte imbalances
  - Uremic frost (urea in sweat)
  - Uremic pericarditis

Complications
- Drug toxicity
- Endocrine/metabolic abnormalities (anemia, acidosis)
- CVD risk
- Infection risk
- Cognitive impairment

Interventions
- Drug dosage adjustments
- Avoid nephrotoxic agents (contrast, aminoglycosides, NSAIDS)
- Restrict progressive risk factors (smoking, uncontrolled diabetes, protein)
- Renal replacement therapy (dialysis, CRRT)
- Renal transplant (best for ESRD)

Dialysis

Indication for renal replacement therapy (RRT) tends to begin when complications arise. The greatest urgency exists in states of **pulmonary edema** that cannot be controlled with diuretics. Severe increasing hyperkalemia, refractory acidosis, and uremia are additional indications for RRT.

When patients cannot tolerate rapid fluid removal via hemodialysis, continuous therapy is oftentimes used in the ICU. A certain degree of anticoagulation therapy is required for CRRT, increasing bleeding risk. Citrate use also entails risks:

Dialysis Lines

- Extracorporeal dialysis catheters
    - Short-term/emergencies (IJ, subclavian, femoral)
    - Long-term/chronic (arteriovenous fistula; months to mature for use)
- Peritoneal dialysis catheters

Complications

- Disequilibrium syndrome → fluid shifts leading to cerebral edema (headache, nausea, seizure activity, hypotension)

Continuous Therapies

- **Continuous renal replacement therapy (CRRT)** → electrolyte, waste, and fluid correction
- **Continuous veno-venous hemofiltration (CVVH)** → fluid correction

> **CCRN Tip**
>
> Dialysis lines carry many of the same risks as central lines: infection and thrombosis. With peritoneal catheters, peritonitis may occur and/or failure of the line. This would necessitate the switch to extracorporeal measures.

Acute Genitourinary Trauma

During assessment of the trauma patient, abnormalities from a physical exam, labs, urinalysis, and imaging (CT, retrograde urethrogram, retrograde cystoscopy) may show trauma to the genitourinary structures. Trauma to the kidneys, ureters, bladder, and urethra are considered genitourinary in nature. Prompt management is necessary to reduce morbidity.

Etiologies

- Blunt abdominal trauma
- Perineal trauma/sexual assault
- Penetrating trauma

> **CCRN Tip**
>
> The most common genitourinary complications following trauma include urinary extravasation, the collection of urine outside the urinary tract, and delayed urethral strictures. This is in addition to the obvious and possible AKIs that may develop.

Signs and Symptoms

- **Hematuria** (most common)
- Pain
    - Lower abdomen → bladder trauma
    - Flank → kidneys/ureters trauma
    - Suprapubic → urethral trauma
- Inability to void (bladder)
- Hematoma/bruising (kidneys)

Treatments

- Stent placements (obstructions)
- Surgical repairs
- Foley catheter (*one attempt*, if resistance is met, urethral injury suspected)
- Suprapubic catheter (bladder trauma)
- Nephrectomy (emergency—excessive bleeding)

Acute Incontinence

A new addition to the CCRN blueprint, incontinence in the ICU has many potential consequences. A large portion of the critically ill have some degree of urinary or fecal incontinence due to acute illness not history. If incontinence is not properly managed, it risks increasing hospital stay and overall morbidity. For the purpose of this section, Table 6-5 discusses the acute nature of incontinence in the ICU, not chronic incontinence briefly mentioned below for urge and stress urinary incontinence.

- **Urge incontinence:** urgency with loss of urine
- **Stress incontinence:** sphincter dysfunction causing loss of urine during laughing, coughing, or sneezing

Table 6-5   Urinary vs. Fecal Incontinence

	URINARY INCONTINENCE	**FECAL INCONTINENCE**
Etiologies	Elderly	Antibiotic use → C. diff colitis
	Frequent UTIs	Liquid stool/diarrhea
	Neurogenic overactivity	Tube feeding intolerance
	Diuretic use	Prokinetic agents/laxatives
	Sedation/coma	Sedation/coma
Interventions	Frequent (timed) voiding	Daily bath/skin assessment
	External catheters	Skin protectant/barrier cream
	Daily bath/skin assessment	Frequent assessments/clean-ups
	Skin protectant/barrier cream	Pads, diapers, etc.
	Indwelling catheter (last resort)	Fecal management system (Flexi-Seal)
Complications	Skin excoriation Incontinence-associated dermatitis Pressure ulcers (low Braden scale) Repeated UTIs Sepsis	

Renal Infections

Urinary tract infections (UTIs) may include anything from the urethra up the tract to the kidneys, making the entire catalog of urinary-based infections is quite large. Acute kidney infections and urosepsis were recently added to the CCRN blueprint in 2020. For this purpose, do not memorize the differences between each type of kidney infection, but rather the common findings among them.

Kidney Infections/Urosepsis

Sepsis caused by urogenital infections make up roughly 25% of known sepsis cases, *E. coli* being the most common insulting pathogen. *Obstructive uropathy* is a known common cause. Prompt recognition and treatment remains a continued problem in the ICU. Any delay in treatment is linked to increased mortality (triggered by organ dysfunction). High-risk patients include the elderly, diabetics, and those experiencing immunosuppression.

Signs and Symptoms
- Flank pain/costovertebral tenderness
- Underlying UTI (polyuria, hematuria, dysuria, urinalysis)
- SIRS (hyperthermia, tachycardia, tachypnea, changes in WBC count)
- Ultrasound/CT → hydronephrosis
- Acute encephalopathy

Complications
- ARDS, DIC, AKI
- Assess lactate levels (end-organ function)

Interventions
- Immediate start of empirical antibiotic therapy (urine and blood culture first)
- Supportive care
  - Hemodynamic support (fluids—crystalloids, vasopressors)
  - Pulmonary stabilization
- Adjunctive therapies
  - Glucose management
  - Indwelling catheter placement (post-renal obstruction/retention)

Life-Threatening Electrolyte Imbalances

As part of the renal blueprint for the CCRN exam, it is important to understand how electrolyte imbalances occur due to AKI and CKD in addition to a multitude of other causes. If these imbalances are not treated promptly, emergencies and death may occur.

Sodium (Na$^+$) Imbalances

Natremic changes are often difficult to correct in the critically ill due to multiple influencing causes and the delicate nature of correcting the imbalance. It is the most common electrolyte imbalance in the hospital, more so in the ICU. Remember the basics of osmosis; water follows salt, so many natremic changes mimic changes to serum osmolality. In general, fluid intake should equal fluid loss (I&O).

Physiological Control
- Changes in thirst mechanism
- ADH control
- Filtering by kidneys

Table 6-6 displays severe hyponatremia and hypernatremia.

Table 6-6   Severe Natremic Changes

HYPONATREMIA SEVERE: <120 MEQ/L	NORMAL: 135–145 MEQ/L	HYPERNATREMIA SEVERE: >160 MEQ/L
Etiologies • Water intoxication (polydipsia) • Fluid overload (SIADH, heart failure) **SEVERE signs and symptoms** • Mental status changes • Seizures → coma • Cerebral edema → herniation **Interventions** • Isotonic or hypertonic solutions (NS, 3% NaCl) • Water restriction • Loop diuretics (hypervolemic)		**Etiologies** • Dehydration, hypovolemic • Diabetes insipidus • Hyperglycemia (DKA, HHS) • Mannitol **SEVERE signs and symptoms** • LOC changes (somnolence → coma) • Brain shrinkage → vascular rupture → intracranial bleeding **Interventions** • Close monitoring (q2–4hr draws) • Isotonic or hypotonic (D5W, 0.45 NS) • Sodium restriction • Vasopressin • Free water correction (oral, NG tube)

CCRN Tip

It is crucial to not correct sodium imbalances too quickly. Any rapid change may lead to cerebral edema, seizures, and death; 8–12 mEq/L changes per 24-hour period are generally considered the maximum speed of change for sodium per day.

Potassium (K+) Imbalances

Nearly every cell in the body relies on potassium to some degree due to the sodium–potassium pump. Changes in natremia and kalemia have overarching problems for body function, especially in the nerves and muscles due to this "pump." This process may ultimately affect conduction in the heart—hence dysrhythmias.

Physiological Control

- Changes in potassium intake (diet)
- Filtering by kidneys
- Changes in insulin and catecholamines
- Aldosterone regulation (mineralocorticoid)

Table 6-7 displays severe hypokalemia and hyperkalemia

Table 6-7   Severe Kalemic Changes

HYPOKALEMIA SEVERE: <2.5 MEQ/L	NORMAL: 3.5–5.0 MEQ/L	HYPERKALEMIA SEVERE: >6.5 MEQ/L

Etiologies
 • Diuretics (loop, thiazide)
 • Excessive loss (urine, GI, sweat)
 • Primary hyperaldosteronism
 • Concomitant hypomagnesemia
 SEVERE signs and symptoms
 • Ascending paralysis
 • Respiratory failure
 • ECG/dysrhythmias
   • U waves
   • PVCs
   • VT/VF
 • Predisposes digoxin toxicity
 Interventions
 • Reduce K⁺ losses
   • Treat vomiting, diarrhea, NG suctioning
 • Replace K⁺ losses
   • KCl (10 mEq/hr—central line preferred)
 • Evaluate for toxicities
 • Treat underlying cause
		Etiologies
		 • Renal failure (AKI, CKD)
		 • Hemolytic process (rhabdo, burns, tumor lysis syndrome)
		 • Adrenal insufficiency (Addison's)
		 • Metabolic acidosis
		 • Medications (ACEi, ARBs, K-sparing diuretics)
		 SEVERE signs and symptoms
		 • ECG/dysrhythmias
		   • Peaked T waves (early)
		   • Wide QRS (late)
		   • PVCs/VT (severe)
		 Interventions
		 • Calcium gluconate (protect myocardium) → **priority first**
		 • Insulin & dextrose
		 • Potassium-binding resins (polystyrene sulfonates)
		 • Beta-2 adrenergic agent (high-dose albuterol)
		 • Dialysis

CCRN Tip

Do not forget to address low magnesium levels when dealing with potassium.

Calcium (Ca⁺⁺) Imbalances

The majority of calcium exists in our bones as calcium phosphate; some exists in the cells and extracellular fluid. When assessing laboratory values, do not confuse total serum calcium with ionized calcium. Ionized calcium, or free calcium not attached to proteins, is readily available for use. There are times hypocalcemia can be missed in the critically ill due to this fact. Most nurses witness an ionized calcium on an ABG unless it is independently ordered as an add-on lab. Remember that phosphorus plays a role in the level of calcium; the two electrolytes have an inverted effect on each other; one goes up, the other goes down.

Physiological Control

▪ Changes in parathyroid function (bone absorption)
▪ Calcitonin and vitamin D

Table 6-8 displays severe hypocalcemia and hypercalcemia.

Table 6-8   Severe Calcemic Changes

HYPOCALCEMIA SEVERE: <7.5 MEQ/L	NORMAL: 8.5–10.5 MG/DL	HYPERCALCEMIA MODERATE: >12 MG/DL CRISIS: >14 MG/DL

Etiologies
 • Acute/chronic renal failure
 • Massive transfusions/plasmapheresis (citrated blood)
 • Severe sepsis
 • Severe alkalosis
 • Low parathyroid hormone/damage to PT gland during surgery
 SEVERE signs and symptoms
 • Neuromuscular irritability
   • Paresthesias
   • Muscle spasms (Chvostek/ Trousseau)
 • Seizures
 • Bronchospasm (stridor)
 • ECG/Arrhythmias
   • Prolonged QT
 Interventions
 • Calcium gluconate
 • Calcium chloride (emergency)
		Etiologies
		 • Malignancy (renal carcinoma, rhabdomyosarcoma)
		 • Severe acidosis
		 • Excess parathyroid hormone
		 SEVERE signs and symptoms
		 • Muscle weakness
		 • ECG/arrhythmias
		   • T-wave flat or inverted
		   • Prolonged PR interval
		   • Widened QRS
		 • Mental status changes
		 • Encephalopathy (emergency)
		 Interventions
		 • 0.9 NS infusion (encourage diuresis)
		 • Bisphosphonates (etidronate, alendronate)
		 • Mithracin IV (malignancy)
		 • Surgery (lectomy)

CCRN Tip

Malignancies make up the vast majority of emergency cases of hypercalcemic crisis. These calcium changes can be acute and rapid in onset.

Magnesium (Mg^{++}) Imbalances

Magnesium plays an important role in certain body functions like cellular function and nerve conduction. Historically it has been fairly underappreciated; however, in a critical care setting, its importance is critical.

Physiological Control
- Changes in cellular shifts
- Reuptake and filtration by kidneys

Table 6-9 displays severe hypomagnesemia and hypermagnesemia.

Table 6-9 Severe Magnesium Changes

HYPOMAGNESEMIA SEVERE: < 2.5 MEQ/L	NORMAL: 1.6–2.5 MEQ/L	HYPERMAGNESEMIA SEVERE: > 5.0 MG/DL
Etiologies • Chronic alcoholism • Malabsorptive states • GI losses (vomiting, diarrhea, NG suctioning) • Cardiopulmonary bypass surgeries (CAB) • Renal-wasting—hyperfiltration (diabetes) **SEVERE signs and symptoms** • Neuromuscular excitability • Tetany/seizures • Ventricular arrhythmias • Torsades de pointes • Delirium, coma **Interventions** • MgSO$_4$ • Correct underlying wasting		**Etiologies** • Decreased renal excretion (AKI, CKD) • Hemolysis syndromes (tumor lysis, rhabdomyolysis) **SEVERE signs and symptoms** • Respiratory depression/arrest • Hypotension • Bradycardia → arrest • Decreased reflexes • Worsening mental status • Muscle paralysis **Interventions** • IV 0.9 NS • Calcium gluconate (antagonist to Mg) • IV loop diuretics • Dialysis

CCRN Tip

Magnesium has many combined effects with the other electrolytes. Oftentimes, they must be corrected together to have a substantive effect.

Phosphorus (Ph^{++}) Imbalances

Table 6-10 displays severe hypophosphatemia and hyperphosphatemia.

Table 6-10 Severe Phosphorus Changes

HYPOPHOSPHATEMIA SEVERE: <2.4 MG/DL	NORMAL: 2.5–4.5 MG/DL	HYPERPHOSPHATEMIA SEVERE: >4.5 MG/DL
Etiologies • Increased excretion (antacid use, diarrhea, kidneys) • Shifts between extracellular to intracellular space (TPN use, refeeding syndrome) **SEVERE signs and symptoms** • Similar to hypercalcemia **Interventions** • IV phosphate replacement		**Etiologies** • Renal failure **SEVERE signs and symptoms** • Similar to hypocalcemia **Interventions** • Saline infusion/diuretics • Phosphate binders (aluminum and calcium based)

Renal Procedures

The main purpose of a renal biopsy is to visualize the glomeruli. The more cells extracted, the better the chance of successfully identifying a diseased glomeruli. A renal ultrasound has many uses across a wide spectrum from infection to trauma. See Table 6-11.

Table 6-11   Renal Procedures

	RENAL BIOPSY	RENAL ULTRASOUND
Indications	AKI (rapid with unknown cause) CKD (assess for degree of end-stage) Renal mass Renal transplantation (assess for rejection)	**Diagnostic Use** Hydronephrosis Renal calculi/colic Urolithiasis AKI/CKD
Risks	**Intra-procedural** • Moderate sedation effects **Post-procedural** Renal hematoma (most common) Arteriovenous fistula (typically asymptomatic) Hemorrhage • Correct coagulation parameters prior • Hold anticoagulants prior (hours to days depending on medication) • Treat hypertension prior Loss of kidney due to complications is very rare	Renal masses Polycystic kidney disease Renal cell carcinoma **Procedural Use** Biopsy Nephrostomy (tube placement) Renal ablation Abscess removal

CCRN Tip

A certain amount of hematuria (microscopic) is expected after a renal biopsy. Drops in hemoglobin and/or continued bleeding after 3 days indicate a much larger problem or if it is fast and large in amount. Understand that *microscopic* and *gross* hematuria mean two different things.

Review Questions

1. A patient with chronic kidney disease is currently undergoing hemodialysis. Prior to the initiation of dialysis, it was noted the current hemoglobin level as 9 g/dL. What is the best explanation for the hemoglobin level?

   A. Hemolytic anemia due to destruction of RBCs in the kidneys

   B. Aplastic anemia due to dysfunctional kidneys

   C. Aplastic anemia due to increased erythropoietin hormone

   D. Destruction of RBCs inside the circuitry of the dialysis machine

2. While in the emergency department a patient coded and achieved a return of spontaneous circulation (ROSC) after 14 minutes. After the code, the nurse notes an ST elevation on the monitor. The patient was transferred to the ICU for treatment. Labs are drawn; the renal panel shows creatinine 3.0 mEq/L and BUN 30 mEq/L. Current blood pressure is 85/40 mmHg. Which of the following is an appropriate intervention at this time?

   A. Administer loop diuretics to improve urine output

   B. Plan for immediate renal replacement therapy

   C. Administer a 1000 mL bolus over 30 min

   D. Assess and optimize cardiac output

Questions 3–5 refer to the following case.

> After a motor vehicle accident, a patient is brought into the emergency department. A crush injury is noted to the right femur. An indwelling catheter is placed and dark urine begins to flow out into the collection bag.

3. Which of the following laboratory findings would the nurse expect at this time?

   A. Potassium 6.0 mEq/L, creatinine 1.0 mEq/L, BUN 20 mEq/L

   B. Urinalysis positive for ketones, metabolic acidosis

   C. CK 35,000, potassium 5.8 mEq/L, azotemia

   D. Sodium 150 mEq/L, calcium 14 mg/dL

4. Fluid resuscitation with 0.9 normal saline was begun to "flush" the kidneys. What compound is often added to the IV bags in this situation to prevent further complications?

   A. Calcium

   B. Bicarbonate

   C. Bumetanide

   D. Potassium

5. The patient in the above scenario begins experiencing multiple PVCs per minute. What interventions are the most appropriate to correct this new complication?

   A. 10 units regular insulin, dextrose, calcium gluconate

   B. 30 units aspart insulin, dextrose, hemodialysis

   C. 40 mg furosemide, hold IV fluids

   D. Assess bowel function, administer sodium polystyrene sulfonate

6. A patient is recently admitted to the ICU with an acute on chronic (superimposed) kidney injury and a history of heart failure. The patient has generalized edema and current blood pressure of 94/55 mmHg. There has been no urine output for the past six hours. Which treatment modality would the nurse expect at this time?

   A. Continuous renal replacement therapy (CRRT)

   B. Hemodialysis with midodrine therapy

   C. 500 mL bolus of lactated Ringer's and albumin

   D. Assessment and consultation for transplant

7. A patient with chronic kidney disease is being assessed for nutritional therapy. Which combinations of nutrients and electrolytes is best for this patient?

   A. High healthy proteins, low potassium, high phosphorus

   B. Low potassium, low phosphorus, low protein

   C. Low carbohydrate, low protein, low potassium

   D. High carbohydrate, low potassium

8. A patient is recently admitted to the ICU due to multiple injuries. Internal damage is suspected. Which of the following would alert the nurse most accurately for potential genitourinary trauma?

   A. Lower abdominal pain

   B. Oliguria and glucosuria

   C. Hematuria

   D. Leukocytosis and flank pain

Questions 9 and 10 refer to the following case.

A patient in end-stage renal disease (ESRD) was recently brought to the emergency department when found unconscious in the kitchen by the patient's wife. The wife states the patient has not felt well the past week and has been unable to travel to dialysis appointments.

9. Which of the following symptoms reflects a potential complication due to missing multiple dialysis appointments?

   A. Shortness of breath and lung crackles

   B. Dizziness and bradycardia

   C. Pruritus and white crystal flakes on the skin

   D. Anemia and bleeding

10. After admission, it became known the patient took medications at home to treat the symptoms of feeling ill. Which of the following medications would worsen GFR and should have been avoided by this patient at home?

   A. Acetaminophen, loratadine

   B. Ibuprofen, losartan

   C. Oxycodone, melatonin

   D. Bismuth subsalicylate, metoclopramide

Answer Key

Question 1

Answer: B

Rationale: The kidneys are responsible for the creation of the hormone erythropoietin. Without this hormone stimulating RBC development in the bone marrow, aplastic anemia occurs. When epoetin alfa is administered, evaluate reticulocyte count to gauge effectiveness. Hemolysis of RBCs by the dialysis machine may occur, but the low hemoglobin here was identified before dialysis even began.

Question 2

Answer: C

Rationale: Preload considerations often come first when considering correcting a patient's blood pressure. In this case, a prerenal AKI is likely and a fluid challenge should be performed. The other decent answer is to assess and optimize cardiac output. With the ST elevations and hypotension, it is possible this patient is experiencing myocardial stunning. Loop diuretics will worsen the blood pressure. Renal replacement therapy is not indicated yet.

Question 3

Answer: C

Rationale: Elevated CK and hyperkalemia are laboratory findings in rhabdomyolysis. The creatinine and BUN in answer "A" are normal findings. A urinalysis may be positive for hemoglobin, not ketones. Hypernatremia and hypercalcemia are not common findings with rhabdomyolysis.

Question 4

Answer: B

Rationale: Bicarbonate is often added to IV bags treating rhabdomyolysis. The goal is to stabilize any underlying acidosis. Remember that fluids should be administered to maintain urine output of 300 mL/hr. Calcium abnormalities may occur in rhabdomyolysis; treatment may occur with calcium gluconate, not in IV bags, if dysrhythmias or tremors occur. Bumetanide is a sister drug of furosemide, a loop diuretic. It is given as an IV infusion. Bumetanide may be given as treatment to encourage increased urine output. The patient will likely be hyperkalemic; adding potassium to treatment will worsen the abnormality.

Question 5

Answer: A

Rationale: Calcium gluconate is given in these situations (hyperkalemia especially) to stabilize the myocardium; the goal to prevent fatal dysrhythmias. It will buy time to correct the problem itself; the hyperkalemia. The standard "first-dose" for hyperkalemia is 10 units of *regular insulin* followed by dextrose; it is given by IV push, not subcutaneously. The effects typically begin in 10–20 minutes.

Insulin aspart is not used for this purpose; aspart and lispro are for sliding-scale or prandial doses subcutaneously. Hemodialysis may be used for severe hyperkalemia if other treatments have not worked. Diuretics may be used in the treatment of rhabdomyolysis; mannitol is more common than loop diuretics. Fluids would **not** be held; fluids continue until myoglobin is completely passed by the urine. Administering sodium polystyrene sulfonate (Kayexalate) may help treat the hyperkalemia, but it would not be the initial treatment. The goal is to immediately correct the problem and reduce the risk of life-threatening dysrhythmias. Kayexalate takes time to work.

Question 6

Answer: A

Rationale: CRRT is the treatment of choice when people do not remain hemodynamically stable on hemodialysis (HD). Given the patient's blood pressure of 94/55 mmHg, it is unlikely they can tolerate HD. Midodrine is sometimes used to prevent hypotension in patients receiving dialysis, but more often in the prevention of orthostatic hypotension. This patient already has low blood pressure prior to dialysis, so CRRT is the safer option. A fluid bolus is unlikely at this time given the underlying problem of the hypotension is contractility of the heart. The preload should be optimized in this situation; adding fluids will likely make the problem worse. If fluids are to be given, albumin is protein (a bad idea for CKD), and LR contains potassium (another bad idea for CKD). A renal transplant would be the final resort if other measures have failed, but it is also not an immediate answer for the problem at hand.

Question 7

Answer: B

Rationale: The theory behind a low protein intake for CKD is to slow the decline in GFR. The other components, like potassium and phosphorus, are restricted due to decreased filtering by the kidneys themselves. The other diets listed do not reflect a renal diet.

Question 8

Answer: C

Rationale: Hematuria is the *most common* sign of genitourinary (GU) trauma regardless of the location of the trauma in the genitourinary tract. Lower abdominal pain is a symptom of a great many things; when associated with GU trauma, the bladder may be involved. Oliguria is a symptom of AKI, which may occur secondary to trauma. Glucosuria may be due to a number of issues, typically hyperglycemia, but not GU trauma. Leukocytosis and flank pain would be due to infection or inflammation, not the GU trauma itself. Do not confuse primary and secondary problems. The primary problem and what this question is asking is to locate symptoms of the trauma itself, not secondary problems that may occur after the fact.

Question 9

Answer: A

Rationale: Since ESRD patients are unable to filter water, electrolytes, and waste products, missing dialysis appointments can be catastrophic. Fluid overload inevitably occurs with the potential for pulmonary edema, the complication noted above with shortness of breath and crackles. There are a number of potential complications due to missed dialysis appointments, many of which are life-threatening.

While a patient may experience dizziness due to metabolic dysfunction as the result of missed dialysis, a patient would become tachycardic, not bradycardic, due to body system dysfunction. White crystal flakes on the skin are describing uremic frost, a symptom of uremia in general. Uremic frost is a late-stage symptom and could occur due to missed dialysis; pruritus, however, is unlikely and more associated with allergic responses or liver failure. Anemia and bleeding due to thrombocytopenia are signs of late-stage kidney failure, not a cause from missed dialysis. Remember that the question is specifically asking complications from missed dialysis, not ESRD in general.

Question 10

Answer: B

Rationale: ACEi/ARBs and NSAIDS are important to avoid when kidney disease exists in any case. Eschewing them is most commonly taught to CKD patients to avoid worsening chronic disease and GFR; however, acute or chronic, any of the above medications are to be avoided in kidney disease. Acetaminophen and antihistamines, such as loratadine, do not affect kidney function. These over-the-counter medications are safe to use. Oxycodone or other pain pills do not need to be avoided in kidney disease, but they may have the dosage lowered to reflect a renal dose. Bismuth and metoclopramide are safe to use; a component is salicylate, or aspirin, technically an NSAID, but aspirin is safe to use in kidney disease.

CHAPTER 7

Integumentary

The integumentary section makes up roughly 3 questions on your CCRN exam, so approximately 2% of the exam is devoted to this topic, making it one of the smaller areas to study. The topic is fairly straightforward, with many of these issues likely already known to you.

Cellulitis

The vast majority of ICU admissions from cellulitis are due to the infection becoming more severe, aka sepsis or septic shock. It is one of the more common dermatological issues leading to an ICU admission.

Etiology

- Immunosuppression
- Surgical wounds
- Staph or strep bacteria
- IV drug users
- Diabetes mellitus
- Animal or human bites

Signs and Symptoms

Cellulitis most commonly affects the lower extremities, but it may occur anywhere. It is a bacterial skin infection either superficial or deep into the tissues. The more serious infections move to the lymph and blood, becoming a systemic problem. (See Table 7-1.)

Table 7-1   Presentation of Cellulitis

EARLY (LOCALIZED)	LATE (SYSTEMIC)
Pain, redness, swelling, fever	Positive blood culture (sepsis)
Fast growing rash	Changes in LOC or mental status
Abscess with pus	Hypotension (septic shock)
	Tachypnea, shortness of breath

Interventions

- Fluid resuscitation
- IV antibiotics
- Surgical procedures
  - Debridement
  - Drainage of abscess

Necrotizing Fasciitis (NF)

A particularly rare but severe and rapidly progressing infection of the fascia and soft tissues, necrotizing fasciitis requires prompt identification to lower morbidity and mortality risk. Sometimes called the "flesh-eating" disease, any delay in diagnosis and treatment drastically increases the risk of potential amputation and death. This is a surgical emergency. It most commonly affects the extremities and the perineum.

CCRN Tip

Memorizing scoring systems is incredibly difficult and pretty much unnecessary in cases like the LRINEC scoring. You likely already know what the normal value for these labs are. It helps to connect the dots and say, "Discolored wound plus pain plus elevated WBC count—this looks like it might be NF."

Etiology

- Age above 50 (primary risk)
- Diabetes mellitus (primary risk)
- Peripheral arterial disease
- Immunosuppression
- IV drug use

Signs and Symptoms

Table 7-2 outlines the classic presentation and laboratory risk indicator for necrotizing fasciitis (LRINEC) scoring of NF.

Table 7-2   Presentation of NF

CLASSIC SYMPTOMS	LRINEC SCORING
Color changes (**red to purple to black**)	C-reactive protein (CRP): ↑
Fever and flu-like symptoms	White blood cell count: ↑
Pain (worsening, unrelenting)	Hemoglobin: ↓
Blistering of the extremity	Sodium level: ↓
Swelling and heat of the extremity	Creatinine: ↑
	Glucose: ↑

Interventions

- Early identification via imaging
- Surgical debridement (**IMMEDIATE**)
  - Wet-to-dry dressings
  - Wound VAC
- IV antibiotics (**IMMEDIATE**)
- Amputation if necessary
- Stabilize hemodynamics
- Supportive treatments
  - Frequent dressing changes
  - Nutritional support

SOFA Scores

Another commonly used tool in the setting of sepsis and potential organ failure is the sequential organ failure assessment score, also called a SOFA score. You do not need to memorize the scoring system itself; just the factors involved listed below. Many of which you likely are familiar with.

- PaO_2/FiO_2 ratio
- Platelet count
- Bilirubin level
- Glasgow Coma Score
- Mean arterial pressure (MAP)
- Vasopressor use
- Creatinine level and urine output

> **CCRN Tip**
>
> A SOFA score is used for organ failure in general, not just necrotizing fasciitis.

IV Infiltration

Infiltration occurs when the catheter slips out of the vein and continues to administer fluids or medication into the interstitial space. Every patient in the ICU has at least one IV catheter if not more. Infiltration is incredibly common. It is not inherently dangerous unless a vesicant or causative agent was used and extravasation occurs.

The common order of treatment for infiltration and extravasation is presented in Table 7-3.

> **CCRN Tip**
>
> **DO NOT** use warm compresses for vesicants. It will cause vasodilation and increase the rate of absorption.

Table 7-3   Treatment of Infiltration vs. Extravasation

INFILTRATION	EXTRAVASATION
1. Stop the infusion	1. Stop the infusion
2. Discontinue the IV	2. KEEP the IV (for now)
3. Apply warm compress	3. Aspirate the IV cannula
4. Elevate extremity	4. Immobilize limb
	5. Elevate the extremity
	6. Administer antidote medication (if ordered)—phentolamine

Extravasation Injury

Depending on the infusion utilized through the IV, damage may occur to not just tissues but also surrounding nerves, muscles, and joints. The damage or symptoms (pain, swelling, skin discoloration), if not caught early enough, may result in needed debridement, skin grafting, or amputation.

This is why cytotoxic medications should be administered through a *central line,* and not a peripheral line, whenever possible. It is also why frequent site assessments and careful monitoring of a vesicant solution is important for nurses to follow.

Diseases of the vasculature or surrounding tissues increase the risk of extravasation. This may include diabetes mellitus, IV drug users, lymphedema, and peripheral vascular disease, among others.

Common Causative Vesicants/Factors

- Chemotherapy
- Dopamine and vasopressors (vasoconstriction → tissue necrosis)
- Agents with pH outside 5.5 to 8.5
- Osmolarity greater than plasma (>290 mmol/L)
- Potassium (10 mEq per hour)

Pressure Ulcers/Injuries

Critically ill patients face a higher incidence of pressure ulcers, now called pressure injuries, for a multitude of reasons. Remember to assess the skin upon admission to rule out any pre-admission issues. Most institutions follow the Braden scale to assess risk (see Table 7-4). It is updated and charted every shift by the nurses. Understand the risk factors for pressure ulcers, patients at high risk, and the nursing considerations to prevent them.

Pressure Ulcers

- Stage 1: Intact skin, nonblanchable redness
- Stage 2: Partial thickness into dermis, red and pink wound bed
- Stage 3: Full thickness, adipose tissue visible
- Stage 4: Full thickness, bone/muscle/tendons visible
- Unstageable: unable to visualize base (black or purple cover)

Table 7-4   Braden Scale Assessment

Sensory Perception	1 point Completely limited	2 points Very limited	3 points Slightly limited	4 points No impairment
Moisture	1 point Constantly moist	2 points Very moist	3 points Occasionally moist	4 points Rarely moist
Activity	1 point Bedfast	2 points Chairfast	3 points Walks occasionally	4 points Walks frequently
Mobility	1 point Completely immobile	2 points Very limited	3 points Slightly limited	4 points No limitation
Nutrition	1 point Very poor	2 points Probably inadequate	3 points Adequate	4 points Excellent
Friction & Sheer	1 point Problem	2 points Potential problem	3 points No apparent problem	

Etiology/Risk Factors
- Bedridden for long periods of time
- Ventilated and sedated
- Medical devices
  - BiPAP/CPAP
  - Feeding tubes, oxygen delivery tubes
  - Restraints
  - Bedpans
  - ID bands

Interventions
- Standard nursing interventions
  - Turn every 2 hours
  - Pressure-relieving mattress
  - Change bed linens (ensure straight, no lines)
  - Daily sponge baths
- Additional considerations
  - Device care (rotation of endotracheal tube)
  - Pressure-sensitive dressings
  - Mepilex foam dressing
  - Rectal-drainage bags (FlexiSeal)

Wounds

Table 7-5 outlines the characteristics of various types of wounds (infectious, surgical, and traumatic).

Basics of Wound Healing

- Primary Intention → wound is closed, skin is joined together (sutures, staples)
  - Sterile semipermeable wound dressing
  - Silver nylon may be used
- Secondary Intention → wound is open, granulation tissue forms naturally (not purposefully closed via sutures, etc.)
  - Preserve moisture in the wound bed (wet dressing)
  - Negative pressure wound therapy (VAC)
- Tertiary Intention → wound is purposefully left open after being cleaned out, inflammation subsides

> **CCRN Tip**
>
> Avoid the tight packing of dressings. It inhibits the healing process of all wounds. Remember that for the CCRN exam, word choices matter. The adjectives used to describe things (tight-packing versus loose-packing, severe versus minor, etc.) greatly affect the meaning of the question.

Table 7-5   Types of Wounds

INFECTIOUS WOUNDS	SURGICAL WOUNDS	TRAUMATIC WOUNDS
Includes infected pressure, surgical, and injury wounds	Approximated and closed incisions	Blunt injury wound
Higher rates of bacterial resistance	Laparoscopic versus open surgery	• No treatment usually necessary
Recognize infectious process	Open surgical wounds → high risk	• Underlying tissues may be damaged
• Erythema, pain, warmth	Colon surgeries → high risk	• Bruises most common
• Purulent drainage (foul-smelling)	Perform a preoperative assessment of potential surgical wound risks	Penetrating injury wound
Test cultures of the wound	• Systemic disease	• Gunshot, stabbing
Recognize biofilms in the wound	• Obesity, smoking, DM	• Pack the wound, change when saturated
• Layer of microbial colonization	• Existing body site infections	
Surgical debridement, pharmacological debridement, mechanical debridement (wet-to-dry dressings)	Nutritional management is crucial to wound healing. Consult a dietitian if necessary.	
	Protect surgical wound integrity	
	• Avoid vigorous cleaning	
	• Keep dressings dry and clean	
	• Assess for dehiscence	
	• Avoid mechanical stress	
	• Coughing, heavy lifting, straining	

Wound Vacs

Negative pressure therapy, or wound vacs, are a commonly used tool in the ICU, acute care in general, and even post-discharge home. For critical care nurses, it is important we understand how to use the technology correctly and monitor for effectiveness and complications.

The two main complications of using wound vacs are bleeding and infection. Depending on the type of wound and the proximity to other things (e.g., blood vessels), it is not unheard of for patients to bleed out (exsanguinate) due to wound vac complications. STOP the wound vac if bright red blood appears in the tubing.

Debridement and Treatment of Wounds

When dealing with wounds, there are four generally accepted approaches to overall treatment. The acronym DIME is universally applied as a general rule of thumb:

Debridement of dead tissue and biofilm
Inflammation and infection
Moisture control
Epithelization assessment (environmental)

There are multiple types of debridements. The specific treatment is dependent on the type of wound (see Table 7-5). Table 7-6 provides a look at the types of debridements and why they are used.

Table 7-6   Types of Debridement

Surgical Debridement	Autolytic Debridement
• Removes necrotic tissue (slough, eschar, necrosis) • Removes biofilm (bacteria) • Stimulate wound bed and prepare for grafting or skin flap • Collection of wound cultures	• Natural process of the body • Allow in noninfected wounds • Requires intact immune system • Requires moist wound bed
Mechanical Debridement	**Alternative Debridement**
• Wet-to-dry • Wet-to-damp (moist) • Irrigation	• Biological (larvae) • Enzymatic (exogenous enzyme)

Wound Management

The entire practice of caring for wounds is enormous. An entire specialty in nursing exists for it: wound, ostomy, and continence nursing (WOCN), aka wound care nurses. There are quite a few interventions we can administer as providers to correct or assist in the healing of either simple or complex wounds. Table 7-7 provides a brief review.

Table 7-7   Types of Dressings

Wet-to-Dry and Moist Gauze	Hydrocolloid Dressings (DuoDerm)
• Deep wounds/moist wound bed • Mechanical debridement • May cause pain/damage *Moist is preferred, not dry*	• Dry wounds • Impermeable to oxygen, moisture, and bacteria • Supports autolytic debridement
Polyvinyl Film (TegaDerm)	**Absorptive Dressings (impregnated gauze, alginates, hydrofibers, lyofoam/alleryn)**
• Semipermeable to oxygen • Impermeable to bacteria • Supports autolytic debridement	• Exudative (fluid) wounds • Absorbs exudate • Packing of wounds
Silver Sulfadiazine/Bacitracin • Infected wounds	

CCRN Tip

Unstageable pressure ulcers and wounds with intact eschar are not good candidates for debridement of any sort. The cover is protecting what lies beneath from infection.

Review Questions

1. A patient with suspected necrotizing fasciitis (NF) was recently admitted to the ICU for close observation. Which of the following laboratory values would be expected in NF?

   A. Sodium 150 mEq/L

   B. Glucose 190 mg/dL

   C. WBC count 4000 cells/uL

   D. Potassium 6.0 mEq/L

2. A patient with cellulitis of the arm is a known IV drug user. They were admitted to the ICU for suspected sepsis after being found unconscious in a park. The physician is placing a central line for antibiotics and the potential future need for pressors. The nurse hooks up a CVP monitor and it displays 2 mmHg. What intervention is likely at this time?

   A. Fluid resuscitation

   B. Norepinephrine

   C. Immediate debridement of the wound

   D. Assessment for opioid withdrawal

3. Which of the following patients would NOT be at high risk for developing cellulitis?

   A. A patient who was throwing out the trash and was bitten by a raccoon

   B. A homeless person who is malnourished and an IV drug user

   C. An HIV patient with a CD4 count of 650

   D. A rheumatoid arthritis patient who has been on methylprednisolone treatment

4. A nurse has recently rounded on an elderly patient. Swelling of the right arm near an IV was noted. Normal saline has been infusing at 75 mL/hr for hydration. Which of the following provides the best care by the nurse for this situation?

   A. Slow down the infusion, notify the physician, start a new IV

   B. Stop the infusion, saline lock the IV, elevate the extremity

   C. Stop the infusion, discontinue the IV, apply a warm compress

   D. Stop the infusion, discontinue the IV, apply a cold compress

5. Which of the following interventions is contraindicated in a patient where a vesicant accidentally infused through an infiltrated IV line?

   A. Discontinuation of the IV

   B. Application of a warm compress

   C. Aspiration of the IV line

   D. Infusion of normal saline in a nearby IV

6. When infusing with an IV line, the nurse must be aware of the functionality of the IV and be cautious with solutions that may cause irritation or vesication at the site. Out of the following solutions and infusion rates, which one would preferably be given via central line to avoid causative damage at the IV site?

   A. Potassium chloride 60 mEq in 100 mL

   B. 0.45% sodium chloride 50 mL/hr

   C. Heparin infusions 1000 units/hr

   D. Insulin infusions 10 units/hr

7. Many wounds require surgical debridement so proper healing may take place. Which of the following is NOT a goal of debridement?

   A. Removal of necrotic tissue to improve formation of granulation tissue

   B. Reduce biofilm and bioburden, improve re-epithelialization

   C. Prevention of angiogenesis, improve re-epithelialization

   D. Preparing for skin grafting after cleaning the wound

Questions 8–10 refer to the following case.

A trauma patient was recently admitted to the ICU after surgery. Multiple diagnoses are present requiring complex monitoring and treatment by the nurse. The patient is intubated on mechanical ventilation. An NG was placed and is to low-intermittent suction. Propofol and fentanyl are infusing for sedation. The patient is resting comfortably. A c-collar is in place for cervical spine protection. Multiple external fixation devices are present after surgery in the limbs. The patient remains a logroll only for potential spinal surgery.

8. Which of the following would the nurse include as preventive treatments for pressure ulcers in this critically ill patient? (SELECT ALL THAT APPLY!)

   A. Assessment of the nares and lips

   B. Placement of a mepilex on the sacral border

   C. Application of heel boots

   D. Rotation of the endotracheal tube

   E. Passive range of motion of the neck

9. There are multiple factors that go into pressure injury risk and prevention in hospitalized patients. Which of the following patients would be considered the highest risk for pressure injuries?

    A. An NPO patient in DKA incontinent to urine, ambulates occasionally (17 points)

    B. An intubated patient in a coma post stroke, foley and stool collection device in place (12 points)

    C. An intubated patient alert and following commands, incontinent to urine and stool, currently receiving tube feedings (13 points)

    D. An elderly patient with friable skin, admitted for dehydration and malnutrition, too weak to leave the bed (8 points)

10. The trauma patient requires another surgery, a small bowel resection. Upon return to the unit, the nurse notices the surgical wound is left open with a wound vac. One hour later, the nurse returns to the room and assesses the wound. Which of the following would prompt the nurse to immediately notify the surgeon?

    A. Whitish purulent drainage into the wound vac

    B. Uneven edges of the black foam used in the wound vac

    C. Red drainage inside the wound vac container

    D. The black foam is not compressed, the wound vac is alarming

Answer Key

Question 1

Answer: B

Rationale: Certain laboratory values are expected in NF. In the chapter, you can see the directions in the LRINEC scoring. Hyperglycemia is one of those findings. As a reminder, do not memorize the exact marker for point for each value, just if it is increased or decreased. Sodium would be decreased, the WBC would be increased, and potassium has no bearing in NF.

Question 2

Answer: A

Rationale: Central venous pressure or right atrial pressures reflect overall fluid status. A CVP of 2 mmHg indicates hypovolemia and dehydration. This patient was found unconscious and in likely sepsis; hypovolemia is likely here. The patient requires fluid resuscitation. Norepinephrine is used to increase blood pressure. This question does not display a blood pressure, and a CVP does not necessitate the need for the medication either. Debridement is not necessary unless the tissue is diseased and devitalized. Cellulitis may advance to that stage, but this question does not offer that information. Do not make assumptions. Debridement would also not help improve a CVP. This patient may certainly go through opioid withdrawal, but it is not the immediate priority. ABCs come first as always.

Question 3

Answer: C

Rationale: The point of concern for immunosuppression in an HIV patient is a CD4 count of 200 or lower. That is when an official CDC defined AIDS diagnosis is made. This CD4 count is still adequate to support the immune system. Animal bites, IV drug use, and steroid treatment causing immunosuppression are all risk factors for development of cellulitis.

Question 4

Answer: C

Rationale: The immediate action when infiltration is suspected for any fluid is to stop the drip. If the infiltration is benign, such as with normal saline, the line should be discontinued, a warm compress applied, and the extremity elevated. A cold compress is a good thought when swelling is due to inflammation. In this case, the swelling is mostly due to fluid and not inflammation.

Question 5

Answer: B

Rationale: A warm compress will cause vasodilation and increase the amount of vesicant absorbed. The goal is to remove as much vesicant as possible and minimize the damage to the surrounding tissues. The IV line is saved initially to attempt aspiration of the vesicant fluid; eventually, it is discontinued. Infusing into a separate IV line that is nearby is not contraindicated. It would be preferable to be infused elsewhere, but it is not contraindicated.

Question 6

Answer: A

Rationale: Potassium chloride (KCL) is irritation to tissues when administered peripherally. A central line is preferred. As we know, a central line is not always available. If the patient complains of discomfort at the IV site of potassium chloride, slow down the drip. Remember 10 mEq/hr is the maximum speed for KCL. Hypertonic solutions can cause irritation, not hypotonic solutions such as 0.45 NS (half-normal saline). Insulin and heparin can be administered either peripherally or centrally; they do not cause irritation.

Question 7

Answer: C

Rationale: One of the main goals of debridement is to improve blood flow to the tissues and improve healing. We do not want to "prevent" angiogenesis; we want to stimulate it. Removal of necrotic tissue and biofilms are crucial to wound healing and are considered a main goal of surgical debridement. If the wound is deep enough, debridement also offers the benefit of creating a clean wound bed ready for skin grafting.

Question 8

Answer: A, B, C, D

Rationale: All of these answers are excellent at preventing pressure injuries EXCEPT rotating a neck that is in a cervical collar. At times we may want to carefully remove the c-collar with help stabilizing the neck to simply relieve pressure from the device itself. Most institutions require a doctor's order to do this. Passive range of motion on extremities would be an encouraged intervention. Do not underestimate the possibility of pressure injuries from devices itself, such as NG tubes and ETTs.

Question 9

Answer: D

Rationale: The best way to go about questions like this is to think about the Braden scale and the factors that are involved. It's not entirely necessary to memorize the point system, but simply understand ballparks. This elderly patient with friable skin is at risk for skin shearing. They are also malnourished, causing risk in the nutrition row. They are also bedridden. The points would come to roughly 8 or 9. The other patients here do have certain risks such as incontinence or malnourishment, but none are as great a risk as the patient in answer D.

Question 10

Answer: C

Rationale: The most immediate risk would be bleeding into the wound vac. It is possible that a vessel was damaged during surgery and the patient could bleed out. The black foam should be compressed and the alarm also needs to be addressed; this should be assessed by the nurse first. The immediate action would not be to call the physician; attempt to fix the problem within your scope of practice first. Whitish purulent drainage is likely expected for this patient given the nature of the surgery. The physician should be told of the drainage, but it is not life-threatening at this time. A good seal on the wound vac is important. Black foam that has uneven edges to the wound may make it difficult for the wound vac to work properly, but it is not an immediate priority as long as the foam is compressed and the wound vac is working.

CHAPTER 8

Hematology/ Immunology

The hematology section makes up roughly 3 questions on your CCRN exam, so approximately 2% of the exam is devoted to this topic, making it one of the smaller areas to study. Coagulopathy largely dictates need-to-know content (DIC, HIT). If necessary, review coagulation panel lab values. The abnormal lab values will also be listed for disease explanation.

Coagulopathies

Learning and applying the entire clotting cascade is a huge undertaking that is really not required of you for the CCRN exam. You *do* need to understand the basics of why and how the human body may clot or break up clots. Understanding where certain medications have effect in the clotting cascade may also be helpful. They are listed in Table 8-1 for a quick review.

Table 8-1   Medications Affecting the Clotting Cascade

HEPARIN	WARFARIN	CLOPIDOGREL/ASPIRIN
• Inhibits thrombin formation	• Inhibits vitamin K • Inhibits prothrombin formation	• Inhibits platelet adhesion
Monitor APTT	Monitor PT/INR	

CCRN Tip

It is important to note that many confuse the difference between bleeding and clotting. In diseases like hemophilia or DIC, the patient does not bleed any faster than a normal person, they CLOT SLOWER.

Coagulation

- Primary hemostasis: platelet clot formation
- Secondary hemostasis: intrinsic/extrinsic pathways (see Table 8-2)
- Fibrinolytic pathway: breaks down fibrin

Table 8-2   Intrinsic Coagulation vs. Extrinsic Coagulation

INTRINSIC PATHWAY	EXTRINSIC PATHWAY
• Endothelial damage (damage inside vascular system) • Measured by partial thromboplastin time (PTT)	• Tissue damage (damage outside vascular system) • Measured by prothrombin time (PT)

Disseminated Intravascular Coagulation (DIC)

Overactivation of the fibrinolytic pathway leads to DIC. This occurs secondary to other problems that cause the overuse of clotting factors (infection, trauma).

Etiology

- **Sepsis**
- ARDS
- Trauma
- Hematological cancers/Solid tumors

Signs and Symptoms

- Increased coag panel values (PT, PTT, INR)
- Increased D-dimer (released upon clot dissolving)
- **Increased fibrin split products (FSP):** *>10 mcg/mL*
- Decreased fibrinogen: <200 mg/dL
- Abnormal bleeding (petechiae, purpura, IV site bleeding, nose, urine, stool)

Interventions

- Treat the underlying cause (may spontaneously resolve)
  - Antibiotics
  - Surgery
- FFP and platelets
- Cryoprecipitate (high in fibrinogen)
- Give anticoagulants (stop clotting → stop DIC)
  - Heparin inhibits thrombin
- Fibrinolytic inhibitors (aminocaproic acid)

Heparin-Induced Thrombocytopenia (HIT)

Anyone who is exposed to heparin of any amount may develop HIT. It is relatively rare (5% of exposed), but it is a serious complication that requires close monitoring. Up to 50% of these patients may develop a thromboembolic event increasing the risk of mortality. Any platelet count below 150,000 is considered thrombocytopenia. A count below 40,000 is considered serious with even lower numbers, less than 20,000, potentially leading to complications such as spontaneous bleeding (intracranial).

Etiology

Table 8-3 compares the two types of HIT.

Table 8-3   Type 1 vs. Type 2 HIT

TYPE 1 HIT	TYPE 2 HIT
• Non-immune reaction	• Immune-antibody (IgG) reaction
• More common	• Slow onset (5–14 days)
• Fast onset (1 day)	• Severe reaction → hypercoagulability
• Mild reaction	• White clot syndrome (thrombosis)

HIT may occur with any type of heparin-based medication and is not dependent on the dose. HIT may develop even with small doses. It is, however, more common in patients with larger doses and for longer periods of time.

Types of Heparin

- Unfractionated heparin (UFH)
- Low-molecular-weight heparin (LMWH)

Signs and Symptoms

- Thrombocytopenia
  - Unexplained drop in platelets with heparin use
- Hypercoagulability (DVT, PE, skin necrosis)
- Assay confirmation of HIT
  - 1st → Enzyme-linked immunosorbent assay (ELISA)
  - 2nd → Serotonin release assay (SRA)

> **CCRN Tip**
>
> As with any type of anticoagulant, be acutely aware of current coagulation lab values. Many of these meds can cause a dangerous increase in these values. For example, argatroban may dangerously increase the PTT.

Interventions

- Discontinue all heparin use (injections, line flushes, etc.).
- List heparin as patient allergy
- Do NOT administer platelets (worsens hypercoagulability)
- Switch to replacement anticoagulant
  - Argatroban/Bivalirudin—direct thrombin inhibitor
  - Fondaparinux (less common)
  - Warfarin—start once platelet count normalizes

Idiopathic Thrombocytopenic Purpura (ITP)

Thrombocytopenia that cannot be linked to any direct cause can be considered idiopathic (unknown). Many of the cases are in fact discovered to be immune in nature, so the term *immune thrombocytopenic purpura* may be used. Unless ITP is severe, the majority of asymptomatic patients do not require treatment, only monitoring.

Etiology

- **Primary rule out**
  - No other blood irregularities (only platelets)
- **Secondary rule out**
  - No causes due to medications (heparin)
  - No causes due to conditions (leukemia, lupus, cirrhosis)

Signs and Symptoms

- Often asymptomatic
- Bruising, petechiae, purpura (expected findings)
- Epistaxis, bleeding gums (common findings)
- GI bleeding, gross hematuria (uncommon findings)
- SERIOUS: intracranial bleeding (platelet count <20,000)

Interventions

- Avoid trauma (contact sports, etc.)
- Avoid aspirin and NSAIDS
- Avoid IM injections
- IV steroids (prednisone)
- Intravenous immunoglobulin (IVIG)

> **CCRN Tip**
>
> Platelet infusions are generally unsuccessful in cases of ITP. The body will continue to destroy the platelets if the underlying problem is not solved. Infusions are generally reserved for patients who have active bleeding.

Anemia

Historically, anemia was treated rather aggressively; however, today research shows better outcomes with a more prohibitive approach. Transfusion is not typically performed until a hemoglobin drops below 7 g/dL or the patient is severely symptomatic. A certain degree of anemia is very common in the critically ill. How it is managed depends on the cause of the anemia (see Table 8-4).

Table 8-4   Common Causes of Anemia in the Critically Ill

Blood loss	Aplastic
• Phlebotomy/labs	• Erythropoietin decrease (renal disease)
• Vascular catheter bleeding	• Bone marrow suppression
• Surgical site (drains, etc.)	• Blood dyscrasias (medication adverse effects)
• Diagnosis (GI bleed)	
Nutritional	**Hemolytic**
• Iron	• Disease process
• Vitamin B12	• Machinery (bypass, VADs)

Epoetin alfa is found to be beneficial in patients where anemia is due to renal disease, but the medication does not come without potential problems. Thrombosis risk increases with administration of this drug. Transfusions also come with risks of their own. They also do not likely solve the underlying problem. See the additional section below regarding transfusions.

Blood Products and Transfusions

Generally speaking, a hemoglobin below 7.0 g/dL triggers the need for transfusion. These patients are anemic to be sure, however other complications may begin to arise such as myocardial ischemia.

Nursing Considerations

- Transfuse FFP, platelets, and cryoprecipitate when multiple units of PRBCs are required; PRBCs do not contain coagulation factors
  - Assess coagulation of patient
  - One unit of PRBCs typically equals 350 mL
  - Massive transfusion = 10 units or more within 24 hours
- Hypothermia → warm blood when multiple units are required
- Hypocalcemia → citrate binds to ionized calcium
- Hypomagnesemia → citrate binds to magnesium
- 2,3-DPG deficiency → oxyhemoglobin dissociation curve shift to the **left**

Transfusion Reactions

Understand the basics on what to look out for and how to fix it. A reaction itself can be acute (during the transfusion) to delayed (days to weeks later). The presentation of the patient and cause of the reaction will dictate the treatment plan. Table 8-5 shows the types of transfusion reactions.

Table 8-5   Types of Transfusion Reactions

Allergic Reaction	Hemolytic Reaction
• Minor	• Immune-mediated (mismatched blood antibody mediated) → potentially **FATAL**
• Urticaria, pruritus	• Fever, chills
• Severe (anaphylactic)	• Hypotension
• Hypotension, shock	• Renal failure
• Dyspnea	• Dark red (Coca-Cola colored) urine
• Airway closure	• Non-immune-mediated (less serious)
Transfusion-Related Acute Lung Injury (TRALI)	**Transfusion-Associated Circulatory Overload (TACO)**
• Fast onset (immediately up to 6 hours post)	• Underlying cardiac issues present (heart failure, renal failure, respiratory failure)
• Lung infiltrates (chest x-ray)	• Dyspnea, tachypnea
• Hypoxia, respiratory distress	• Hypertension and JVD

CCRN Tip

Any increase in temperature of more than 1 degree Celsius is a problem. This would be a point of concern and trigger stopping the transfusion and order listed below.

Anytime a transfusion reaction is suspected, the primary interventions are the same. Stop the transfusion. Disconnect the blood and tubing. Establish new tubing with normal saline to keep the vein open. Closely monitor the patient for compromise (q15min vitals). The physician should be notified. Additional orders may follow. Save the tubing and blood. It will be sent to the blood bank after you confirm the right blood went to the right patient (clerical check).

Interventions

- Diphenhydramine (Benadryl) and steroids → allergic reactions
- Diuretics → fluid overload and hemolytic reactions
- Acetaminophen → febrile reaction
- Epinephrine → anaphylaxis

> **CCRN Tip**
>
> Any hemodynamic or oxygenation requirements are treated accordingly. Many transfusion reactions present differently, not just with the type of reaction, but patient to patient. The nurse must be focused and diligent when assessing the patient given the wide array of possible symptoms.

Immune Deficiencies

The entire spectrum of immunodeficiency disorders is quite large; many of which, the result of genetics. The most important thing to keep in mind is the risk for infection in these patients. How do we manage these risks as nurses? Can you recognize a high-risk patient? A brief review of the immune system is presented in Figure 8-1. The types of immune deficiencies are outlined in Table 8-6.

Figure 8-1   Overview of the immune system

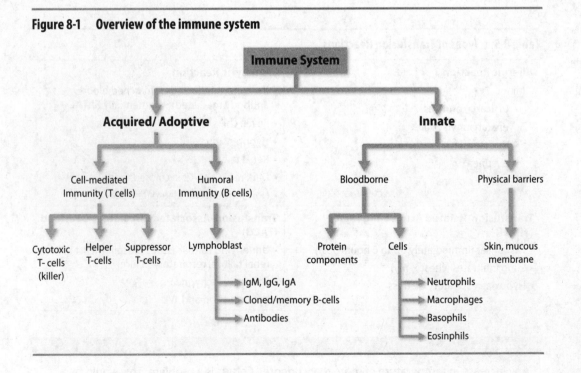

Table 8-6   Types of Immune Deficiencies

B cell dysfunction	T cell dysfunction

• Antibody/immunoglobulin deficiency
• Hypogammaglobulinemia
	• Glucocorticoid therapy
	• HIV Infection
	   • AIDS (CD4 <200)
	   • Pneumocystic pneumonia
	• Comorbidity risk of HepB/HepC

	Leukopenia/neutropenia • Low WBC (especially granulocytes)

Signs and Symptoms

- Frequent recurrent infections (respiratory, sinuses, ears)

Interventions

- IVIG therapy → B cell dysfunctions
- Antibiotic prophylaxis → B or T cell dysfunctions
- Antifungal prophylaxis → B or T cell dysfunctions
- Vaccinations (no live vaccines—flu-intranasal, MMR, etc.)
- Antiviral medications
  - Antiretrovirals for HIV

> **CCRN Tip**
>
> General nursing care should always be included in these patients. Appropriate use of PPE, washing of hands, avoiding contaminated products, food, and water. Remember that neutropenic precautions include avoiding fresh fruits and vegetables, no plants or pets, etc.

Oncologic Complications

The main oncologic complications on the CCRN exam are tumor lysis syndrome and pericardial effusion. Pericardial effusion is covered in more detail in Chapter 2, "Cardiovascular." It is mentioned here as a potential complication to either the cancer itself metastasizing to the area or treatment (radiation and chemo).

Tumor Lysis Syndrome (TLS)

The "lysing" or breaking down of the cancer cells causes the release of contents inside. These materials get into the blood and can cause a variety of problems. It is potentially fatal, making it crucial for nurses to monitor closely when TLS is a risk. A helpful way to remember TLS symptoms is to compare it to rhabdomyolysis; both are quite similar but with very different causes.

Etiology

- Hematological cancers (leukemias and lymphomas)
- Release of tumor cell contents into the bloodstream
  - Uric acid crystals
  - Potassium, phosphorus
- Predisposing factors
  - Previous kidney disease
  - Dehydration/hypotension

Signs and Symptoms

- Laboratory findings
    - Hyperkalemia
    - Hypocalcemia
    - Azotemia (BUN)
    - Hyperuricemia
    - Hyperphosphatemia
- Clinical findings
    - Acute kidney injury
        - Elevated creatinine
        - **Oliguria (ominous sign)**
    - Cardiac dysrhythmias
    - Seizures
    - Multisystem organ failure

Interventions

- Prevent/manage dysrhythmias
    - Q4hr potassium draws
    - Telemetry
    - Sodium polystyrene sulfonate (Kayexalate)
    - Calcium gluconate (protect myocardium)
- Preserve renal function/urine output
    - IV hydration
    - Allopurinol/rasburicase (excrete uric acid)
    - Diuretics (loop) → furosemide
    - CRRT if necessary

CCRN Tip

At times, the uric crystals may be seen in the urine itself.

CCRN Tip

There are multiple ways to address severe hyperkalemia in the ICU. In an emergency, hemodialysis may be the treatment of choice. Insulin (regular) with D50 can also help temporize the situation.

Review Questions

1. A patient with an active DVT has been on a heparin drip in the ICU for the past 24 hours. The morning labs from today suggest heparin induced thrombocytopenia (HIT). Which of the following interventions would the nurse immediately implement for this patient?

   A. Stop the heparin infusion, begin argatroban

   B. Notify the surgeon for emergency thrombectomy

   C. Administer platelets to increase platelet count

   D. Contact pharmacy, decrease the drip rate on the heparin infusion

2. A patient with endocarditis is newly admitted to the ICU. The patient has a platelet count of 50,000. There are no other blood irregularities and the cause of the thrombocytopenia remains unknown. While collecting the morning medications for this patient, which of the following administrations would the nurse question?

   A. Ketorolac

   B. Prednisone

   C. Ondesteron

   D. IV ciprofloxacin

3. The patient in question two is being prepared for a surgery. Current platelet count on the morning labs is 30,000/mm³. Which of the following interventions should the nurse perform at this time?

   A. Contact the charge nurse and cancel the surgery

   B. Contact the surgeon for potential platelet transfusion

   C. Hold all morning medications until the surgeon sees the patient

   D. Redraw the morning labs closer to surgery

Questions 4–6 refer to the following case.

A patient in the ICU is on post-op day 1 from an uncomplicated coronary bypass surgery. They are now extubated on 2 L nasal cannula. The morning labs show a hemoglobin of 7 g/dL. The physician decides to transfuse one unit of PRBCs. Two hours after the transfusion begins, the patient complains of shortness of breath. The current vitals and hemodynamics are as follows:

BP = 105/80 MAP = 88	RR = 24	SpO_2 = 90% 2L = NC
Temp = 37.5°C	CVP = 4	CO = 6L/min
Pain = 2/10 at incisional site		

4. Which of the following complications of transfusion is likely happening in this patient given the information above?

   A. Hemolytic reaction (immune-mediated)

   B. Anaphylaxis

   C. Transfusion-associated circulatory overload (TACO)

   D. Transfusion-related acute lung injury (TRALI)

5. With the suspected complication in question 4 in mind, which nursing action is most appropriate?

   A. Slow down the transfusion, administer diphenhydramine and steroids

   B. Stop the transfusion, obtain an order for chest-x ray

   C. Stop the transfusion, administer furosemide

   D. Continue the transfusion, increase the oxygen delivery

6. Which of the following interventions would be appropriate for the nurse to do and continue for this patient in the coming hours?

   A. Monitor vital signs q1hr

   B. Discard tubing and send remaining blood to blood bank

   C. Administer normal saline through new tubing

   D. Draw blood for ELISA assay

7. A patient with leukemia has begun a second round of chemotherapy. The patient has a history of hypertension, acute kidney injury, and hyperlipidemia. Which of the following signs would warn the nurse of potential tumor lysis syndrome?

   A. Urine output 30 mL over the last two hours

   B. Sinus tachycardia, 120 BPM

   C. Serum potassium 3.0 mEq/L

   D. Serum calcium 10 mg/dL

8. Tumor lysis syndrome can be a potentially life-threatening complication. It is important for the nurse to understand predisposing factors that may place patients at higher risk of developing TLS. Which of the following would be one of the predisposing factors?

   A. Chronic kidney disease

   B. Hypertension, BP 160/90 mmHg

   C. Anemia, hemoglobin 9 g/dL

   D. Fluid overload

9. A patient was recently admitted to the ICU from the floor due to advancing shortness of breath and desaturations requiring oxygen therapy. The patient has a diagnosis of *Pneumocystis jiroveci* pneumonia secondary to AIDS. The most recent CD4 level was 40 cells/uL. Which of the following treatments would be appropriate for this patient?

   A. Administration of acyclovir

   B. Administer the pneumococcal and flu (intranasal) vaccines

   C. Administer prophylactic antibiotics

   D. Place the patient on airborne precautions and test for HepC

10. A patient recently diagnosed with HIT is transferred to the ICU due to bleeding. When reviewing the eMAR, the nurse would hold which of the following medications?

    A. Lovenox

    B. Acetaminophen

    C. Fondaparinux

    D. Bactrim

Answer Key

Question 1

Answer: A

Rationale: The most important thing to do when HIT is suspected is to discontinue all heparin drips and heparin-based products. Alternate anticoagulation should be used, such as argabatran, fondaparinux, or warfarin. As with any active coagulopathy issue, routine coagulation panel draws should be included in the plan of care. Monitoring of improvement or worsening status is important, but in addition to that, argabatran can adversely affect the PTT.

Emergency thrombectomy is not warranted at this time. It would also not be the first thing or immediate intervention the nurse would do. Some physicians and surgeons decide to place an inferior vena cava (IVC) filter to prevent pulmonary embolism. This hasn't been known to be overly successful, but the decision may still be made for high-risk patients. Platelets should NOT be given in moments of HIT. Similar to ITP, platelets should not be administered unless absolutely necessary, such as in the case of severe bleeding. Contacting the pharmacy at this time will not aid in the current problem. The heparin drip should be discontinued.

Question 2

Answer: A

Rationale: Aspirin and other NSAIDS like ketorolac are held in moments of ITP. They can worsen the thrombocytopenia. Steroids like prednisone are a common mode of treatment for ITP. Ondesteron is not contraindicated in patients with ITP. It is worth noting that IV ciprofloxacin is a perfectly valid treatment for many types of infections, but there are certain antibiotics that may cause blood dyscrasias. Part of an ITP diagnosis is the rule-out of medications that are causing the drop in platelets. In this case it is highly unlikely, but be aware of this potential adverse effect of some antibiotics.

Question 3

Answer: B

Rationale: The surgeon will likely cancel the surgery if the platelet count cannot be improved. The risk of bleeding is too high. This severe thrombocytopenia may be corrected by platelet infusions. It is not the job of the nurse to cancel surgeries. Any concerning lab values should be elevated to the appropriate level—in this case, the surgeon. Holding all medications would be bad practice without a reason to do so. Certain medications that would increase the risk of bleeding in this patient may be held if they were not already held pre-operatively. The platelet number is unlikely to improve in the short period of time between the present and the surgery. The issue of thrombocytopenia needs to be elevated to the surgeon.

Question 4

Answer: D

Rationale: The vital signs and hemodynamics show a potential TRALI reaction. The shortness of breath may be attributed to many types of transfusion reactions; however, the normal CVP and cardiac output can rule out TACO. The stable blood pressure can rule out anaphylaxis. The patient is normothermic with no new-onset pain and no signs of discolored urine. A hemolytic reaction is unlikely.

Question 5

Answer: B

Rationale: Anytime a severe transfusion reaction is occurring, stop the transfusion immediately. A chest x-ray would show infiltrates suggesting a TRALI reaction. Steroids and diphenhydramine would be interventions for an allergic reaction. Diuretics such as furosemide would be interventions for fluid overload like TACO. The oxygen will surely be increased to treat the current hypoxia, but the transfusion will not continue.

Question 6

Answer: C

Rationale: Anytime a transfusion reaction occurs, the physician will be notified. Regardless of the severity of the symptoms, this information needs to be shared. New tubing and a drip of normal saline establish an open vein. Vital signs will be monitored frequently—every 15 minutes. One hour is too long. Tubing and the blood together are sent to the blood bank for testing. Do not throw away the tubing or the blood. An ELISA assay tests for HIT. It is not used to test types of transfusion reactions.

Question 7

Answer: A

Rationale: Oliguria is an ominous sign of TLS. This patient is not making enough urine. There is a predisposition due to the AKI diagnosis already present. This is a known risk factor for TLS. The chemotherapy may cause an intrarenal AKI, which further increases the risk for TLS.

Sinus tachycardia may be a sign of a multitude of things, not just TLS. Dysrhythmias would certainly suggest potential TLS, but this manifests due to the hyperkalemia; PVCs may be present along with other ECG changes. Hyperkalemia is a symptom, not hypokalemia. When the cancer cells are destroyed, potassium is released. The calcium value listed in answer D is a normal lab value.

Question 8

Answer: A

Rationale: Kidney disease, acute or chronic, predisposes a patient to TLS. Renal excretion is the body's main mechanism of urate and many types of electrolytes and particles. Hypertension and anemia are not known risk factors for TLS. Fluid volume does have a correlation to TLS, but it would be dehydration, not fluid overload, that increases the risk.

Question 9

Answer: C

Rationale: A CD4 level below 200 cells/uL defines an AIDS diagnosis. A level even lower like in this patient seriously increases their risk of opportunistic infections like *jiroveci*. It is important to begin prophylactic treatment in patients with a severe reduction in T cell levels. The same rule applies to B cell immune deficiencies.

Antivirals like acyclovir will not benefit this patient. *Pneumocystis jiroveci* is a fungal infection. Immunocompromised patients often receive vaccines to prevent infections. A pneumococcal vaccine may be administered to this patient; however, live vaccines (flu-intranasal, MMR) are best held until the immune system improves. Hep C comorbidity is not uncommon in these patients; however, *Pneumocystis jiroveci* is not an airborne precaution. The infection is rarely seen in patients with adequate immune systems.

Question 10

Answer: A

Rationale: Lovenox is the brand name for enoxaparin, a heparin derivative. All heparin-based products need to be discontinued upon HIT suspicion or diagnosis. Acetaminophen, fondaparinux, and Bactrim are all safe to administer to this patient at this time.

CHAPTER 9

Musculoskeletal

The musculoskeletal section is comparatively much smaller than other areas of study for the CCRN exam. Roughly two questions may come up regarding these topics, or about 2% of the exam. Many of the issues noted in this chapter are connected to other diseases as well—for example, rhabdomyolysis often causing acute kidney injury.

Compartment Syndrome

There are not many true orthopaedic emergencies, but compartment syndrome is one of them. When a buildup of interstitial fluid occurs in the fascial compartment, a loss of circulation may occur. The emergency manifests most frequently in the legs, but it may affect other areas. Without prompt attention, typically by fasciotomy, ischemic damage may become permanent (necrosis) and amputation may become inevitable.

> **CCRN Tip**
>
> An early tool to use for symptomatology is the 5 P's: pain, paresthesias, pallor, paralysis, and pressure.

Etiologies

- Crush injuries (soft tissue trauma)
- Fractures (most common)
  - Long bone (femur, tibia)
- Rhabdomyolysis
- Burns

Signs and Symptoms

- Early signs
  - Numbness
  - Tingling
  - Paresthesias
  - Tense "wood-like" limb
- Late signs
  - Severe pain ("out of proportion")
  - Paralysis (nerve damage)

- Pulselessness → not absolute, patient may still have a pulse
- Elevated compartment pressures
  - **30 *mmHg or greater* than diastolic**
  - <10 mmHg → normal pressure

Interventions

- Remove constricting devices and clothing
  - Casts, dressings, clothes, etc.
- Maintain limb at the level of the heart
- **Fasciotomy**
- The wound typically remains open to allow swelling and inflammation to decrease. Maintain sterility and be cautious for signs of infection.

Rhabdomyolysis

There are a number of causes that lead to this state of severe muscle damage. As the contents of destroyed myocytes leak into the intravascular space, a number of complications may arise.

<table>
<tr><td>CCRN Tip</td></tr>
<tr><td>Components of a Myocyte

• Potassium, phosphates, acids

• Myoglobin (nephrotoxic)

• Creatine kinase</td></tr>
</table>

Etiologies

- Trauma (crush injuries)
- Extreme physical activity
- Prolonged immobility
- Compartment syndrome
- Hypo/hyperthermia states
- Drugs, medications, toxins

Signs and Symptoms

- Classic triad
  - Weakness
  - Myalgia
  - Tea-colored urine
- AKI
  - Azotemia
  - Low urine output
- Urinalysis
  - Tea-colored urine
  - Myoglobin
- Hyperkalemia (dysrhythmias)
- Metabolic acidosis
- Elevated CK: >10,000 U/L, or 5 times the normal

<table>
<tr><td>CCRN Tip</td></tr>
<tr><td>For reference, a normal CK is <200 U/L. Unrelated but important, a common dipstick test often is positive for hemoglobin; however, the test is mistaking myoglobin for hemoglobin. It is a false positive.</td></tr>
</table>

Interventions

- Early and aggressive *fluid therapy* (maintain 300mL/hr of urine output)
- Sodium bicarbonate, mannitol, and furosemide (acidosis and oliguria)
- Manage electrolyte imbalances (hyperkalemia)

Fractures

The section here on fractures covers the life-threatening sequelae and damage by femur and pelvic fractures. This implies unstable fractures (displaced), not stable. High-impact trauma and falls (elderly) make up the vast majority of these injuries. Table 9-1 outlines the complications and interventions involving long bone and pelvic fractures.

Table 9-1   Fractures

	FEMUR/LONG BONE FRACTURES	PELVIC FRACTURES

Complications	Pulmonary (fat embolism)
	  • **Life over limb**
	  • Assess for petechiae
	Hemorrhage
	Wound infections (open fracture)
	Compartment syndrome
	Neurological injuries
	Deep vein thrombosis
		Hemorrhage
		Neurological injuries (lumbar, sacral)
		  • Bowel, bladder incontinence
		Wound infections (open fracture)
		Muscle ruptures, increased DVT risk, hernias, erectile dysfunction

Interventions	Prompt antibiotics (open fracture)
	Immobilization (stabilize)
	Skeletal traction
	Nail, plate, external fixators
	Pain management
	Treat muscle spasms
		External compression → stop bleeding
		Stabilization (do not move)
		Surgical intervention
		  • Open reduction internal fixation (ORIF)
		  • External fixation
		Skeletal traction
		Pain management

> **CCRN Tip**
>
> Fractures may be defined as open or closed. An open fracture (breaking through the skin) is a risk for infection of either the bone or the wound itself.

Infections

Osteomyelitis is the inflammation and/or infection of the bone or bone marrow. Healthy bone rarely becomes infected; however, when a breach occurs in the integrity of the bone (trauma, open fractures, surgery), infection is possible. In older patients, decubitus ulcers down to the bone are a leading cause. Patients with diabetes mellitus or peripheral vascular disease are at increased risk of osteomyelitis.

Signs and Symptoms

- Erythema, swelling, dull pain
- Fever, elevated inflammatory markers (sedimentation rate, c-reactive protein)
- Septic arthritis (spread from osteomyelitis → **complication**)
- Periosteum pressure → ischemia → necrosis

CCRN Tip

As with many infections, if left untreated, sepsis and systemic infection is an increasing risk.

Interventions

- Biopsy → pathogen recognition → antibiotics (long-term)
- Removal of implanted hardware (if necessary)
- Surgical containment/debridement
- Manage or correct underlying peripheral perfusion issues

Functional Issues

Functional issues related to critical care largely point to the safety components and risk factors our patients may experience. Many of these issues prolong hospital stay and increase overall morbidity and mortality. Table 9-2 outlines these functional issues.

Table 9-2   Nursing Considerations of Functional Issues

IMMOBILITY	FALLS	GAIT DISORDERS
Complications	**Complications**	**Risk Factors**
Cardiovascular compromise	Monitor minimum of 24 hours post-fall	Physical factors
• Increase in resting HR	**Minor**: dressings, ice, topical medications	• Old age
• Decrease in EF	**Moderate**: suture, splint	• Poor vision
• Orthostasis	**Major**: surgery, casting, neuro consultation	Neurological factors
Respiratory compromise	**Death**	• Sensory issues (visual, proprioception, vestibular)
• Atelectasis	**Risks**	• Neuromotor issues (spasticity, choreic, dystonia)
• Pneumonia	Morse Falls Scale (MFS)**	• Cognition (depression, slow gait, anxiety, cautious gait)
Thromboembolic events	Gait disorders	Orthopaedic factors
Pressure ulcer formation		• Myelopathy (spondylosis)
Muscle wasting (ICU-AW)*		• Osteoarthritis
Bone demineralization		Medical conditions
Contractures		• Heart failure (orthostasis)
Hyperglycemia		• Respiratory disease
Changes in sleep patterns		• Obesity
Delirium		
Interventions		
Interdisciplinary approach; may include turning, ROM, etc. Think global.		

*See CCRN Tip
**See Figure 9-1

> **CCRN Tip**
>
> ICU-AW, or intensive care unit–acquired weakness, is clinically observable weakness due to prolonged immobility in the ICU with no other cause. It is often assessed and charted in the EMR. Some key factors are presence of sepsis, length of mechanical ventilation, and presence of organ failure, among others.

Grades of Muscle Weakness

- Grade 0: No movement
- Grade 1: Minimal movement (no movement with contraction)
- Grade 2: Movement with no gravity
- Grade 3: Movement against gravity, but not resistance
- Grade 4: Movement against gravity, and some resistance
- Grade 5: Normal strength

Morse Falls Scale (MFS)

The MFS is a rapid and simple method of assessing and rating a patient's likelihood of falling. This is a new addition to the CCRN; understand the risk factors, ranking system, and how to prevent falls via standard and high risk protocols.

Figure 9-1   Morse Fall Score

History of falling	NO	0
	YES	25
Secondary diagnosis (more than one diagnosis)	NO	0
	YES	15
Ambulatory aid	None, on bed rest, uses W/C, or nurse assists	0
	Crutches, cane(s), walker	15
	Furniture	30
IV/Heparin lock or saline	NO	0
PIID	YES	20
Gait/transferring	Normal, on bed rest, immobile	0
	Weak (Uses touch for balance)	10
	Impaired (Unsteady, difficulty rising to stand)	20
Mental status	Oriented to own ability	0
	Forgets limitation	15

RISK LEVEL	MFS SCORE	ACTION
No risk	0–24	Good basic nursing care
Low risk	25–50	Implement standard fall prevention interventions
High risk	≥51	Implement high risk fall prevention interventions

Review Questions

1. A patient in a motor vehicle accident had his legs pinned in the door before being rescued by first responders. Upon arrival to the emergency room, the nurse performs a rapid assessment for injuries. Which of the following late findings would lead the nurse to believe of impending compartment syndrome of the legs?

    A. Numbness and tingling
    B. Pain unresponsive to opioids
    C. Diminished peripheral pulses
    D. Compartment pressure of 8 mmHg

2. Which of the following is TRUE regarding compartment syndrome?

    A. Compartment syndrome is possible without complete occlusion
    B. The affected body part is best elevated above the level of the heart
    C. Compartment syndrome occurs when muscle tissues swell and become necrotic
    D. Loss of motor function is one of the earliest symptoms of compartment syndrome

Questions 3–5 refer to the following case.

An elderly patient was admitted to the ICU 2 hours ago. The emergency room states the patient was found lying down in her kitchen, they suspect for longer than 24 hours. The patient was unconscious in the ED, not protecting the airway, and subsequently intubated. A CT of the head was performed showing likely ischemic stroke. Upon admission to the ICU, an indwelling catheter was placed revealing dark-colored urine. Labs reveal an elevated CK and hyperkalemia.

3. What is the best explanation for the color of the urine in this patient?

    A. Presence of hemoglobin in the urine
    B. Poor perfusion leading to myolysis
    C. Elevated creatine kinase leading to acute kidney injury
    D. Destruction of myocytes causing myoglobinuria

4. The most likely cause of rhabdomyolysis in this patient is what?

    A. Excessive aerobic exercise
    B. Drug toxicity
    C. Prolonged immobilization
    D. Anemia and hypotension

5. Which of the following are priority interventions for patients with rhabdomyolysis?

    A. Intravenous fluids and rhythm monitoring

    B. Pain management and furosemide

    C. Restrict fluids and administer diuretics

    D. Assess and manage metabolic alkalosis

6. A 45-year-old male patient is being treated for an obvious open fracture of the radius after a fall from a ladder. The bone is visible. Which nursing interventions should be performed first for this type of fracture?

    A. Apply hard pressure to reset the bone

    B. Apply a sterile dressing and immobilize the limb

    C. Irrigate with sterile saline and debride the wound

    D. Administer morphine and warm compresses to treat muscle cramps

7. After a complicated fracture of the femur, a patient in the ICU develops shortness of breath, tachypnea, and restlessness. The nurse enters the room to perform a rapid assessment. Visible pinpoint red spots are across the patient's chest? Which of the following is the most likely explanation for these changes in the patient?

    A. Small adipose particles are causing occlusions in lung and dermal capillaries

    B. Hypertension and severe pain related to the fracture

    C. Rapid breathing is likely due to severe acidosis

    D. Rhabdomyolysis leading to increased exhalation of carbon dioxide

8. A patient was recently admitted to the ICU directly from a nursing home. Nursing home staff state the patient was difficult to arouse this morning, had a fever of 102°F, and was visibly soaked in sweat. Immediate assessment by the nurse in the ICU reveals a large stage 4 pressure ulcer on the sacrum. Which of the following findings would suggest the wound has advanced causing osteomyelitis?

    A. Erythema and tenderness of the surrounding skin

    B. Fever of 102°F and localized paresthesias

    C. Elevated erythrocyte sedimentation rate and pain

    D. Hypercalcemia, fever, and tremors

9. Which of the following patients would be the highest risk for falls according to the Morse Falls Scale?

   A. A COPD patient with no history of falls; has two peripheral IV's heplocked

   B. Post-op knee replacement; patient remains confused with IV continuous 0.9 NS

   C. A patient in septic shock intubated, sedated, and on pressors

   D. An oriented patient with diabetes, requires a cane to walk, fell a month ago

10. A patient in the MICU diagnosed with severe COPD exacerbation has remained intubated for the past 5 days; a tracheostomy is likely. Due to prolonged bed rest, which of the following complications would result in a PaO_2 of 55%?

    A. Orthostatic hypotension

    B. Atelectasis

    C. Ventilator-associated pneumonia

    D. Bronchial inflammation

Answer Key

Question 1

Answer: B

Rationale: "Pain out of proportion" is a commonly used saying for situations like this. Pain should be responsive to medications. When it is not, typically something much more serious is going on. Numbness and tingling would be considered an early sign of compartment syndrome, not a late sign of impending emergency. The same would apply to pulses, but it is worth noting that a person can have compartment syndrome and still have pulses. A compartment pressure less than 10 mmHg is considered normal.

Question 2

Answer: A

Rationale: Compartment syndrome may occur without a complete occlusion of arteries. This is why a patient may still have pulses even in the setting of the emergency—granted absent pulses always indicates a problem. Whatever body part is being affected, it should be at the level of the heart, not higher or lower. A buildup of interstitial fluid that pushes on the vasculature affecting blood flow describes compartment syndrome. While swelling within the muscle compartment would be a fair wording, almost all cases are caused by bleeding or swelling after an injury, not of the muscle tissue itself. Paralysis would be considered a late sign of compartment syndrome.

Question 3

Answer: D

Rationale: The dark or "tea-colored" urine commonly seen in rhabdomyolysis is due to myoglobin in the urine (not hemoglobin). Hemoglobin in the urine would give a dark appearance, but that would be seen in hemolytic diseases, not this. Ischemia is a known cause of rhabdomyolysis, albeit rare, but it would be more important to focus on what the question is asking regarding the "color" of the urine and why. Neither poor perfusion nor creatine kinase explains the color.

Question 4

Answer: C

Rationale: Given the patient was found unconscious on the floor for likely more than 24 hours, prolonged immobilization makes the most sense. It is unlikely an elderly patient exercised to the point of rhabdomyolysis before collapse. Drug toxicity is a known cause of rhabdomyolysis, but with no information regarding the current medicine regimen of this patient, it would be considered a stretch in a question like this. The same rule would apply for anemia and hypotension. The precipitating event was likely the stroke, then the prolonged immobilization caused rhabdomyolysis.

Question 5

Answer: A

Rationale: Aggressive intravenous fluid therapy is the mainstay and priority treatment for patients with rhabdomyolysis. Given the risk for hyperkalemia, telemetry is common for close monitoring of the heart rhythm. Pain management is important, but like previous nursing exams, prioritization runs down an ABC/medical emergency thought process. Diuretics, like furosemide, may be used in certain circumstances but are secondary to fluid therapy. Restriction of fluids is the complete opposite of the goal. Flush the kidneys to prevent worsening AKI. Patients with rhabdomyolysis experience metabolic acidosis, not alkalosis.

Question 6

Answer: B

Rationale: Immobilization or stabilization is a common priority infection for all fractures. Until advanced diagnostics and treatment can be initiated, the scope of practice for the nurse is limited. The same thought for resetting the bone and debridement; this is NOT the scope of a registered nurse. A sterile dressing will help prevent infection, a common complication of open/compound fractures. Nurses may irrigate wounds from time to time, but these are typically chronic wounds or wounds that have been assessed by a specialist first. Morphine may be appropriate, but not warm compresses. Heat will make the problem worse by precipitating vasodilation and swelling.

Question 7

Answer: A

Rationale: Fat embolism syndrome is a common complication and risk factor for fractures of the long bones whether open or closed. Pulmonary embolism and petechiae both develop due to occlusions in the capillaries. Hypertension and severe pain would not explain the shortness of breath and petechiae. Rapid breathing may occur during states of acidosis like in DKA, but it does not answer the current state of this patient. The symptoms in this question do not match rhabdomyolysis. The breathing off of carbon dioxide is again an explanation for a state of compensation due to acidosis, like Kussmaul breathing in a DKA patient.

Question 8

Answer: C

Rationale: The best indicators of osteomyelitis include elevated inflammatory markers (ESR, CRP), fever, and dull pain. Erythema and tenderness around the skin would be an indicator or a wound infection, not of the bone itself. Paresthesias typically describe a dysfunction of the peripheral nerves. A more central injury like a sacral pressure wound would exhibit pain due to the osteomyelitis, not paresthesias. Hypercalcemia is not common in osteomyelitis; the bone is infected, not breaking down.

Question 9

Answer: D

Rationale: These types of questions are tricky without the scale directly next to the question. This requires a baseline understanding of the Morse Falls Scale and how risk factors are ranked. Review this knowledge in the chapter. The patient in answer "D" has the highest score. This is a new addition to the CCRN exam.

Question 10

Answer: B

Rationale: Prolonged immobility has many consequences. The patient in this question is hypoxemic. While COPD would certainly lower the expected range of arterial oxygenation, 55% is too low. The most likely cause due to immobility would be atelectasis, or the partial collapsing of the alveoli decreasing ventilation. The question is asking the cause of the hypoxemia due to prolonged immobilization, neither orthostatic hypotension, VAP, nor bronchial inflammation answers this question. They may all be causes of hypoxemia, but not in the context of prolonged immobilization.

CHAPTER 10

Neurology

The neurology section makes up roughly 10 questions on your CCRN exam, so approximately 8% of the exam is devoted to this topic, making it one of the larger areas to study. Understanding neurology can be difficult without a strong foundation in anatomy and physiology. It may be advisable to do a brief review of your A&P on this topic. Below there is a brief introduction to common terminology in neuro assessments. You will see many of these assessments throughout the chapter.

Neurology Assessment

Level of Consciousness (LOC)

Any change in LOC is cause for concern. It is oftentimes one of the earliest signs of something going wrong neurologically. The CCRN could use the following definitions and the Glasgow Coma Scale (see Figure 10-1 and Table 10-1) to test and compare severity of patients in answers (who is worse off?).

LOC Assessment: Noxious Stimuli (painful)
- Shaking, sternal friction rub, trapezius squeeze, lunula (nail) pressure

Figure 10-1   Levels of consciousness

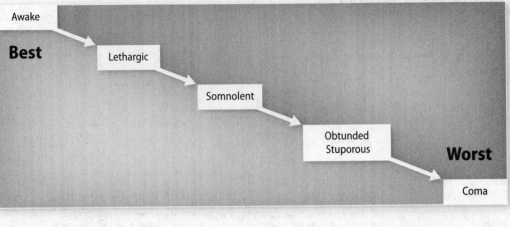

Table 10-1   Glasgow Coma Scale

FEATURE	RESPONSE	SCORE
Best eye response	Opens spontaneously	4
	Opens to speech	3
	Opens to pain	2
	No eye opening	1
Best verbal response	Oriented	5
	Confused	4
	Inappropriate words	3
	Incomprehensible sounds	2
	No verbal response	1
Best motor response	Obeys commands	6
	Localizes pain	5
	Withdraws from pain	4
	Flexion to pain (decorticate)	3
	Extension to pain (decerebrate)	2
	No motor response	1

Cranial Nerve Assessment

Not much needs to be known about cranial nerves for the CCRN exam, luckily, but you should be able to name them and count them out. Reminder: There are 12; many people use mnemonics to memorize them. The CCRN may take it one step further regarding specific assessments for certain cranial nerves (see Table 10-2).

Table 10-2 Cranial Nerves and Assessment

CRANIAL NERVE	ASSESSMENT/PROBLEM
I. Olfactory	Smell

II. Optic	Sight
	• Damage to cranial nerve II may lead to loss of visual field
	• Homonymous hemianopsia
	  • Loss of visual field opposite location of damage (contralateral)
	  • Assess for neglect; patients may need to "scan" the area to be aware of objects

III. Oculomotor	Movement of the eye and pupils • Damage may cause abnormal gaze and pupillary abnormality • Results in dilated pupils and/or diplopia • Herniation causes ipsilateral dilation first
IV. Trochlear	Controls eye movement • Damage may result in diplopia
V. Trigeminal	Sensation and motor function of the face • Trigeminal neuralgia (tic douloureux) • Damage may cause difficulty biting and chewing
VI. Abducens	Extraocular motor functions
VII. Facial	Facial expression and anterior taste
VIII. Vestibulocochlear	Sound and equilibrium from inner ear • Damage may result in abnormal Doll's eye test and cold caloric tests • **Doll's eyes** → eyes turn toward same side as head turned or no movement • **Cold caloric** → eyes should move toward side water injected
IX. Glossopharyngeal	Swallowing and gag reflex
X. Vagus	Parasympathetic innervation to the heart • Vaso-vagal stimulation may lead to drop in heart rate and blood pressure Swallowing and gag reflex
XI. Accessory	Rotation of neck and shoulders • Damage may occur during neck surgery causing loss of function
XII. Hypoglossal	Speech and swallowing

Figure 10-2   Lobes of the brain

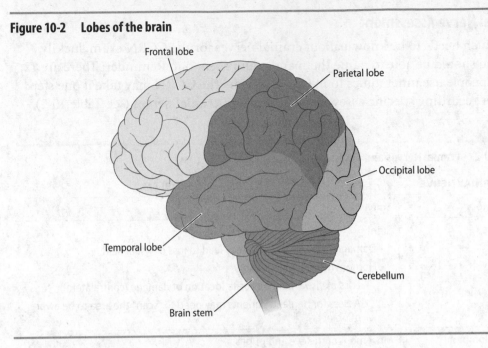

Lobes of the Brain and Brain Stem

Figure 10-2 shows the lobes of the brain.

- Frontal lobe
  - Broca's area → aphasia → large risk in ischemic strokes
    - Be cautious of interventions—no need to talk louder (especially in expressive aphasia)
  - Personality → assess behavior (patient may be abnormally aggressive)
  - Memory → inability to form new memories
- Temporal lobe
  - Processes sensory information (hearing, taste, smell)
- Parietal lobe
  - Perception → proprioception (position, location, interpretation of objects)
- Occipital lobe
  - Vision → damage may lead to homonymous hemianopsia or blindness
- Cerebellum
  - Balance and coordination
  - Ataxia → dysfunction in voluntary movements
- Brain stem
  - Midbrain and pons
  - Medulla → heart rate, breathing, blood pressure

Acute Spinal Cord Injury (SCI)

Spinal cord injuries may occur due to a number of issues. SCI is complicated by a complex post-traumatic set of issues from neuropathic pain and numbness to paralysis. The immediate goal in many cases is to immediately stabilize and decompress the spinal cord. The phrase "time is spine" is an often-used tool to direct goals through the immediate, acute, and sub-acute stages of SCI.

- **Primary SCI**
  - Direct physical trauma (penetrating or blunt injury)
- **Secondary SCI**
  - Post-injury decompensation (hemorrhage, spinal cord ischemia, inflammation)

Signs and Symptoms

- Dependent on location of injury
  - Cervical: cardiovascular and respiratory compromise (neurogenic shock, loss of phrenic nerve innervation to diaphragm)
  - Thoracic
  - Lumbar
  - Sacral
- Spinal shock: loss of motor and sensory function (temporary loss may last up to 12 months; early signs of recovery involve spasticity and regaining reflexes)
- Neurogenic bladder

Interventions

- "Time is spine"
  - Immediate: ABCs, immobilization
  - Acute: early diagnostics (CT, MRI), surgical decompression
    - Consider steroid use within 8 hours unless contraindicated
    - Maintain elevated blood pressure, MAP goals 85–90 mmHg
  - Sub-acute: rehabilitation (PT, OT), avoid autonomic dysreflexia, bladder and bowel care, prevent pressure ulcers and pneumonia
- Increased risk for pneumonia due to impaired gag and cough; encourage pulmonary clearance and incentive spirometry use
- Manage increased DVT and pressure ulcer risk
- Bladder and indwelling catheter care if appropriate; straight cath is preferred

Autonomic dysreflexia (AD) is a potentially life-threatening complication of SCI typically seen in injuries at or above T6. It is caused by a trigger below the level of injury, oftentimes the bladder or bowel via distention. It is critical to manage bladder or bowel dysfunction for this purpose. Hypertension that is not correct may be treated with antihypertensives such as nifedipine or nitroglycerin.

- Sudden hypertension
- Diaphoresis
- Headache

Encephalopathy

Any disease state that affects brain function can be defined as encephalopathy. There are a multitude of causes, many of which are covered in areas of this book like hepatic encephalopathy in liver failure or sepsis-associated encephalopathy. For the purposes of this section, neurology, the CCRN blueprint places importance on understanding **delirium**; an acute onset of symptoms.

Combined Symptoms of Delirium

- Disturbance in attention (inability to direct or focus the patient)
- Reduced orientation (lack of focus on environmental cues)
- Disorganized thinking
- Sleep–wake cycle disruptions

    Severe cases of encephalopathy may lead to seizures or death.

CCRN Tip
Hyperactive delirium
• Increase in psychomotor activity
Hypoactive delirium
• Decrease in psychomotor activity

Interventions

- Tailored monitoring
    - CAM-ICU monitoring—patient must be AWAKE
    - Mini-mental (COG) analysis for cognitive impairment
    - CIWA for alcohol withdrawal
- Treat the underlying pathology of the delirium (infection, ammonia, drugs, etc.)
- Consider use and need for pharmacological and nonpharmacological interventions
- Ensure safety, reorient the patient, provide supportive environment, ensure adequate sleep

Dementia

When comparing and contrasting dementia and delirium, remember that dementia is progressive and chronic, whereas delirium is acute and reversible. Alzheimer's disease makes up the largest portion of dementia patients. Dementia may also be caused by vascular disease or more atypical causes such as infections (tertiary syphilis).

Signs and Symptoms

- Loss of cognitive function in multiple areas (memory, reasoning, visual-spatial)
    - Agnosia: inability to recognize objects
    - Apraxia: inability to perform previously learned tasks
- Changes in behavioral (agitation, apathy, aggression, hallucinations)

Interventions

- Diagnostic assessments
  - Montreal Cognitive Assessment (MoCa)
    - Word, animal, object recall
    - Tests executive functions and judgment
  - Mini-Cog: common tool is drawing a clock
- Nonpharmacological
  - Priority is always **safety first**
  - Cognitive stimulating activities (communication, exercise, family exposure)
- Pharmacological
  - Acetylcholinesterase inhibitors (donepezil, memantine, rivastigmine)

Traumatic Brain Injury (TBI)

TBI occurs when an external traumatic force causes physiological damage and/or dysfunction to the brain. This may be in the form of a blunt (closed) trauma or penetrating trauma. Despite the severity of TBI, temporary or long-term physical, behavioral, emotional, and cognitive changes may be seen in varying degrees. Some terminologies to know follow.

- **Primary Brain Injury**
  - The initial traumatic event, direct physical damage
- **Secondary Brain Injury**
  - The delayed aftermath; may include hypotension, hypoxic damage, cerebral edema and increased ICP, and infection

Table 10-3 contrasts the characteristics of focal versus diffuse TBIs.

> **CCRN Tip**
>
> Cerebral blood flow is a common concern with secondary injury. Goals include maintaining perfusion without allowing ICP to increase, a delicate dance of interventions.

Table 10-3   Differences in Focal and Diffuse Traumatic Brain Injuries

FOCAL INJURIES	DIFFUSE INJURIES

Skull fractures
• High-impact etiologies
• Higher likelihood of hemorrhages
• Basilar skull fractures: CSF leakage
   • Do not pack to prevent drainage, may lead to increased ICP
   • Meningeal tear
     • Otorrhea
     • Rhinorrhea (avoid trauma and blowing of nose)
• Raccoon eyes (bruising around eyes)
• Battle's sign (bruising back of ear)
To confirm the presence of CSF, test for glucose. CSF contains glucose. Alternate test is "halo," which appears yellow on gauze.
Contusion and lacerations
• Damage to small blood vessels near bony prominences
• Includes coup and contrecoup injuries
Hemorrhage and hematomas
• Covered in more detail below
	Diffuse vascular injury
	• Petechial hemorrhages: shearing of blood vessels
	• Common in severe TBI
	Diffuse brain swelling
	• Edema and vascular swelling
	• Cytotoxic swelling: extracellular fluid shifts into cells
	• Vasogenic swelling: extracellular fluid from broken down blood–brain barrier
	• Leads to increased ICP
	Diffuse axonal injury
	• Transection or shearing of axons
	• Acute axonal swelling (3–6 hours)
	• Degeneration of axons may occur and persist leading to increased disability

Ranking of TBI

The Glasgow Coma Scale is the most widely used method of an immediate TBI assessment. It does not give a complete clinical picture, but given its ease of use, it is fast and effective. A very common question and statement in the setting of a TBI is "Was there a loss of consciousness?" The duration of LOC and post-traumatic amnesia are also commonly used tools.

- Mild: GCS of 13–15 (most common)
- Moderate: GCS of 9–12
- Severe: GCS of 3–8

Concussion

Concussions are classified as a type of mild TBI. They are also the most common type of TBI, with the majority of patients making a full recovery. There are, however, patients who retain certain deficits.

- Wide variety of causes (sports, banging of the head, abuse)
- Force causes an acceleration–deceleration injury. Neurometabolic changes increase glucose demand of the brain without adequate supply.
  - Complicated → abnormal head CT
  - Uncomplicated → normal head CT

> **CCRN Tip**
>
> It seems that 5 mm is a common number when it comes to TBIs. For example, 5 mm in brain shifts often triggers the need for a surgical intervention. And 5 mm of depression in a skull fracture often triggers the need for surgical intervention.

- Glasgow Coma Scale of 13–15 (mild TBI)
- Immediate 24 to 48 hours should include strict rest followed by gradual increase in activity
- Post-concussive syndrome (PCS)
    - Cognitive deficits in attention or memory
    - Fatigue, sleep issues, headache, dizziness, irritability

Hematomas

Table 10-4 compares types of hematomas (epidural vs. subdural).

Table 10-4   Epidural vs. Subdural Hematomas

TYPE OF HEMATOMA	CLINICAL PICTURE

Epidural	**Signs and Symptoms**
	• Most common in the temporal region resulting from meningeal arterial bleed. Skull fractures are common.
	• Life-threatening condition
	• **Initial LOC** loss → transient recovery → neurological decline
	• Decreasing level of consciousness
	• Increasing ICP
	   • Ipsilateral pupil dilation → anisocoria (result from **uncal herniation**)
	   • Contralateral paresis or plegia
	   • Cushing reflex/triad
	Interventions
	• Immediate head CT scan
	• Laboratory tests (CBC, coag panel, liver panel)
	• NEUROSURGICAL EMERGENCY → immediate decompression required
	   • Burr holes
	   • Craniotomy with evacuation
	• External ventricular drain (EVD) with ICP monitoring

Subdural	**Signs and Symptoms** • Nontraumatic injury may be abuse (shaken baby syndrome) • Similar symptoms to epidural hematomas, however, potentially delayed due to acute, sub-acute, and chronic presentation of injury **Interventions** • Early identification of underlying anticoagulation therapy (poorer outcomes → delayed bleeds) • Hourly neuro checks → complications like ICP may be delayed • ICP monitoring → surgery if ICP 20 mmHG or higher

Intracranial Hemorrhage

A separation of terminology not to be confused, hemorrhage, in the neurological sense, may also be subdefined as a hemorrhagic stroke. The terminology used typically dictates the location of the bleed: intracerebral, intraventricular, subarachnoid, and brain stem. The location of the bleed also largely explains many of the symptoms.

Subarachnoid Hemorrhage (SAH)

SAH is a life-threatening emergency requiring prompt assessment and treatment.

Etiology

- Traumatic head injury
- Aneurysm (saccular) rupture (oftentimes within the Circle of Willis)
- Contributing factors may include cocaine abuse, anticoagulation, smoking, hypertension, and alcohol abuse

Signs and Symptoms

- **Early**: severe rapidly progressing headache, neck pain, N/V, photophobia
- **Late**: LOC changes, nuchal rigidity, increasing ICP
  - May include positive Brudzinski and Kernig's signs
- Seizures are commonly associated with aneurysm rupture and AVM malformations
- Delayed complications
  - Rebleeds
  - Vasospasms typically occur 3–5 days after onset of SAH

Interventions

- ABC priority → decreased LOC may prompt intubation
- EVD drain with ICP monitoring
- Prevention strategies
  - Vasospasms → nicardipine/nimodipine, intravenous fluids, balloon stenting
    - Hypervolemia to prevent
  - Seizures → antiepileptics
  - Rebleeds → blood pressure management → SBT 140–160 mmHg → labetalol
- Surgical intervention
  - Coiling and clipping → reduce further bleeding
  - Craniotomy → evacuate bleeding

ICP Monitoring and Treatment

Within the human skull there is 80% brain tissue, 10% blood, and 10% cerebrospinal fluid. Given the rigid nature of the skull and the finite space, an increase in any component leads to intracranial pressure (ICP). This is a very common topic on the CCRN exam. The Monro-Kellie hypothesis works off of this concept of limited space. If one volume goes up, the other two must go down to avoid ICP.

Cerebral Edema

- **Cytotoxic (intracellular) cerebral edema**
  - Hypoosmolality (water intoxication), ischemia
- **Vasogenic (blood–brain barrier failure) cerebral edema**
  - Space-occupying lesions, TBIs

Early vs. Late Increased ICP

- Early signs and symptoms
  - Level of consciousness changes
  - Headache
  - Nausea/vomiting
  - Diplopia
  - Papilledema
  - Pupillary changes
- Late signs and symptoms
  - Decorticate/decerebrate positioning
  - Coma/flaccidity of muscles
  - Cushing's triad (impending herniation)
    - Cushing's triad (impending herniation)
    - Irregular breathing
    - Bradycardia
  - Herniation and death

ICP/CPP Monitoring

- Intracranial pressure
  - Normal: 0 to 10 mmHg
  - Elevated: 10 to 20 mmHg
  - Severe: 20 mmHg or greater
- Cerebral perfusion pressure (MAP minus ICP)
  - Normal: 80 to 100 mmHg
  - Decreased: 50 to 80 mmHg
  - Severe: 50 mmHg or less

Nursing Considerations for ICP Monitoring

- Maintain the transducer at the level of the ear (Foramen of Monro → external auditory meatus)
- Understand differences between ICP waves
  - A (plateau) waves → severely elevated ICP
  - B waves → slightly elevated ICP
  - C waves → expected
  - Dampening may indicate impending obstruction of the catheter or positioning clamping
- Take into account nursing care actions that may temporarily increase ICP
  - Turning, suctioning, stimulation

CCRN Tip

Most studies encourage maintenance of **CPP above 60 mmHg**. Some encourage a range of 50 to 70 mmHg. The minimum to understand is certainly **50 mmHg**. This is achieved through IV fluids and vasopressors. Monitor blood pressure and MAP closely since this is one of the main factors in CPP. Prevention of secondary injury is key.

Treatment of Increased ICP

- Osmotic diuretics → mannitol → typically given when ICP is 20 mmHg or greater
  - Monitor serum osmolality, stop treatment if osmolality reaches 320 mOsm or higher, assess every 4–6 hours
  - Inspect for crystallization
- Hypertonic crystalloids (3% saline)
  - Secondary use in patients with elevated osmolality not eligible for mannitol administration
- Treat pain and anxiety → propofol if intubated
- Maintain midline neck position and semi-Fowler's body position
  - Encourages venous outflow from the cranium
- Maintain normal acid/base balances; acidity causes vasodilation
- The conversation of hyperventilation and induced respiratory alkalosis is a debated topic. Most research states it may be used only in acute deterioration (herniation), never prophylactically, and only temporary to bridge a gap in treatment. Alkalosis may also cause vasoconstriction and cerebral ischemia.
- External ventricular drain (EVD)—see Figure 10-3
  - Ensure proper zeroing, height (cmH_2O), sterility, CSF inspection, and ICP waveform analysis
  - Protocol is often neurosurgeon or institutionally driven
    - Clamp unless ICP above 20 mmHg, delayed clamping when absent blood in CSF, etc.
  - Drain cerebrospinal fluid through the EVD; the neurosurgeon will specify orders of amount removed per hour
  - Assess orders to clamp or obtain an order to clamp temporarily if transporting a patient to CT or elsewhere
- Patients may be put into a medically induced coma if the above measures do not adequately manage ICP

Figure 10-3   External ventricular drainage

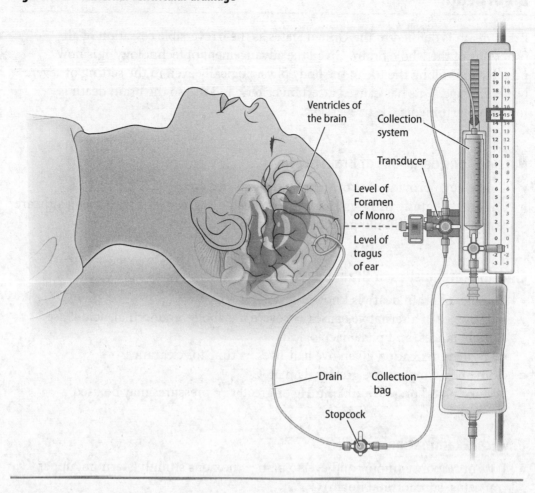

Ventricles of the brain

Collection system

Transducer

Level of Foramen of Monro

Level of tragus of ear

Drain

Collection bag

Stopcock

Brain Herniation

Brain herniation is the inevitable result of expanding brain tissue. As the brain components herniate, blood flow is lost and death often occurs.

Uncal vs. Central Herniation

- Uncal herniation
  - Often the result of epidural hematomas
  - LATERAL (side-to-side) shift
  - Uncus (medial temporal lobe) swelling toward the brain stem and oculomotor nerve (cranial nerve III) → leads to dilation and nonreactive pupil
    - 1st symptoms → pupils
- Central herniation
  - Swelling of both sides of the brain
  - Brain shifts DOWNWARD
  - Pressure pushes downward on the reticular activating system
  - 1st symptoms → LOC changes
    - Bilateral symptoms → pupils, Babinski

Brain Death

Brain death is defined in the United States as the irreversible cessation of all functions of the whole brain. Given the advancement of technology, it is now possible to prolong the life of the body physiologically even in the setting of severe brain damage. This has caused a certain criteria to arise so the brain death is indeed determined to be irreversible.

Nursing Considerations of Brain Death

- Continue to provide care until brain death is declared
- Engage the family through the entire process; disagreements with the healthcare team and family should prompt ethics team involvement

Clinical Prerequisites of Brain Death

- Etiology of brain death is known
  - Absence of alternative causes → severe metabolic, endocrinal, acid–base imbalances, and pharmacological
  - Drug intoxication given five half-lives → time for clearance
- Core body temperature greater than 36°C
- Systolic blood pressure 100 mmHg or greater → pressures may be used

Physical Examination

- Loss of response (motor and eye) to pain → noxious stimuli (sternum, upper trapezius, supraorbital notch)
- Loss of brain stem reflexes
  - Absent pupillary reflex (light reflex)
  - Absent eye motion (Doll's eyes)
  - Absent corneal reflex
  - Absent oculovestibular reflex (Caloric test) → irrigation of ear with ice water
  - Absent gag reflex
  - Absent cough reflex

Apnea Test

Assesses pulmonary drive triggered by the brain; monitor $PaCO_2$.

- Repeat ABG 8–10 minutes after initiation of apnea test → **$PaCO_2$ greater than 60 mmHg** or rise of 20 mmHg from baseline is indicative of brain death
- Hypotension, cardiac dysrhythmias, and hypoxia below 85% SpO_2 should discontinue the test

Ancillary Tests

Ancillary tests are performed when an apnea test is not possible or brain death remains inconclusive.

- Loss of cerebral blood flow (angiography, transcranial ultrasound)
- Loss of cerebral electrical activity (EEG)

Stroke

Cerebrovascular accidents account any acute compromise in perfusion of the brain via the vasculature. It remains a leading problem in the United States and for healthcare professionals in critical care. Recognizing the differences between the types of strokes and treatment protocols is critical for the CCRN exam. Common knowledge dictates an early FAST exam and typically triggers an institutional code for stroke.

Table 10-5 contrasts ischemic and hemorrhagic stroke.

Table 10-5   Ischemic vs. Hemorrhagic Stroke

ISCHEMIC STROKE	HEMORRHAGIC STROKE
Etiology • More common than hemorrhagic • Risk factors include hypertension, diabetes, smoking, obesity, and atrial fibrillation **Signs and symptoms** • Contralateral presentation (left-sided infarct leads to right-sided weakness, hemianopsia, Babinski) **Interventions** "Time is brain" • Immediate CT scan • Rule out other causes of symptoms (hypoglycemia, electrolyte imbalances, circulatory issues, etc.) • Tissue plasminogen activator (tPA) up to 4.5 hours post, less than 3 hours is best • Mechanical thrombectomy up to 6 hours post Permissible hypertension allows blood pressure significantly higher than normal • Do not treat unless above 220 mmHg • Preferred less than 180 mmHg • Beta blockers first-line drug (labetalol) Modifiable factors • Weight loss and diet • Manage risk factors (antihypertensives, antihyperlipidemics)	**Etiology** • Hypertension, aneurysm rupture, arteriovenous malformation, illicit drug use among others • Includes intracranial hemorrhage covered earlier in this chapter (subarachnoid hemorrhage) **Signs and symptoms** • Similar to ischemic stroke **Interventions** • Blood pressure management • Beta blockers, ACE inhibitors, calcium-channel blockers, hydralazine • Surgical decompression • Monitor for delayed seizures and ICP

tPA Administration

Administration of tPA comes with a rather large body of understood information from contraindications and post-administration considerations. Here are the hard hitters.

- Contraindications
    - Current hemorrhage or hypercoagulative state (current blood thinner use, thrombocytopenia, elevated INR, etc.)
    - Advanced age (>80 years)
    - Recent head trauma, stroke, or surgery
- Post-administration considerations
    - Hemorrhagic transformation → serial neuro exams (LOC)

> **CCRN Tip**
>
> **NIHSS Exam**
> - Level of consciousness
> - Language
> - Dysarthria (slurred words)
> - Motor function
> - Visual field deficits
> - Eye movement abnormalities
> - Facial paralysis
> - Ataxia (finger to nose)

Neurological Infectious Disease

The overall cases of meningitis have declined in the past decades largely due to vaccination. High-risk groups still warrant particular attention—children, the immunocompromised, and those who live in high-population close quarters. The entire spectrum of infectious disease in this sense is not needed for the CCRN; however, a solid approach is to split meningitis into viral, bacterial, and fungal causes (see Table 10-6).

Table 10-6 Types of Meningitis

BACTERIAL	VIRAL	FUNGAL
Spread via respiratory route (common)	Spread via the bloodstream from an infected area	Spread via respiratory route, transported via blood (hematogenous), and oral route
• *Neisseria, Streptococcal, E. coli*	• *Enteroviruses (Coxsacksie)*	• *Candida, Histoplasmosis, Cryptococcus*
Petechiae (meningococcus)	Low-grade or no fever	Lumbar puncture
Lumbar puncture	Lumbar puncture	• Increased lymphocytes
• Cloudy CSF	• Clear CSF	• Increased protein count
• Increased protein count	• Increased protein count	• Decreased glucose count
• Decreased glucose count (60% or less of serum)	• Normal glucose count (100% of serum or slightly below)	Treat with amphotericin B and fluconazole
Treat with IV cephalosporins (ceftriaxone) → vancomycin may be added	Treat with supportive care → fluid and electrolytes, pain management; antivirals not common unless specifically indicated	

Shared Symptoms of Meningitis

- Positive lumbar puncture culture (pathogen and increased WBCs)
- Nuchal rigidity, fever, headache, photophobia
- Positive Brudzinski's sign → chin to chest, flexed knees
- Positive Kernig's sign → straighten leg out from flexed position

> **CCRN Tip**
>
> Lumbar puncture is contraindicated with increased ICP—it may lead to brain herniation.

Neuromuscular Disorders

Dysfunction of the peripheral nerves or muscles is a simplified explanation of the pathophysiology of neuromuscular disorders. Each of the following diseases in this section have certain unique issues found potentially on the CCRN example.

Muscular Dystrophy

Muscular dystrophies are genetic disorders that result in progressive muscle wasting and weakness.

> **CCRN Tip**
>
> Muscle wasting eventually leads to cardiomyopathy in both DMD and BMD, although it is much faster in DMD.

Etiology
- Inherited
- Deficient in dystrophin protein
- The greater the amount of dystrophin, the less severe the muscular dystrophy

Signs and Symptoms
- **Duchenne (DMD)**
  - Early childhood onset
  - X-linked recessive disorder
  - Severe weakness and wasting (atrophy)
  - Respiratory failure
- Becker (BMD)
- Adolescent or adulthood onset
- Less severe and slower progression than DMD
- Muscles affected: legs, spine, heart, shoulders, hip

Interventions
- **Nonpharmacological**
  - Physical therapy
  - Muscle training
  - Monitor for scoliosis
- **Pharmacological**
  - Reduce inflammation due to muscle damage
  - Corticosteroid (prednisone)
- Eventually, ventilation support will be required due to progressive muscle weakness
- Patients are at increased risk for certain infections due to weakened muscles → pneumonia

Cerebral Palsy (CP)

Cerebral palsy is a common pediatric condition causing abnormal muscle tone and movement.

Etiologies
- Abnormal development of the fetal brain or injury to the infant brain

Signs and Symptoms
- Spastic diplegia, hemiplegia, quadriplegia
- Dyskinetic/hyperkinetic

Interventions
- Screen for neuromuscular disorders that may mimic CP
- Medications for spasticity
  - Baclofen, benzos, dantrolene
- Interdisciplinary approach to care

Guillain–Barre Syndrome (GBS)

GBS is a post-infectious, immune-mediated neuromuscular disorder. The most common trigger of GBS are viral infections like the flu or other respiratory illnesses and gastrointestinal infections. More recently, the Zika virus was shown to cause GBS. Contrary to popular belief, the flu vaccine very rarely (one in one million) causes GBS.

Pathophysiology
- Demyelination of neuronal axons
- Antibodies bind to peripheral motor neuron synapses

Signs and Symptoms
- Proximal and distal weakness → typically begins proximally
  - Ascending paralysis → flaccidity
- Once the diaphragm is affected, intubation and ventilation is likely
- CSF shows normal WBC and elevated protein; if WBC is elevated, infectious processes that mimic GBS should be considered

Interventions
- ABCs → intubation with respiratory failure
- Intravenous immunoglobulin (IVIG)
- Plasma exchange (plasmapheresis) → removes antibodies
- Corticosteroids have shown no benefit in research although is continued to be given in many cases

Myasthenia Gravis (MG)

MG is an autoimmune disorder that affects neuromuscular junctions. Antibodies affect the function of acetylcholine at the synapse.

CCRN Tip

Differentiating between MG and other neuromuscular conditions may be required on the exam. MG typically begins with *facial weakness*, this allows for easy differentiation, since Guillain-Barre, for example, begins distally.

Signs and Symptoms

- Fluctuating muscle weakness progressing throughout the day
- Ocular weakness (ptosis, diplopia) → most common symptom
- Electrodiagnostic testing and positive antibody test
- Respiratory failure → myasthenia gravis crisis → ventilation

Understand the difference between myasthenia gravis crisis and cholinergic crisis. This may come up on the CCRN exam. MG crisis comes from a decrease in acetylcholine whereas cholinergic crisis comes from a dangerous elevation in the neurotransmitter. When questioned, a *tensilon test* is performed. When tensilon is administered, the following occur:

- Myasthenia crisis → improvement
- Cholinergic crisis → increased weakness

Interventions

- Immunosuppressive treatment (prednisone, cyclosporine)
- Cholinesterase inhibitors (pyridostigmine/Mestinon)
- Antibody treatment (rituximab)
- IVIG and plasmapheresis → if no response to immunosuppressive therapy, especially used in MG crisis
- Thymectomy for MG with thymoma

Seizure Disorders

A seizure itself may have multiple etiologies, but all originate from the central nervous system; the brain. Certain conditions increase the susceptibility to have a seizure or what is commonly known as a seizure threshold. Epileptic seizures (often simply known as seizures) are transient, typically lasting less than 2 minutes. The spectrum of seizure disorders is rather large; however, for the CCRN exam focus on the hard-hitting points and nursing considerations.

- **Partial seizure**: singular area triggers in the brain
- **Generalized seizure**: diffuse triggers in the brain

Nursing Considerations for Seizures

- Airway is the priority; ensure a clear airway
  - Turn if patient has copious secretions or is vomiting
  - Abnormal breathing leading to respiratory acidosis
- Post-ictal periods
  - Decreased LOC, headache, nausea
  - May last hours in some cases
- Drug therapy for seizure disorders
  - Sodium channel blockers (phenytoin, carbamazepine)
  - GABA agonists (benzodiazepines, barbiturates)
  - Alternatives (gabapentin, levetiracetam)

- **Status epilepticus** → medical emergency (generalized convulsive)
  - Single generalized convulsion lasting longer than 5 minutes or repeated seizures without regaining consciousness
    - Eventually leads to brain damage affecting the cells themselves → increased metabolic demand during the seizure
    - This hypermetabolism may lead to death
  - Seizure must be interrupted with medication → lorazepam

Signs and Symptoms Profile of Status Epilepticus

- Respiratory compromise → increased $PaCO_2$, decreased PaO_2
- Catecholamine release → tachycardia, hypertension, hyperglycemia
- Destruction of muscle tissue → lactic acidosis and hyperkalemia
- Disruption in thermoregulation → hyperthermia

Space-Occupying Lesions

Tumors that press against adjacent brain tissue may be defined as a space-occupying lesion. If the legion grows, as is the case in metastatic disease, eventually intracranial pressure will increase causing further complications. Monitor for new-onset *seizures* or epileptic episodes and signs of increased ICP. Early CT or MRI scans will display severity of the lesion or lesions and dictate the course of treatment.

Interventions

- Surgical interventions to evacuate lesion and improve edema and ICP
  - Transsphenoidal hypophysectomy (pituitary tumor) may result in slight CSF drainage for 48 hours. The nose should not be packed; place a loose dressing.
- Pharmacological treatment
  - ICP → mannitol, **steroids** (dexamethasone)
  - Abscess → antibiotics

Review Questions

1. A patient with a traumatic brain injury was admitted to the ICU 6 hours ago for close monitoring. New assessment reveals a trending increase in systolic blood pressure and decrease in diastolic blood pressure. The current heart rate is 50 BPM down from 75 BPM 2 hours ago. Which of the following findings would the nurse expect in addition to the above if Cushing's triad was of concern?

   A. Narrowing pulse pressure
   B. Irregularity in breathing
   C. Pupils not reactive to light
   D. Abnormal posturing with flexed arms

2. When assessing Glasgow Coma Scale in multiple patients in the neurological unit, which patient is of the most concern?

   A. Eyes open to pain, confused speech, localizes pain
   B. Eyes open spontaneously, oriented speech, obeys commands
   C. Eyes do not open, incomprehensible noises, withdraws from pain
   D. Eyes open to pain, no verbal response, extension to pain

3. Which of the following would the nurse witness as early signs of neurological problems?

   A. Lethargy and pupillary changes
   B. Hypertension with a widening pulse pressure
   C. Elevated lactic acid and positive Babinski reflex
   D. Loss of gag reflex and posturing

4. A 46-year-old female patient was recently admitted to the ICU for close monitoring after a motor vehicle accident. She lost consciousness en route to the hospital in the ambulance. In the emergency room she regained consciousness and was able to describe the events of the accident. Hours later in the ICU, the patient develops anisocoria with the right pupil larger than the left. She is also hypertensive with signs of posturing. Given the presentation and progression of this patient, which of the following is the most likely neurological cause?

   A. Epidural hematoma
   B. Subdural hematoma
   C. Subarachnoid hemorrhage
   D. Basilar skull fracture

5. A 65-year-old male was brought to the emergency room after being hit in the head with a bat. There is bruising around the back of the ears with clear fluid leaking from the ears themselves. A basilar skull fracture is considered likely. The healthcare team would like to test the clear liquid for being potentially cerebrospinal fluid. How would the nurse differentiate and test the CSF?

   A. Place the liquid on gauze and assess for a red halo

   B. Assess for the presence of glucose

   C. Assess for the presence of leukocytes

   D. Place the liquid in water and assess for separation

6. A 75-year-old patient in the neurological unit is being prepared for discharge 12 hours after experiencing dizziness and left-sided weakness. Supportive therapy was provided, but no tPA or further interventions were warranted. Which of the following most likely describes this patient's clinical diagnosis?

   A. The patient experienced a right-sided stroke

   B. The patient experienced a transient ischemic attack

   C. The patient will require follow-up CT scans for a potential brain tumor

   D. The patient experienced minor bruising on the spine

7. A 65-year-old male patient was admitted to the neuro ICU due to a hemorrhagic stroke. He now exhibits stupor when previously awake. Recent abnormalities in his breathing is also noted. There is concern for central brain herniation and potential impending death. Changes in levels of consciousness in central brain herniation is due to which of the following?

   A. Lateral swelling on the brain and brain stem

   B. Lateral displacement of the brain on cranial nerve III

   C. Downward swelling on the reticular activating system

   D. Downward swelling of the brain on the brain stem

8. Two days after a patient was admitted to the neuro ICU due to a traumatic brain injury, the nurse is monitoring the ICP and notes a pressure of 22 mmHg. The patient has previously received mannitol for acute episodes of increased ICP. Which of the following orders is appropriate at this time?

   A. Administration of mannitol; current serum osmolality 340 mOsm

   B. Unclamp the EVD and allow CSF drainage

   C. Evaluate positioning, ensure supine midline position

   D. Administer bicarbonate; current arterial pH 7.35

9. While assessing ICP pressure in a traumatic brain injury patient, which of the following waveforms does the nurse understand to require immediate intervention?

   A. A waves
   B. C waves
   C. B waves
   D. Z waves

10. A 86-year-old male is diagnosed with a left epidural hematoma. The nurse notes right-sided weakness in the arm and leg. Which other findings would the nurse expect with this type of bleeding?

   A. Dilated and nonreactive right pupil, central brain herniation
   B. Dilated and nonreactive left pupil, central brain herniation
   C. Dilated and nonreactive right pupil, uncal brain herniation
   D. Dilated and nonreactive left pupil, uncal brain herniation

11. A 65-year-old patient arrives at the emergency department. He has a known history of drug and alcohol abuse. He is experiencing severe pulsating headache, photophobia, nuchal rigidity, and a positive Kernig's sign. The patient is immediately taken to radiology for a CT of the head. While in CT the patient experiences a seizure and is given 1 mg lorazepam for relief. Which diagnosis is likely given the signs and symptoms?

   A. Epidural hematoma
   B. Subdural hematoma
   C. Basilar skull fracture
   D. Subarachnoid hemorrhage

12. Many neuromuscular disorders share similar symptoms. Which disorder is caused by antibodies that affect the function of acetylcholine and may lead to respiratory distress?

   A. Myasthenia gravis
   B. Guillain–Barre syndrome
   C. Muscular dystrophy
   D. Cerebral palsy

13. A 35-year-old male patient was previously admitted to the neuro ICU from an occupational-related injury to his head. An external ventricular drain (EVD) was placed immediately upon arrival to the ICU by the neurosurgeon. The nurse has orders to maintain cerebral perfusion pressure at or above 60 mmHg and to keep the EVD drain open. If the current ICP is 15 mmHg and the current MAP is 70, which of the following is needed of the nurse?

   A. Continue to monitor, CPP is adequate

   B. Clamp the drain and place the patient supine

   C. Initiate vasopressors as ordered and titrate to increase CPP

   D. Administer mannitol, monitor intake and output

14. The nurse is about to perform an apnea test on a potentially brain-dead patient with the physician and respiratory therapy bedside. Current vital signs include BP 100/70 mmHg, HR 95, and SpO_2 93% with preoxygenation. When would the healthcare team immediately discontinue the apnea test due to complications?

   A. BP 120/90 mmHg, HR 110

   B. BP 80/50 mmHg, HR 120

   C. SpO_2 88%, HR 115

   D. $PaCO_2$ 60 mmHg

15. A 65-year-old female was recently evaluated in the emergency room for new-onset lower leg weakness. In the ER, the patient states not feeling well over the past couple weeks with a low-grade fever and cough. She denies any trauma. Without a clear diagnosis, the patient was discharged home with instructions. One week later the patient arrives back at the ER with paralysis of both legs. Given the above case, what is the most likely explanation for the patient's progressive weakness?

   A. Guillain–Barre syndrome triggered by viral illness

   B. Spinal cord damage resulting in neuropathy

   C. Motor neuron dysfunction in myasthenia gravis

   D. Undiagnosed amyotrophic lateral sclerosis

16. An epileptic patient on the neurological unit develops a seizure that has not ceased after more than 5 minutes. The nurse attempts to obtain vitals, but is unable to due to the violent seizing. Which of the following signs and symptoms would the nurse expect in this state of status epilepticus?

   A. Elevated $PaCO_2$ and hyperglycemia

   B. Respiratory alkalosis and bradycardia

   C. Hypokalemia and bradycardia

   D. SpO_2 93% and PaO_2 85%

17. A 75-year-old male is admitted to the neuro ICU with aphasia and right-sided hemiplegia. History given by staff at the nursing home state the symptoms began 2 hours prior. Recombinant tissue plasminogen activator (tPA) is being considered. Which of the following contraindicate the use of tPA?

    A. 75 years of age
    B. Heart valve replacement surgery three months ago
    C. Platelet count of 150,000
    D. Current INR 1.2

18. A 22-year-old male patient is admitted with nuchal rigidity. Which of the following would lead the nurse to suspect bacterial meningitis instead of bacterial or fungal meningitis?

    A. Cerebrospinal fluid that is clear with an elevated protein count
    B. Cerebrospinal fluid that is cloudy with an elevated protein count
    C. Cerebrospinal fluid that is clear with a normal glucose count
    D. Cerebrospinal fluid that is cloudy with an elevated glucose count

Answer Key

Question 1

Answer: B

Rationale: Cushing's triad includes hypertension with widening pulse pressure, bradycardia, and irregular breathing. The other findings do indicate worsening ICP and condition, but they are not part of Cushing's triad.

Question 2

Answer: D

Rationale: Utilizing Glasgow Coma Scale, the patient with eyes opening to pain with no verbal response and extension to pain adds to a count of 6. The other answers have higher GCS. This is a generalized question about GSC; there may be an explanation of the behavior as well instead of simply saying "extension to pain." It may be written as *a patient exhibits downward pointing of the toes.*

Question 3

Answer: A

Rationale: Early signs of neurological decline include pupillary changes and decreasing levels of consciousness. The other answers are symptoms of late neurological decline with increasing lactate levels pointing to poor perfusion and potential organ failure.

Question 4

Answer: A

Rationale: Loss of consciousness followed by a period of transient recovery followed by neurological decline is characteristic of epidural hematoma. Initial loss of consciousness is indicative of a large problem in most cases. Subdural hematomas are not as rapid as their epidural counterparts. In SAH, LOC changes are typically seen later on, not immediately. Basilar skull fractures typically present with CSF leakage either otorrhea or rhinorrhea.

Question 5

Answer: B

Rationale: CSF contains glucose at roughly 60% of what is normally found in the serum. A halo test would display a yellow ring, not a red ring. Leukocytes would indicate an infectious process such as meningitis. Placing the clear liquid in water is not a known test.

Question 6

Answer: B

Rationale: The main feature of a transient ischemic attack (TIA) is the short-term "transient" nature, typically less than 24 hours in length (usually far less). A stroke itself would require and warrant a longer hospital stay and would likely include interventions to some degree. A brain tumor as well would not be transient; the symptoms would continue until corrected. Bruising of the spine may explain some peripheral weakness, more typically bilateral, however. Dizziness is also not common with a spinal injury.

Question 7

Answer: C

Rationale: Central brain herniation causes downward pressure on the reticular activating system. This pressure manifests with changes in levels of consciousness with eventual respiratory depression when the pressure reaches the brain stem. Uncal herniations cause lateral displacement on cranial nerve III (oculomotor) leading to pupillary changes.

Question 8

Answer: B

Rationale: The question states out of the following orders which to follow, so the question is not a matter of the validity of the order, but rather which order you wish to follow. While directed by institutional policy and neurosurgeon orders, unclamping the EVD to allow for CSF drainage is a valid treatment for elevated ICP—when it is ordered as such. Mannitol is often given in states such as this; however, it should not be administered when serum osmolality reach 320 mOsm or higher. Patient position should be semi-Fowler's with the neck midline; this allows for venous drainage. Bicarb may be administered to avoid acidotic states that increase ICP; the pH is normal here, so the bicarb is not needed.

Question 9

Answer: A

Rationale: Plateau waves, also called "A" waves, are rapid-onset waves that are clinically dangerous and require immediate interventions. With spikes in ICP in A waves, ischemia may occur or, worse, brain herniation. A handy mnemonic often used is *A = awful, B = bad, C = cool.* Z waves do not exist in ICP monitoring.

Question 10

Answer: D

Rationale: Pressure on the oculomotor cranial nerve (III) leads to ipsilateral pupil dilation and contralateral weakness or plegia. This lateral pressure leads to uncal brain herniation. Central herniation occurs when there is downward pressure due to swelling, not lateral.

Question 11

Answer: D

Rationale: The signs and symptoms of this patient are most in line with subarachnoid hemorrhage. Given the history of drug and alcohol abuse with the seizure in CT, an aneurysm rupture is most likely. When the aneurysm ruptures, blood floats around the meninges causing irritation; this explains the nuchal rigidity and positive Kernig's sign. The other answers do not correlate with the sign and symptoms in this question.

Question 12

Answer: A

Rationale: Myasthenia gravis is an autoimmune disorder where antibodies cause severe dysfunction in synapse communication—specifically, the neurotransmitter acetylcholine. If severe enough, it may lead to a crisis, respiratory distress, and intubation. The other answers do not reflect an autoimmune disorder of this nature.

Question 13

Answer: C

Rationale: CPP is calculated by subtracting ICP from MAP. In this case, the current CPP is 55 (70 − 15 = 55). With a minimum CPP order of 60, the nurse must work to increase the MAP. Out of the potential answers, the best way to accomplish this is by administering vasopressors to maintain CPP.

Question 14

Answer: B

Rationale: An apnea test should be immediately discontinued when hypotension, cardiac dysrhythmias, and/or a SpO_2 85% or lower occurs. A slight increase in blood pressure can be expected as well as a mild increase in HR. A $PaCO_2$ of 60 mmHg correlates with brain death, not a complication itself.

Question 15

Answer: A

Rationale: Guillain–Barre is most commonly triggered by viral illness such as the flu or cold. Weakness begins peripherally, then works its way up and central. Eventually it may affect the diaphragm, affecting breathing; this eventually requires intubation and ventilation. The patient reports no previous trauma so spinal cord injury is unlikely. The symptoms of SCI are typically not delayed; this patient did not arrive to the ER until one to two weeks after the onset of symptoms. Myasthenia gravis begins in the face and works its way down. ALS is also unlikely as the progression of ALS occurs over months and years, not weeks.

Question 16

Answer: A

Rationale: A simplified triad approach can make learning what happens during status epilepticus: respiratory compromise, catecholamine release, and destruction of muscle tissue. From this pathophysiology signs and symptoms are more easily approached. Catecholamine release causes tachycardia and hypertension. Muscle destruction causes lactic acidosis and hyperkalemia. Respiratory compromise results in an increase in $PaCO_2$.

Question 17

Answer: B

Rationale: Recent surgery is a contraindication to tPA use as it can precipitate bleeding. Age is a factor, but the cut-off is typically 80 years of age. Thrombocytopenia and elevated coagulation panels are contraindications to tPA use; in this case, however, those values are normal.

Question 18

Answer: B

Rationale: In bacterial meningitis, cerebrospinal fluid is cloudy with an elevated protein count and decreased glucose count. In viral meningitis, CSF is clear with an elevated protein count, and normal glucose count.

CHAPTER 11

Behavioral/ Psychosocial

The behavioral/psychosocial section makes up roughly five questions on your CCRN exam, so approximately 4% of the exam is devoted to this topic. While psychiatry as a whole is an incredibly large area of study, the CCRN exam has fairly directed topics of interest—anxiety and depression, suicide and substance abuse. This section also includes how to manage patients receiving medications like antipsychotics and antidepressants. Delirium and dementia were moved to the neurology chapter (Chapter 10) with the new 2020 changes to the blueprint.

Abuse/Neglect

Healthcare professionals often encounter situations where abuse is suspected. It is important to approach sensitive situations with therapeutic communication and compassion as well as how to recognize those patients that may be at risk.

Elder Abuse

Abuse toward the elderly has been a vastly underreported problem. New laws have established mandatory reporting for healthcare professionals among other safeguards. Risk factors for elder abuse include cognitive impairment, functional dependence, frailty, and psychological problems, among many others.

Types of Elder Abuse
- Physical: may include misuse of medications and restraints
- Psychological: may include isolation and threats
- Sexual: may include inability to give consent or pressure into giving consent
- Financial: misappropriation of money, fraud, theft, changes in wills
- Neglect: failure to meet or withholding of care

Signs
- Abrasions, lacerations, bruises, burns
- Spiral fractures

- Pressure ulcers
- Emotionally withdrawn
- Poor medication compliance

Interventions

- Mandatory reporting to adult protective authorities
- *Elder Abuse Suspicion Index* is a tool utilized to screen for potential abuse. It includes a series of questions with the goal of assessing need for assistance, fear of retaliation, and withholding of needs like food.
- Communication to family, social services, and appropriate agencies

Domestic Abuse

A complicated issue in its own right, domestic abuse is more common than people think. Roughly one-third of women will experience abuse, and one-fifth of men. All pregnant women upon admission should be assessed for abuse. The following table outlines the risks, signs and symptoms, and interventions of domestic abuse.

Risks

- Female gender (80%+)
- Homelessness
- History of violence
- Lower education
- Pregnancy
- Alcohol and drug abuse

Signs and Symptoms

- Physical violence
  - Inconsistent story with injuries
  - Head, neck, face (most common)
- Sexual violence
- Psychological
  - Anxiety, depression, withdrawn

Interventions

- Establish a safe environment with privacy
- Assess for life and limb issues
- Assessment, screening, and referrals for abuse (establish voluntary nature → NOT mandatory)
- Evaluate emotional state and treat (therapeutic communication)
- Take into account cultural differences
- Be cognizant of verbal tone and body language when communicating with all patients

Agitation/Aggression/Violence

Most if not all healthcare professionals will witness and manage agitation, aggression, or violent behavior in a patient at some point. Proper communication and management are key to these situations. Many cases of these behaviors are a reflection of a current medical state, such as drug or alcohol intoxication, psychological stress, and head trauma, among many others.

- **Agitation:** restlessness and excessive movement associated with mental distress
- **Aggression:** physical or verbal directed at objects or peoples, including themselves (suicide attempts or ideations)
- **Violence:** extreme aggression with the intent to injure

Interventions

A "least invasive to most" mentality is best utilized when dealing with these behaviors.

- De-escalation methods (therapeutic communication)
  - Ask simple, nonjudgmental *open-ended* questions targeted to the "why" of the behavior
  - Questions regarding potential medical or psychological issues
    - Psychosis → questions about hallucinations or delusions
- Seclusion → restraints → medications
- Body awareness
  - Stand close to an escape/keep distance from the patient
  - Provide care in teams
  - Call security if necessary

> **CCRN Tip**
>
> Restraints are often audited by agencies federal and state. Caution must be utilized to protect patient safety. Death of a patient in restraints is an automatic autopsy.

Medical Management of Aggressive Behavior

When medications are utilized, the primary goal is to correct the behavior, NOT overly sedate. When possible, allow the patient to choose medication and route of administration.

- Mild to moderate agitation → benzodiazepines
- Severe agitation → antipsychotics
  - First-generation: haloperidol
  - Second-generation: olanzapine, risperidone
- If the agitation is due to alcohol withdrawal, fast-acting benzodiazepines like lorazepam are indicated. CIWA protocol is covered later in this chapter.
- If the agitation is due to delirium, assess the cause, often medical. Antipsychotics are first-line for agitation due to delirium.

> **CCRN Tip**
>
> New studies suggest second-generation medications are preferable. The thought being to minimize side effects like *prolonged QT interval*, sedation, and extrapyramidal symptoms (EPS). A prolonged QT may lead to torsades de pointes. Be aware that multiple other medications may prolong the QT, such as certain antibiotics and antiemetics.

Anxiety

Anxiety has a variety of associations, from panic disorders to phobias. It is one of the most common psychiatric problems in the United States. As critical care nurses, anxiety is often witnessed due to fear associated with illness or treatment. As you may see in Figure 11-1, a GABA receptor is affected by both benzodiazepines and alcohol. This may create a compounding effect in pharmacology.

> **CCRN Tip**
>
> In the ICU, anxiety is often confused for pain. Use appropriate pain scales to assess appropriate management. Precedex (dexmedetomidine) is a commonly used medication in critical care and is often preferred over benzodiazepines, sedation, or first-line antipsychotics.

Anxiety

Etiologies

- Panic disorder
- Generalized anxiety disorder
- Specific phobias
- Social anxiety disorder
- Substance-induced anxiety
  - In the ICU, assess for potential triggers caused by care or treatment

Signs and symptoms

- Cognitive
  - Fear of injury or death
  - Poor concentration
- Physical
  - Tachycardia, shortness of breath, chest pain
- Behavioral
  - Restlessness and agitation

Interventions

- Assess for underlying medical causes (metabolic, respiratory, etc.)
- Pharmacotherapy
  - Benzodiazepines (fast acting)
  - SSRIs/SNRIs/TCAs
  - Beta blockers
- Psychotherapy
  - Cognative-behavioral
  - Exposure therapy

Figure 11-1   GABA receptor

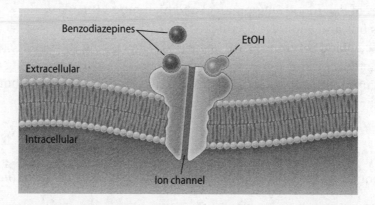

*Note that alcohol and benzodiazepines utilize the same receptor. This results in a compounding effect with polysubstance abuse.

Mood Disorders

There are many subsets of mood disorders, but the main two are major depressive disorder and bipolar disorder. Many cases of depression may go undiagnosed in the ICU, including situational issues the patient may be experiencing due to illness. It often affects recovery and motivation to heal. Due to heavy research on the topic, it is known women are twice as likely to be diagnosed with major depression than men.

Mood disorders are diagnosed and categorized in the *Diagnostic and Statistical Manual of Mental Disorders* (DSM-5). The majority of disorders have a collection of symptoms required to make a formal diagnosis. In addition to the classic types of disorders, consider alcohol and substance abuse factors (use and withdrawal) that may affect mood.

Medical Conditions Linked to Depression
- Cardiovascular disorders (heart attack)
- Cancer
- Metabolic/endocrine dysfunction (thyroid disorders)
- Neurological disorders (dementia)

Signs and Symptoms
- Major depressive disorder (MDD)
  - Low depressed mood
  - Anhedonia (lack of interest in activities)
  - Appetite and weight changes
  - Psychomotor retardation (slowing down of movement and thought)
  - Fatigue or loss of energy
  - Feelings of worthlessness or guilt
  - Diminished ability to concentrate
  - Recurrent thoughts of death/suicide

CCRN Tip

The symptoms of MDD may also be used as criteria for hypomania in bipolar disorder. Diagnosis requires a collection of depressed mood and four other symptoms in the list.

- Bipolar disorder
  - Cycles of low mood (hypomania) and high mood (mania)
  - Delusions and euphoria (mania)
  - **Manic episodes** (grandiosity, decreased sleep, racing thoughts, easily distractible, lack of concern for consequences—reckless spending of money)
  - Bipolar I: manic episodes with or without hypomania and psychotic episodes
  - Bipolar II: hypomania (typically less severe)

Interventions

- Continuously assess suicidal thoughts and ideation (*see suicide, in the following section*)
- Nonpharmacological measures (therapeutic)
  - Types of therapy
    - Behavioral, cognitive, interpersonal, psychotherapy
  - Complementary and alternative therapy (CAM)
    - Acupuncture to yoga
    - Homeopathy to reflexology
  - Provide emotional support and safe environment (engage the patient)
- Pharmacological interventions for depression
  - Selective serotonin reuptake inhibitors (SSRIs)/SNRIs
    - Paroxetine, sertraline, citalopram, etc.
    - **Black Box Warning**—increased energy at onset of use increases the risk for suicide
    - Primary treatment (starting point) for depression treatment
    - Side effects (GI upset, sexual dysfunction, sleep disturbances)
  - Tricyclic antidepressants (amitriptyline)
    - Less commonly used (when other medications do give relief)
    - **Risk for toxicity** and **prolonged QT** (dysrhythmias, hypotension)
    - Anticholinergic side effects (dry mouth, constipation, etc.)
  - Monoamine oxidase inhibitors (MAOIs)
    - Rarely used
    - **Drug interactions common** (perform a medication reconciliation)
- Pharmacological interventions for bipolar disorder
  - Antipsychotics
    - Typical antipsychotics (haloperidol)
    - Atypical antipsychotics (clozapine, risperidone, aripiprazole)
    - Risk for **neuroleptic malignant syndrome (NMS)**: hyperthermia, muscle rigidity, changing hemodynamics
    - Side effects: prolonged QT, extrapyramidal symptoms (tardive dyskinesia)
  - Mood stabilizers
    - Lithium → assess fluid volume status (osmolality) → risk for toxicity
  - Anticonvulsants (valproate, lamictal, carbamazepine)

Medication Nonadherence

Patients with major psychiatric disorders have been known to be at increased risk for noncompliance or nonadherence to medication regimens. It remains a challenging issue for treatment and overall morbidity of the patient. Without adherence to medication, the likelihood of repeat hospitalization increases.

Factors of Nonadherence

- Intentional vs. unintentional
- Failing to fill or refill prescriptions
- Incorrect dosing and timing
- Beliefs and fear of side effects
- *Education and follow-up* remain the best solution for nonadherence
- Provider–client relationship and rapport increases adherence

Suicidal Ideation

Suicide remains an enormous public health problem, being the 11th most leading cause of death in the nation. Assessment of suicidal ideation in patients and management in those identified to be at risk, is crucial for healthcare professionals. Hospital admissions and patients admitted to the ICU due to suicide attempts is in the hundreds of thousands per year. The following factors all influence a person's risk.

- **Protective factors** → family, support, access to healthcare
- **Resilience** → the ability to protect oneself from crisis and stressful situations
- **Coping** → assess positive versus negative coping mechanisms

Be careful with semantics. There is a difference between suicidal *thoughts* and suicidal *ideation*.

Etiologies/Risk Factors

- Demographic and socioeconomic factors
  - Age → larger risk in *older age*
  - Gender → *men* are more successful at suicide
  - Social status (low income, low education, unemployment)
  - Social change (life changes that may be detrimental → loss of job, homelessness)
- Major depression and other mental health disorders (10 times higher than general public)
- Family history of suicide and abuse
- Risk-taking behaviors
  - Alcohol and substance abuse
  - Delinquent or criminal behavior
  - Violent and nonviolent behavior

Interventions

- Assessment of suicide attempts
  - Intent, injury, lethality
  - These three key areas may offer insight into potential risk for future attempts and reasons for the current attempt

> **CCRN Tip**
>
> While men are more likely to be successful at suicide, women are far more likely to report feelings of suicidal intent and attempt suicide.

- Primary prevention
  - Universal suicide risk screening (every patient, every admission)
    - "Have you had thoughts of hurting yourself?"
    - "Do you have a plan?"
    - Follow-up for patients reporting positive symptoms
  - Blocking of access for means (firearms, pills, etc.)
  - Community resources (online and telephone support, clergy, social services)
  - Strengthen and establish connections, support systems, and new coping abilities
- Secondary prevention
  - Patients who attempt suicide often seek help in a hospital
  - Intervene on immediate medical needs and **safety planning**
    - One-to-one supervision (sitters)
    - Remove plastic bags, sharp objects, rope-like items, etc.
    - Frequent assessment and documentation

> **CCRN Tip**
>
> Remember that gastric lavage (pumping the stomach) is only effective if the contents ingested are still in the stomach. General consideration to perform gastric lavage is if the material was ingested less than **1 hour prior.**

Post-Traumatic Stress Disorder (PTSD)

Etiologies

- Experienced or witnessed a traumatic event
- Repeated exposure to distressing images (deceased bodies, child abuse)

Signs and Symptoms

- Intrusion symptoms
  - Psychological and physiological reactions to triggers
  - Distressing memories and dreams
  - Dissociative reaction (episode of reliving the memory)
- Avoidance of people, activities, places, and reminders of the trauma
- Negative alterations in cognitions and mood
  - Negative feelings of self (esteem)
  - Negative emotions (anger, fear, anxiety)
  - Negative interest (anhedonia, loss of friends)
- Alterations in arousal and reactivity
  - Angry outbursts
  - Exaggerated startle (hypervigilance/hyperarousal)

Interventions

- Immediate psychological help after the incident or trauma
- Assess for comorbid psychological and substance abuse conditions
- Trauma-focused psychological therapies
  - Cognitive-behavioral therapy
  - Exposure therapy
- Pharmacological therapies are similar to depression although not the primary focus in PTSD treatment. Psychological therapies are mainstay.

Substance Dependence or Abuse

Critical care nurses manage patients that may be admitted due to the direct effects of a substance, many times in addition to other conditions. On the other hand, many patients experience symptoms of withdrawal separate from the admitted medical diagnosis. Obtaining a thorough substance history at the beginning of admission, including toxicology, is extremely helpful in minimizing complications during the ICU stay.

A simple approach is to utilize the separation of an acute overdose versus a potential withdrawal. The symptoms are often opposite each other for a given substance.

Potential Substances of Misuse

- **Stimulants**
  - Cocaine
  - Amphetamines (meth, dextroamphetamine, methylphenidate)
  - Nicotine
- **Depressants**
  - Alcohol (most common)
  - Benzodiazepines
  - Barbiturates
  - Opioids (heroin, methadone, buprenorphine)
- **Other**
  - Cannabinoids
  - Hallucinogens

> **CCRN Tip**
>
> One thing of note; do not confuse *overmedicated* for *overdosed*. There are situations where a reversal agent may be used for patients who overdosed on certain substances. An overmedicated patient is commonly given time for the body to naturally process the substances; a good example is sedative substances.

Severe prolonged (chronic) misuse of these substances define **substance abuse disorder**, commonly referred to as addiction. Below are some common terminologies not to be confused with one another.

- **Overdose:** an accidental or intentional poisoning by drugs, medications, or substances
- **Withdrawal:** physical or psychological adverse effects to discontinuing a substance
- **Dependence:** physiological need of a substance or withdrawal will occur
- **Tolerance:** increased need (dosage) of a substance to achieve the same desired effect

Drug-Seeking Behavior

Any behavior with the goal of obtaining drugs and/or substances could define "drug-seeking behavior." Most commonly, the drugs sought after are opioids or benzodiazepines. The following is a list of some common findings among patients who exhibit drug-seeking behavior.

- Requests and complaints
  - Asking for a specific drug or brand by name
  - "Alleged" multiple allergies to different drugs
  - Annoyed when questioned about medication or drug use

- Incorrect use of prescribed medications
- Incorrect use of healthcare services
  - Visiting multiple practitioners (doctor shopping)
- Resistant behavior
  - Does not consider non-addictive alternatives
- Manipulative behavior

Overdose and Withdrawal Comparisons

Before analyzing overdose versus withdrawal symptoms, it may be helpful to learn whether a substance is a *stimulant* or a *depressant*. This often reflects the overall signs and symptoms. Tables 11-1 through 11-3 show common substance abuse seen in the ICU and on the CCRN exam—alcohol, benzodiazepines, and opioids, all three of which are depressants. The priority for all three of these overdoses is airway control and management. Remember trauma ABCDE!

Table 11-1   Alcohol Overdose and Withdrawal

Overdose	Multiple organ systems affected: cardiac, pulmonary, gastrointestinal, neurological.
Withdrawal	CIWA protocol → diaphoresis, sensory disturbances, anxiety, orientation, etc.
	RASS scoring → if intubated, 0 to –2 is sedative goal
	Delirium tremens (DTs)
	• Onset 48–96 hours since last drink
	• Seizure activity may result in death
	Hallucinosis → may occur during or after heavy alcohol use (do not confuse with DTs)
	• Immediate safety priority (hallucinations may be "command")
	Treatment
	• Oral sedatives if possible (lorazepam, chlordiazepoxide/Librium)
	• IV titration of benzos if the patient is intubated or without NG/OG tube
	• Concurrent administration of benzo and phenobarbital
	• IV hydration (saline solutions or "banana bag")
	• Multivitamins, thiamine (B1), nutrition, folate (B9), electrolytes
	• Prevent complications (thiamine for Wernicke's encephalopathy and Korsakoff syndrome)
	• Nutrition (glucose) to prevent hypoglycemia
	• Seizure precautions for DTs

Brief Alcohol Symptomology Review

- Wernicke's encephalopathy → encephalopathy (disorientation), ocular motor dysfunction (nystagmus), ataxia (gait)
- Korsakoff syndrome → memory loss (antero and retro), confabulation, psychosis

Table 11-2   Benzodiazepine Overdose and Withdrawal

Overdose	Similar to alcohol overdose • Dyspnea/hypoxia • Level of consciousness changes (stupor, coma) • Mental status changes (disorientation) Reversal agent → flumazenil
Withdrawal	Symptoms may begin 1–3 days after last dose; symptoms peak around 2 weeks Signs and symptoms are similar to alcohol withdrawal • Tremors or seizure activity • Anxiety and agitation • Changes in cognitive thinking (hallucinations, psychosis) **Treatment** • Administration of previous used benzodiazepine (titrate down slowly) • Assess and manage cardiac, pulmonary, organ complications

Table 11-3   Opioid Overdose and Withdrawal

Overdose	Signs and symptoms include: • Respiratory depression and dyspnea • Pinpoint pupils (miosis) • Hypotension and loss of consciousness Naloxone is a competitive antagonist for the opioid receptor • Multiple administration routes available (oral, intranasal, IV) • Repeated doses may be required
Withdrawal	Signs and symptoms include drug cravings, muscle pain and spasms, N/V/D, chills, dilated pupils (mydriasis) **Treatment** As with many substance withdrawals, prevention is the best course of action Methadone, buprenorphine, or long-acting replacements to opioids are administered then slowly titrated down over time

CCRN Tip

Administration of naloxone may result in a rapid withdrawal syndrome. The patient may experience aggression, diaphoresis, and tachycardia. Dosing of naloxone begins at the smallest rational dose then titrates up for this reason.

Review Questions

1. A patient in the ICU was admitted due to chronic alcohol abuse, liver failure, and severe aggression with changes in mental status. Twelve hours after , the patient begins screaming hysterically; the nurse suspects alcoholic hallucinosis. Which of the following statements reflects the best form of communication to use with the patient at this time?

   A. "Would you like some lorazepam for your anxiety?"

   B. "What you are experiencing is related to your heavy alcohol use"

   C. "Explain to me what you are hearing and seeing"

   D. "Please do not scream, it is not helping"

2. A patient with unstable atrial fibrillation is admitted to the ICU. Repeated PRN doses of haloperidol have been needed for severe aggression. New-onset bradycardia, 45 BPM, and rhythm irregularity is noted on the monitor. Which of the following actions is appropriate by the nurse at this time?

   A. Obtain an ECG and assess for prolonged QT

   B. Obtain a crash cart and anticipate transcutaneous pacing

   C. Obtain a serum potassium level and administer magnesium sulfate

   D. Hold all beta blockers and contact the physician anticipating amiodarone

3. A 82-year-old male patient is admitted from a nursing home. He is diagnosed with a urinary tract infection and has been experiencing delirium with combativeness. The patient is complaining of pain in the right arm and is sent for x-rays. Assessment reveals a spiral fracture of the humerus. Partial bruising is also present on the affected arm and wrist regions. Which of the following actions is most appropriate by the nurse at this time?

   A. Request medical records from the nursing home

   B. Report concerns to adult protective services

   C. Contact the physician to perform a thorough assessment

   D. Question the patient about the injuries

4. A 36-year-old patient was admitted to the ICU 3 days ago due to respiratory distress secondary to severe respiratory viral illness. The patient has improved and the healthcare team is moving to extubate the patient; however, the patient is incredibly anxious and difficult to communicate to. Which of the following pharmacological considerations would be appropriate at this time?

   A. Dexmedetomidine IV infusion

   B. PRN IV lorazepam for agitation

   C. Fentanyl IV infusion with PRN IV midazolam

   D. PRN IV haloperidol

5. A 23-year-old female patient is reporting a depressed mood upon admission. The nurse understands which of the following additional signs and symptoms are NOT associated with major depressive disorder (MDD)?

    A. 5-lbs weight gain in the past month
    B. Increased sensitivity to noise and light
    C. Difficulty focusing at work
    D. Family reports slowed movements when performing tasks

6. Studies have shown that psychiatric patients have a higher degree of medication nonadherence than medical counterparts. A bipolar patient on lithium and risperidone is nearing discharge from the unit. Which of the following interventions would best encourage the patient to adhere to the medication?

    A. Assess for family support that may help with reminders
    B. Discuss the medication and follow-up phone calls
    C. Call the pharmacy to notify about the patient's lack of adherence
    D. Suggest the physician writes an order for longer-acting medications

7. A 55-year-old patient was recently admitted to the ICU due to an overdose of aspirin; suicide intent is suspected. The spouse reports a recent job loss and heavy drinking. The patient is currently sedated due to combative behavior in the emergency room. The spouse is sitting bedside. Which of the following should be implemented to the plan of care at this time?

    A. Perform an immediate gastric lavage with an Ewald tube and consider activated charcoal
    B. Provide privacy for the spouse and the patient
    C. Inform the spouse that involuntary admission to a psychiatric unit is likely after medically cleared
    D. Obtain an order for one-to-one supervision and remove sharp objects from the room

8. A patient with heavy alcohol abuse was intubated in the emergency room from a lack of airway protection. The physician begins a regimen of treatments— fluids and vitamins. The following day, once clinically sober, the patient is extubated. Upon arousal the patient is unable to form new memories. Which of the following best explains the reasoning for the current patient condition?

    A. Vitamin B1 (thiamine) deficiency leading to Wernicke's encephalopathy
    B. Vitamin B9 (folate) deficiency leading to buildup of metabolic toxins
    C. Vitamin B1 (thiamine) deficiency leading to Korsakoff syndrome
    D. Vitamin B3 (niacin) deficiency leading to increased ICP

9. A 46-year-old female patient is in the emergency room waiting for a bed in the hospital. She is being held due to changes in mental status and gross tremors. She reports daily diazepam use for severe anxiety but has not taken her medicine in over 24 hours due to feeling nauseated. What is the best preventive measure to avoid benzodiazepine withdrawal?

A. Administer alternate sedatives such as buspirone

B. Administer low-dose benzodiazepines

C. Administer flumazenil immediately

D. Administer IV fluids with vitamins

10. A patient with chronic alcohol abuse is admitted for close monitoring of likely withdrawal. The patient has frequent admissions for withdrawal in the past. All of the following are symptoms of withdrawal under CIWA protocol, EXCEPT?

A. Anxiety or agitation

B. Paroxysmal sweating

C. Tremors and shaking

D. Lethargy or stupor

Answer Key

Question 1

Answer: C

Rationale: The immediate risk is patient safety. If the hallucinations are "command" in nature, the patient may want to harm themselves or others. Nursing priority is to assess this risk and react accordingly. While lorazepam may be helpful in a situation of acute anxiety or agitation, the question is not pointing to anxiety, but rather hallucinations. It is not appropriate at this time and would likely be unhelpful. Stating the hallucinations are due to the patient's alcohol intake is not helpful at this time and could be construed as judgmental. Furthermore, a patient in acute psychiatric crisis is unable to understand or rationalize current situations. The same rule applies to answer "D" here; the patient would be unable to understand why you might be asking them to cease screaming. To them the hallucinations are real.

Question 2

Answer: A

Rationale: Haloperidol along with other antipsychotics may cause a prolonged QT on the ECG. The immediate risk is impending code blue, most commonly torsades de pointes. Medications causing this prolonged QT need to be immediately stopped. All of the other answers suggested are plausible interventions for a situation like this; however, they all assume the problem. Prolonged QT needs to be identified, not assumed, and then follow-up actions may be taken. If the patient deteriorates further and the blood pressure becomes seriously low, transcutaneous pacing may be in order. Hypokalemia and other electrolyte imbalances may be assessed and corrected after the immediate QT risk is assessed. Holding beta blockers would be appropriate; amiodarone may worsen the bradycardia and should be avoided.

Question 3

Answer: B

Rationale: The nurse is a mandatory reporter of elder abuse, same as child abuse. The nurse does not need to speak with anyone to perform this action, although at times it moves through social workers first. Requesting medical records or contacting the physician is not appropriate at this time. Questioning a dementia patient would likely be unhelpful.

Question 4

Answer: A

Rationale: Given the goal of extubation, medications that induce moderate sedation are avoided; this would include propofol, midazolam, and fentanyl. Dexmedetomidine is often used as a bridge for patients such as this who experience continued anxiety or agitation. One side effect to be cautious of is bradycardia. Haloperidol is also likely to sedate the patient too much to effectively extubate.

Question 5

Answer: B

Rationale: Increased sensitivity to noise and light is more aligned with PTSD or "hypervigilance." This is not a common symptom of depression or part of how major depressive disorder (MDD) is diagnosed in the DSM. Weight gain, difficulty concentrating, and psychomotor retardation are all symptoms of MDD.

Question 6

Answer: B

Rationale: Research shows that education and follow-up are the best mitigating factors to reduce medication nonadherence. This may include the purpose of the medication, common side effects, and scheduled calls with providers regarding progress. Family support is helpful in a number of circumstances, but it cannot be relied on for consistent follow-through. Contacting the pharmacy in regard to nonadherence is likely a breach of HIPAA and would not be helpful since the point of contact only occurs during refills. Long-acting medications are occasionally used as a next step for repeated difficulty in adherence to medications. This may include an IM injection of the medication monthly.

Question 7

Answer: D

Rationale: With safety being the priority concern, suicide precautions should be immediately implemented. One-to-one supervision, removing potentially harmful objects from the room, and frequent assessment are included in the plan of care. Gastric lavage is only useful within a short window of time, typically less than 1 hour. This patient is almost certainly outside of this window. Privacy is not allowed for a suicidal patient given the risk. While an involuntary admission is possible for this patient, this notification is not a priority need right now.

Question 8

Answer: C

Rationale: Antero and retrograde amnesia are symptoms of Korsakoff syndrome. It is caused by thiamine deficiency due to alcohol use. Wernicke's encephalopathy includes symptoms such as gait disturbances and nystagmus. Neither Korsakoff syndrome nor Wernicke's encephalopathy is caused by a folate or niacin deficiency.

Question 9

Answer: B

Rationale: While it may appear counterintuitive to administer benzodiazepines to a person addicted to benzodiazepines, the body is dependent on these medications. Treatment is to administer the benzodiazepine and taper off slowly. Buspar (buspirone) is utilized for anxiety, but it is not a benzodiazepine and would not assist in withdrawal. The medication also can take weeks to show benefit. The reversal drug flumazenil would be appropriate for acute overdose, not withdrawal.

IV fluids and vitamins may certainly be appropriate for this patient, but it would not help with withdrawal symptoms.

Question 10

Answer: D

Rationale: The vast majority of the symptoms of alcohol withdrawal mirror excitement or stimulation, not sedation or depression. Alcohol itself is a depressant, causing symptoms such as lethargy and stupor. Remember that many substances have opposite overdose and withdrawal symptoms. The other symptoms listed are part of CIWA assessment.

CHAPTER 12

Multisystem

The multisystem section makes up roughly 17 questions on your CCRN exam, so approximately 14% of the exam is devoted to this topic. This is an increase from 8% on the previous CCRN exam prior to the March 2020 changes. Multisystem includes a wide variety of topics on the exam blueprint. Certain components are included in alternate chapters in this book. When this occurs, it is noted so you may jump to the section for study. A good example is acid–base imbalances. ABG analysis is crucial in respiratory questions (Chapter 3), but it is also included in multisystem. These doubled-up topics are at the end of this chapter.

Multisystem Trauma

Injuries sustained by trauma that affect multiple systems are often catastrophic and severe in nature. The amount of kinetic energy needed to sustain multisystem damage is typically aggressive, such as in motor vehicle accidents, gunshot wounds, and falls from high altitudes. Two additional potential traumas: drowning and burns.

Triage

Triaging is typically performed in the field or in the emergency room, especially when resources are limited. P1 though P3 is a fairly standard method of triage. Another commonly used tool is the "Emergency Severity Index (ESI)." ESI ranks triage based on the anticipated medical resources required.

- **Priority 1 (P1):** red → immediate life-saving care needed
- **Priority 2 (P2):** orange → urgent care needed within hours
- **Priority 3 (P3):** green → treatment may be safely delayed ("walking wounded")
- **Deceased:** black → no priority, patients beyond saving (severe head injury, significant loss of blood, cervical spine break)

Primary Survey (ABCDE)

- Airway → voice and breath sounds (stridor) → head tilt, chin lift → possible intubation

- Breathing → RR, pulse ox, auscultation → 100% oxygen, bag max ventilation
- Circulation → HR, BP, ECG, skin color → IV access with NS/LR infusion, elevate legs
- Disability → LOC, PERRLA, neuro → assess for hypoglycemia, recovery position
- Expose/environmental → inspect skin, temperature → manage temperature (heat, cool)

Hypotension/Shock

Circulatory failure and hypotension lead to shock. Left untreated, shock leads to cellular death and eventual organ dysfunction. On a cellular level, shock is defined by increased oxygen demand or dysfunctional oxygen use, most commonly caused by poor perfusion and oxygen delivery.

Three Phases of Shock

- Compensatory → stimulation of **sympathetic** response (ACTH release → "fight or flight") and **RAAS**
- Progressive → hypotension as compensation fails
- Refractory → systemic failure and MODS

Distributive Shock

Table 12-1 details the types of distributive shock.

CCRN Tip
Types of Allergic Reactions
• Type I: Anaphylactic → immediate IgE hypersensitivity
• Type II: Cytotoxic → antibody-dependent
• Type III: Immune complex → antigen buildup
• Type IV: Cell-mediated → delayed
Immunoglobulin E (IgE) are antibodies of the immune system that react to certain allergens causing a release of chemicals on the cellular level.

Table 12-1   Types of Distributive Shock

ANAPHYLAXIS	NEUROGENIC/VASOGENIC
Etiology/pathophysiology	**Etiology/pathophysiology**
• Fast (less than 20 minutes) and severe allergic reaction	• Complication of spinal cord injury
• Release of histamine	• Cervical or high thoracic
• Classic signs and symptoms	• Sudden loss of sympathetic/vagal tone
• Urticaria (more delayed than other symptoms)	• Autonomic dysfunction
• Angioedema	• Hypotension
• Hypotension via cardiovascular collapse and vasodilation	• Bradycardia
• Respiratory distress via bronchospasm	• Temperature dysregulation (flushed warm skin)
Interventions	**Bradycardia** typically occurs in neurogenic shock, whereas hypovolemic shock typically has tachycardia
• Removal of offending agent	**Interventions**
• Prepare for impending airway obstruction → intubation/O_2	• First line → IV fluids ("fill up the tank")
• Stridor, tongue swelling, hoarseness	• Second-line → vasopressors and inotropes
• **Epinephrine IM** 0.3–0.5 mg (1:1000) every 5 to 10 minutes	• High MAP goals to aid in spinal perfusion (>80 mmHg)
• Intravenous reserved for cardiovascular collapse or cardiac arrest	• Treatment of bradycardia → atropine
• Aggressive fluid resuscitation with normal saline, multiple liters may be necessary	• Surgery may be required to decompress the spine
• Histamine blockers and steroids	**Do not** confuse with *spinal shock,* a reversible condition not related to blood pressure
• Secondary to prevent worsening down the line	
• Monitor for rebound/biphasic anaphylaxis	

Hypovolemic and Hemorrhagic Shock

For both hemorrhagic and nonhemorrhagic shock, a decrease in intravascular volume and an increase in systemic vascular resistance occurs. Eventually if blood loss is great enough, cardiac output cannot compensate and decreases; hypotension ensues. Table 12-2 compares hypovolemic versus hemorrhagic shock.

Early Signs and Symptoms (minimal loss)

- Increased sympathetic response
  - Increased peripheral vasoconstriction → SVR
  - Increased HR → output
  - Increased cardiac contractility → output
- Increased diastolic BP and narrowed pulse pressure

Late Signs and Symptoms (severe loss)

- Decreased systolic blood pressure
- Increasing lactic acidosis
- Shunting of blood to vital organs → hemodynamic collapse → MODS → death

Table 12-2   Hypovolemic and Hemorrhagic Shock

HYPOVOLEMIC	HEMORRHAGIC

Etiology/pathophysiology
• Third space loss (trauma, cirrhosis)
• Insensible losses/skin (burns, pyrexia)
• Renal losses (diuretic use, endocrine disorders)
• Gastrointestinal losses (vomiting, diarrhea, NG suction)
Interventions
• Assess and treat the underlying cause
• Obtain large-bore IVs or central line
  • Note: most central lines are not large bore, a large peripheral may be preferred
• Trendelenburg position → increase preload
• IV fluid resuscitation (2–4 liters isotonic crystalloids)
  • Rapid bolus
• Passive leg raise tests may help with determining preload (fluid) responsiveness
• DO NOT use vasopressors; worsens SVR
• Monitor electrolytes and acid–base balance
	Etiology/pathophysiology
	• Internal or external
	• Trauma
	  • Penetrating or blunt
	• GI bleeding
	• Vascular bleeding (aneurysm rupture, dissection)
	• Spontaneous bleeding (anticoagulant use)
	• The average 70 kg male has 5 liters of circulating blood
	Interventions
	• Localize and control the bleeding
	• Damage control resuscitation
	  • Avoid death triad
	    • Coagulopathy
	    • Acidosis
	    • Hypothermia
	• Blood transfusion
	  • PRBCs, platelets, cryo
	• Consider and monitor blood transfusion reactions (see Chapter 8)
	• Consideration of antifibrinolytics (aminocaproic acid)
	• Monitor electrolytes and CBC

Goals • MAP >65 mmHg • Urine output >0.5 mL/kg/hr • Normalization of heart rate • CVP is no longer used as an end-goal; use more as an assistive number • Maintain HgB greater than 7.0 g/dL	

American College of Surgeons Advanced Trauma Life Support (ATLS) Hemorrhagic Shock Classification

While this classification system is not hugely important for the CCRN, understand the general flow or worsening condition. Where does a patient start and where might they likely end up? Tachycardia is the first sign of blood loss as the body attempts to compensate.

- **Class I:** Up to 15% blood loss (750 mL or less)
  - Normal blood pressure
  - HR and RR normal to slightly elevated
- **Class II:** 15–30% blood loss (750–1500 mL)
  - Normal or slightly decreased blood pressure
  - HR and RR increasing

- **Class III:** 30–40% blood loss (1500–2000 mL)
    - Significant drop in blood pressure
    - HR and RR increased
- **Class IV:** More than 40% blood loss (2000 mL or greater)
    - Severe hypotension with narrowed pulse pressure
    - Tachycardia >120 BPM
    - Urine output minimal or absent
    - Mental status altered

Types of Fluid Resuscitation

The type of crystalloid used in states of hypovolemic shock may be tailored to individual patients. This determination is made by evaluating patient chemistries, acid–base status, and the amount of volume likely required. Isotonic salines are hyperchloremic; large infusion amounts may lead to a **hyperchloremic acidosis**.

LR and PlasmaLyte are buffered or balanced crystalloids and may be preferred to avoid hyperchloremic acidosis. Assess chemistry panels; a hypernatremic patient should not receive normal saline or a hypertonic solution. LR contains potassium and should be avoided in hyperkalemic patients.

Alternate Types of Shock

Three other types of shock covered elsewhere in the book. The first, **obstructive shock**, is covered in Chapter 2 (cardiovascular) and Chapter 3 (respiratory). This includes tension pneumothorax, pulmonary embolism, and cardiac tamponade. Extracardiac issues lead to a severe decrease in left ventricular cardiac output. The second, **endocrine shock**, covered in Chapter 4 (endrocrine), includes Addisonian crisis and myxedema coma. The third, **cardiogenic shock,** is covered in Chapter 2 as well.

Sepsis Continuum

The overall picture of sepsis and the sepsis continuum (see Table 12-3) displays one of the most common conditions in critical care, accounting for the most deaths and the largest expenditure. Due to increasing research in recent years, overall mortality has improved. Many hospitals now manage sepsis using strict protocol and bundles. Commonalities between bundles are described in more detail in the following sections. This area is relatively common on the CCRN exam; have a high understanding.

Pathophysiology of Sepsis Continuum

- Activation of inflammatory mediators (histamine)
- Risk factors include infectious, neoplastic, and immunosuppressive processes

Table 12-3   The Sepsis Continuum

Systemic Inflammatory Response Syndrome (SIRS)	Sepsis
• Hyperthermia >38°C or Hypothermia <36°C • Tachycardia >90 BPM • Tachypnea >20 RR • Leukocytosis >12,000 or Leukopenia <4000 (with or without bands >10% shift) *Two of the four* above criteria required for a SIRS diagnosis	• After SIRS criteria, identification of an infectious source defines sepsis • Positive culture (not necessarily blood) • May include suspected infections (positive cultures, acute abdomen, infected wounds, etc.)
Severe Sepsis	**Septic Shock**
• Sepsis with organ dysfunction (see MODS section, later in the chapter) • Most common signs → hypotension → tissue hypoxia • Aerobic respiration → anaerobic respiration → lactic acidosis	• Sepsis-induced hypotension **refractory** to fluid resuscitation • Vasopressors required to maintain MAP >65 mmHg • Low cellular VO_2 (oxygen consumption) → ominous sign • Do not confuse with SvO_2, which would be elevated

CCRN Tip

VO_2 describes the uptake of oxygen by cells. DO_2 (oxygen delivery) is often adequate in septic shock. During anaerobic respiration, this number decreases as the cells are no longer using oxygen for ATP production. Both VO_2 and DO_2 are covered on the CCRN exam.

Septic Shock
- Early signs and symptoms (**warm** shock)
  - Dynamic precordium → tachycardia and bounding pulses
    - Flash capillary refill
  - Warm extremities and skin
  - Blood pressure normal → compensated
  - Hyperthermia
- Late signs and symptoms (**cold** shock)
  - Shock progresses → catecholamine release increases
  - Increased peripheral vascular resistance → shunting of blood
    - Cool extremities
  - Blood pressure low
    - Weak and thready pulse
  - Hypothermia
  - Movement into MODS

Treatment and Management of Sepsis and Septic Shock

The treatment guidelines outlined in Table 12-4 follow the *Surviving Sepsis 2016 Guidelines* with changes from the 2018 update. The 2018 update changes the 3- and 6-hour bundle into a **1-hour bundle**.

Table 12-4   Sepsis Guidelines and Bundles

HOUR-1 BUNDLE (RESUSCITATION BUNDLE)	HOUR-24 BUNDLE (MANAGEMENT BUNDLE)

• Measure lactate level
• Obtain blood cultures prior to administration of antibiotics
• Administer broad-spectrum antibiotics (before vancomycin)
• Immediate administration of 30 mL/kg crystalloids
• Initiate vasopressors for refractory hypotension
  • 1st → norepinephrine
  • 2nd → epinephrine and/or vasopressin
  • 3rd → inotropes
Goals
• MAP >65 mmHg and an increase in urine output to 0.5 mL/kg/hr
• CVP >8 mmHg
• Central venous oxygen saturation (ScvO$_2$) >70% or SvO$_2$ >65%
• Adequate resuscitation should result in the **heart rate** returning to normal
	• Administration of low-dose steroids (may be contraindicated)
	• Administration of recombinant human activated protein C (rhAPC)
	• Maintain glucose control: <180 mg/dL
	• Maintain medium inspiratory plateau pressure (IPP) <30 cm H$_2$O for intubated patients

CCRN Tip

Time zero is defined as the first annotation in the chart for sepsis. This may occur in the emergency room or in other care areas such as the floor or ICU.

Multi-Organ Dysfunction Syndrome (MODS)

MODS is a very common cause of mortality in critical care. The spectrum of the syndrome is complex and involves dysfunction of two or more organs. MODS typically begins as infection and **sepsis**; however, shock of any type may lead to this widespread organ dysfunction when homeostasis cannot be maintained without intervention. Changing degrees of severity means that while at some stages an organ may recover, if advanced enough, the organ may not be salvageable.

- **Primary MODS:** organ dysfunction due to a direct and identifiable insult
- **Secondary MODS:** dysfunction due to host response, typically the sepsis continuum

Types of Organ Dysfunction

One hallmark of MODS is an inability for organs to maximize oxygen use. Due to mitochondrial dysfunction, even with adequate perfusion and oxygen supplementation, the dysfunction on a molecular level often causes hypoxia of the organs. This may be seen diagnostically by an increased lactate level.

Cardiovascular Dysfunction
- **Clinical manifestations**
  - Vasodilation with increased permeability → third spacing → **hypotension** and **tachycardia**
  - Reduced secretion of vasopressin → increased vasodilation → **reduced SVR**
  - Myocardial ischemia → elevated troponin
  - Changes in electrophysiological function → dysrhythmias
  - Increased cardiac output until compensation fails and collapse
- **Interventions**
  - Fluid administration (isotonic)
  - Vasopressors
  - Myocardial support and blood thinners
  - Monitor electrolytes (potassium and magnesium)
  - Inotropes if cardiac output collapses

Pulmonary Dysfunction
- **Clinical manifestations**
  - Endothelial/alveolar injury → acute lung injury and ARDS
    - Dyspnea/tachypnea
    - Hypoxemia → $PaO_2/FiO_2 < 300$
    - Hypercapnia
  - Alveolar edema/pulmonary edema
- **Interventions**
  - Assisted ventilation (NIV → intubation)
  - Increased PEEP often required
  - Oxygen supplementation
  - Optimized fluid resuscitation (do not overload)

Gastrointestinal and Hepatic Dysfunction
- **Clinical manifestations**
- Paralytic ileus → intolerance to enteral feedings
- Stress ulcer formation
- Liver dysfunction
  - Elevated liver enzymes
  - Elevated bilirubin with jaundice
  - Elevated coagulation markers
  - Elevated ammonia
  - Decreased albumin
  - Hypoglycemia
- **Interventions**
  - Avoid narcotics and causes of paralytic ileus
  - Administration of PPI
  - Avoid hepatotoxic agents
  - Monitor for bleeding

Renal Dysfunction
- **Clinical manifestations**
- Acute kidney injury
  - Elevated creatinine/BUN (azotemia)
  - Decreased GFR → decreased urine output
- Elevated potassium
- **Interventions**
  - Correct prerenal hypoperfusion
  - Avoid nephrotoxic agents
  - Dialysis
    - HD
    - CRRT

Neurologic Dysfunction
- **Clinical manifestations**
  - Encephalopathy → contusion, delirium
    - Lethargy → coma
  - Peripheral neuropathy → motor and sensory deficit
  - Highest mortality
- **Interventions**
  - Treatment of underlying causes (hypoperfusion, hyperammonemia)
  - Symptom management
  - Seizures, delirium

Hematologic Dysfunction
- **Clinical manifestations**
  - Thrombocytopenia (less than 100,000)
  - Elevated coagulation markers
  - DIC → elevated d-dimer/decreased fibrinogen
  - Activated protein C → decreased serum level
- **Interventions**
  - Monitor bleeding and lab values
  - Blood products may be necessary in certain circumstances (DIC, severe thrombocytopenia)
  - Hemoglobin <7 g/dL → standard trigger for transfusion

Endocrine and Metabolic Dysfunction
- **Clinical manifestations**
  - Decreased serum cortisol → adrenal/corticosteroid insufficiency
  - Glucose intolerance/insulin resistance → hyperglycemia
  - Metabolic acidosis
  - Thyroid abnormalities (less common)
- **Interventions**
  - Steroid administration is not often utilized unless fluids and vasopressors do not maintain blood pressure
  - Correct hyperglycemia to moderate goals → 140–180 mg/dL

End-of-Life

The spectrum of end-of-life and/or terminal disease is fairly large and without any one singular method of approach. The important consideration is palliative care, or initiating the conversation of palliative care, which can be made before a prognosis is determined. The healthcare team and the patient do not need to wait. Table 12-5 notes some consideration regarding palliative care and hospice care.

- **Advance directives:** written desires about medical treatment when unable to advocate for oneself; often includes a living will and a durable power of attorney for healthcare
- **Do not resuscitate order (DNR):** may include some or all life-saving interventions (CPR, intubation, medications)

Table 12-5   Palliative vs. Hospice Care

PALLIATIVE CARE	HOSPICE CARE (END-OF-LIFE)

• Therapeutic interventions
  • Pain and symptom management
  • Physical, psychological, spiritual
• May be administered at the same time as curative therapy
• Appropriate for any patient with serious illness or chronic illness
	• Expected 6 months or less/terminal phase of life
	• Includes palliative care
	• May be provided at home, hospital, or skilled nursing facility
	• Includes bereavement services for family
	• Consider cultural issues

Common Symptoms with Interventions in End-of-Life

- Physical pain → opioids
- Dyspnea → benzodiazepines and low flow nasal cannula
- Nausea, vomiting, anorexia → antiemetics, slow decrease in food intake is expected
- Dry mouth → mouth swabs, IV hydration is curative not palliative
- Terminal delirium (restlessness, anxiety) → haloperidol
- Death rattle → repositioning and anticholinergics (reduce secretions)

Healthcare-Associated Infections (HAIs)

HAIs are an enormous burden on the healthcare system and patients. Many governmental agencies now monitor HAIs and form prevention protocols in the attempt to minimize morbidity and mortality. HAIs share several universal risk factors:

- Elderly
- Immunocompromised
- Chronic illnesses
- Long hospital stays

Be sure to understand the bundles and protocols in Tables 12-6 to 12-8 for three HAIs—central line–associated bloodstream infection (CLABSI), catheter-associated urinary tract infection (CAUTI), and ventilator-associated pneumonia (VAP)—as well as the infectious diseases listed in Table 12-9. **Prevention is the key.**

Table 12-6   Central Line–Associated Bloodstream Infection (CLABSI)

RISK FACTORS	PREVENTION PROTOCOLS

• Rapidly placed central lines (code blue)
  • Especially femoral site or internal jugular
• Questionable sterility during placement procedure
• Parenteral therapy and lipids (includes propofol)
• Multiple lumens on CVC
	• Hand hygiene
	• Chlorhexidine and skin preparation
	• Sterile dressing (transparent) changes
	  • Every 5–7 days
	  • Replace if soiled
	• Remove catheters when no longer needed (nurse driven)
	• Change IV tubing q 4–7 days
	  • Propofol q 6–12 hours
	• Scrub access ports or use disinfection caps
	• Prevent cross-contamination from other areas of the body

Table 12-7   Catheter-Associated Urinary Tract Infection (CAUTI)

RISK FACTORS	PREVENTION PROTOCOLS

• Prolonged placement (>2 days)
• Female gender
• Elevated degree of illness
• Overly accessed catheter ports
  • Irrigation
• Improper or lacking catheter care
• Fecal incontinence
• Immobility and bladder dysfunction
  • Paraplegia
  • Cerebrovascular accidents
	• Hand hygiene
	• Avoid unnecessary catheterization
	• Decrease catheterization days
	  • Nurse driven, protocol driven
	• Cautious aseptic insertion
	• Frequent catheter care
	• Urinary retention protocol (reduce reinsertions)
	• Continued education on prevention

Table 12-8   Ventilator-Associated Pneumonia (VAP)

RISK FACTORS	PREVENTION PROTOCOLS
• Pneumonia developing 48 to 72 hours after intubation (prolonged intubation) • Prehospital intubation/emergency intubation • Chest injury/trauma • Smoking history and COPD • Increased age • Enteral nutrition	• Hand hygiene • Frequent oral care (q4hr minimum) • Oral chlorhexidine • Prevent aspiration • Elevate HOB (30–45 degrees) • Subglottic ETT suction • Gastric residual checks when necessary • Use of pantoprazole and/or sucralfate for antacid prophylaxis • Early ambulation post-extubation • Encourage less invasive ventilation options when appropriate (BiPaP) • Do not break integrity in ventilator circuit • Maintenance of ETT cuff pressure • Prevent condensation in circuitry falling backward into the patient • Avoid oversedation and paralytics when appropriate

Table 12-9   Infectious Diseases

Methicillin-Resistant *Staphylococcis aureus* (MRSA)	Vancomycin-Resistant *Enterococci* (VRE)
• **Risk factors** • Prolonged hospitalization • ICU admission • Antibiotic use • HIV infection • Hemodialysis and central lines • **Infection sites** • Skin and subcutaneous • Osteomyelitis • Meningitis • Pneumonia • Endocarditis • **Treatment** • Vancomycin (most common)	• **Risk factors** • Chronic renal failure • Antibiotic use (vancomycin) • Hemodialysis • ICU admission • **Infection sites** • UTIs • Bacteremia • Endocarditis • **Treatment** • Beta-lactams • Aminoglycosides (gentamicin)

(continued)

Table 12-9   Infectious Diseases (continued)

Carbapenem-Resistant Enterobacteriaceae (CRE)	Influenza
• **Risk factors**	• **Risk factors**
• Multiple hospital admissions (especially ICU)	• Seasonal (August or winter)
• Immunocompromised	• Heavy populated areas (hospitals, cities, nursing homes, prisons)
• Prolonged intubation	• **Clinical presentation**
• Recent travel to endemic area	• Fever and headaches
• **Infection sites**	• Cough and sore throat
• UTIs	• Muscle pains
• Pneumonia	• **High-risk complication groups**
• Surgical sites	• Children and elderly
• Bacteremia	• Immunocompromised
• **Treatment**	• Pregnant women
• Combination therapy with multiple antibiotics	• **Treatment**
	• Vaccination
	• Oseltamivir
	• Amantadine

> **CCRN Tip**
>
> A couple terms to know. **Pandemic** reflects a widespread disease (epidemic) across a country or the world. **Epidemic** reflects the spread of a disease to a community. These terms are commonly associated with the flu on the CCRN blueprint. Odd side note: this book was written during the COVID-19 crisis.

Pain Management

Pain remains a challenge among the critically ill, especially given the frequent difficulty in assessment for such patents. Pain complicates comorbidity and hospital stay when patients are under- or overmedicated. There is also the psychological fear when pain is not appropriately managed. More than 50% of critical patients state having experienced moderate to severe pain in the ICU.

Pain Assessment

Self-reporting pain using a numeric scale is ideal; however, many patient situations make this impossible. Utilize alternate pain scales such as the following to assess for pain in these circumstances. Pain and sedation are assessed routinely in the ICU.

- Behavioral pain scale (BPS)
  - Facial expression
  - Upper limbs
  - Compliance with ventilator
- Critical care pain observation tool (CPOT)
  - Facial expression
  - Body movements

- Muscle tension
- Compliance with ventilator (intubated) or vocalization (extubated)
- FLACC
  - Face, legs, activity, cry, consolability
  - Utilized for children up to 7 years of age

The Pain Spectrum

Pain in the ICU has the potential to turn from acute to chronic. Pain alters the brain chemistry. Higher severity and duration of pain increases the risk. Table 12-10 contrasts acute versus chronic pain.

Table 12-10   Acute vs. Chronic Pain Spectrum

ACUTE PAIN	CHRONIC PAIN
Clinical manifestations • Hypertension • Tachycardia/tachypnea • Agitation **Management** • Systemic opioids (intermittent or continuous) • Multimodal pharmacology (utilization of two or more types of medications) • Central versus peripheral anesthesia (local, spinal blocks)	**Nociceptive pain**: physical damage **Neuropathic pain**: nervous system damage **Nociplastic pain**: nociceptive with no evidence of damage Assess for chronic pain conditions that may be present on top of acute issues; chronic pain sufferers typically have multiple comorbidities

COMPLICATIONS OF POOR PAIN MANAGEMENT
Under-treatment complications • Prolonged mechanical ventilation • Hypoxemia • Self-extubation • Ventilator asynchrony • Delirium, depression, and chronic pain **Over-treatment complications** • Prolonged mechanical ventilation • Ventilator-associated pneumonia • Prolonged cognitive issues (delirium, PTSD) • Respiratory depression • Skin breakdown and pressure ulcers • Impairment of body functions (bowel function, urinary function, circulatory function)

Thermoregulation

Physiologically, the human body regulates core temperature very carefully. The hypothalamus controls the majority of thermoregulation, which is why a number of neurological disorders and pathologies can interrupt normal thermoregulation.

This may include stroke, brain or spinal cord injury, Wernicke's, and tumors. The hypothalamus achieves thermoregulation through the neurotransmitter acetylcholine via motor neurons and glands.

Both low and high body temperature may be encountered in the ICU, but a greater amount of attention is typically paid to the other vital signs. Abnormal temperature is linked to increased mortality and longer recovery times. Careful consideration of temperature in critical care is warranted.

- **Normal core temperature:** 35.5–37.5°C
- **Hypothermia:** <35°C; with severe hypothermia, <28°C
- **Hyperthermia:** >38°C; with severe hyperthermia, ≥41.5°C

Table 12-11   Thermoregulation Spectrum

HYPOTHERMIA	HYPERTHERMIA (FEVER/PYREXIA)

Risk factors
• Drowning
• Surgery (especially if prolonged)
• Trauma
• Endocrine conditions (hypopituitarism, hypoadrenalism, hypothyroidism)
• Burns
• Elderly
Corrective mechanisms
• Shivering (not possible if the patient is paralyzed)
• Peripheral vasoconstriction
• Increased muscle tone/contraction
• Bradycardia → decreased metabolism
	Risk factors
	• Infection
	• Trauma
	• Post-operative inflammatory response
	• Heatstroke
	• Malignant hyperthermia, neuroleptic malignant syndrome, serotonin syndrome
	Corrective mechanisms
	• Diaphoresis (increases based on temperature)
	• Tachycardia → increased metabolism
	• Reflex vasodilation
	• Pharmacology
	  • Acetaminophen
	  • Dantrolene
	  • Cooled IV fluids

Targeted Temperature Management

Previously known as therapeutic hypothermia, targeted temperature management has the primary goal to preserve brain tissue and function, usually following a cardiac arrest. Hypoxic ischemic brain injury due to a collapse in perfusion during arrest may result in coma and brain death. This warrants intervention when the patient achieves *return of spontaneous circulation (ROSC)*.

One thing of note to understand is exclusion criteria of therapeutic hypothermia. Coma may be caused by other events such as overdose, CVA, or head trauma; these cases are contraindications to hypothermia. In the event a patient has cardiogenic shock (<90 mmHg systolic), this patient should not receive hypothermia. Hypothermia itself may cause the blood pressure to decrease.

Targeted Temperature Protocol

The Advanced Life Support Task Force created by the American Heart Association reviewed a collection of studies to answer the question of ideal temperature. While no clear consensus states a temperature, all agree that some degree of hypothermia improves neurological outcomes. These studies recommend cooling to **32°C to 36°C**. This may seem like a wide range, but studies ranging in targeted temperature do not show one benefit over another. Regardless of goal temperature, continuous monitoring is required (bladder, rectal, core via central line). Methods of cooling may include ice packs, cooled IV fluids, and cooling blankets. Studies suggest a **minimum of 24 hours** of hypothermia, with some lasting as long as 72 hours.

Performing Therapeutic Hypothermia

- **Induction** → obtain baseline assessment, labs, glucose, ECG, etc.
- **Maintenance** → paralytics and sedation, hemodynamic monitoring, laboratory monitoring (hyperglycemia, hypokalemia, hypomagnesemia)
- **Rewarming** → warm slowly (**0.5°C to 1°C**) per hour over 8 hours (passive rewarming), assess for hyperkalemia

> **CCRN Tip**
>
> Paralytics inhibit shivering. Always administer sedation with paralytics.

Bariatric Complications

This section does not cover the bariatric surgeries found in Chapter 5, "Gastrointestinal," but rather the complications and physiological changes due to obesity. Obesity is a common comorbidity in the ICU and is not only a risk factor for many diseases but complicates the hospital stay itself. Understand BMI numbers to indicate possible obesity in a patient. (See Figure 12-2.)

Figure 12-2   BMI Ranges

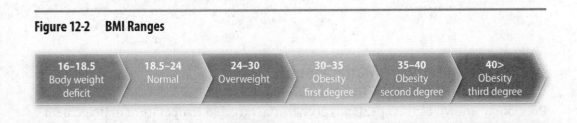

| 16–18.5 Body weight deficit | 18.5–24 Normal | 24–30 Overweight | 30–35 Obesity first degree | 35–40 Obesity second degree | 40> Obesity third degree |

Obesity Considerations

- Lipophilicity of medications—certain medications, like benzodiazepines, take longer to clear the body due to lipophilicity (affinity to adipose tissue)
- Difficulty in vascular access → ultrasound guidance often needed
- Immobility related complications
  - DVT, pressure ulcers, muscle deconditioning
- Difficulty in respiratory management
  - Intubation, prolonged ventilation, extubation)
- Obesity is a chronic inflammatory condition with increased risk for many medical conditions (see Table 12-12)

Table 12-12. Risk Profiles with Obesity

CARDIAC	RESPIRATORY	METABOLIC	GASTROINTESTINAL	ONCOLOGICAL
Hypertension Atherosclerosis CAD	Sleep apnea Hypoxia Hypercapnia	DM type II Dyslipidemia	GERD Cholelithiasis	Colorectal Esophageal Hepatocellular Renal Prostate Breast

> **CCRN Tip**
>
> **Table 12-12** is certainly not all-inclusive; rather, it displays the wide array of factors that may affect bariatric patients. Remember to review Chapter 8 for bariatric surgeries; *anastomotic leaks* are a big risk post-op.

Comorbidity with Transplant History

Understanding all of the factors contributing to ranking systems for people on the transplant list is not needed for the CCRN exam. What is possible is understanding the bigger picture of transplant patients after they have received the transplant itself, specifically, a solid organ. A number of things may be seen in these patients. Strict management is typically performed by the transplant coordinator with appropriate follow-up on the interdisciplinary team.

> **CCRN Tip**
>
> While not a comorbidity, be aware of signs and symptoms for transplant rejection (fever, new organ dysfunction).

- Infection → immunosuppression due to medications (tacrolimus, cyclosporine)
  - Increased risk for nosocomial and community-acquired infections
- Reactivation of latent infections → tuberculosis, MRSA, VRE, etc.
- Cancer → a result of immunosuppression → skin cancer or lymphomas most common
- New-onset diabetes → oftentimes due to anti-rejection medications
- Preexisting comorbidity at the time of transplant
  - Cardiovascular disease (HTN and congestive heart failure [CHF])
  - Kidney disease → common with many types of transplants

Life-Threatening Maternal/Fetal Complications

A handful of pregnancy-related complications may be seen on the CCRN exam. They are new additions to the 2020 exam blueprint. These complications are fairly straightforward in the sense of understanding symptomatology and treatments for the given problems.

Eclampsia/HELLP Syndrome

Pre-eclampsia typically occurs after 20 weeks of gestation. The etiology remains somewhat unknown, but comorbid conditions do increase the risk, such as chronic hypertension, chronic renal failure, and diabetes. Table 12-13 details the signs and symptoms, interventions, and complications for pre-eclampsia/eclampsia.

Table 12-13   Eclampsia

PRE-ECLAMPSIA	ECLAMPSIA
Signs and symptoms	**Signs and symptoms**

• Hypertension (systolic ≥140 mmHg)
• Proteinuria
• Edema (face, hands, feet)
• Abdominal pain (RUQ/epigastric)
Ankle edema is fairly common in pregnant women. Look for edema in abnormal places or if it is *pitting*.
	• Central nervous system abnormalities
	  • Generalized tonic-clonic seizures
	  • Headaches
	  • Vision changes
	• Life-threatening → loss of airway

Interventions	**Interventions**

• Maintain airway and prevent aspiration
• Maternal and fetal monitoring
  • Vital signs, fetal heart monitoring, fluid balances, lab tests
• Post-seizure care → prevent recurrence
  • Maintain oxygenation (supplemental oxygen)
  • Magnesium sulfate and lorazepam
  • Treat severe hypertension → labetalol, hydralazine, nifedipine
  • Assess fetal bradycardia → sustained bradycardia may warrant cesarean
  • Corticosteroid therapy → stimulate fetal lung development prior to delivery
  • Delivery of the fetus within 24 hours → induction
Calcium gluconate may be used in cases of magnesium sulfate toxicity
	• ABC supportive care
	• Immediate delivery of the fetus

Complications	

• Stroke
• Myocardial infarction
• Renal failure → monitor urine output
• Placenta abruptio
• *HELLP Syndrome* (**H**emolysis, **E**levated **L**iver enzymes, **L**ow **P**latelet count)
  • Assess laboratory data
  • Risk for DIC and ARDS → ICU admission
  • Severe changes may require treatment → platelets, transfusions, intubation	

CCRN Tip

Recognize the changes in laboratory data to effectively recognize this complication most commonly associated with the pre-eclampsia spectrum.

Postpartum Hemorrhage (PPH)

PPH is the leading cause of maternal mortality in childbirth. There are varying degrees of severity related to the amount of blood loss and a variety of risk factors and etiologies that may lead to the bleeding. Blood loss amounts are based on information from the American College of Obstetrics and Gynecology.

Etiologies

- *Uterine atony* → poor contraction of the muscle (most common)
  - Risks in prolonged use of oxytocin, multiparity, multiples, polyhydramnios, etc.
- Retained placenta
- Abnormal placentation (previa, accreta, etc.)
- Coagulation disorders

Signs and Symptoms

- Traditional blood loss calculations
  - 500 mL or more for vaginal birth
  - 1000 mL or more for cesarean birth
- New guidelines for blood loss
  - 1000 mL or more with signs and symptoms of hypovolemia within **24 hours**
  - Tachycardia and hypotension (**RED FLAG**)
- Soft boggy uterus → uterine atony

Interventions

- Assess and treat the underlying cause → surgical interventions possible
- CBC, type and screen, crossmatch
- Hemodynamic maintenance
  - Blood and blood products → massive transfusion may be necessary
- Treat uterine atony
  - Uterine massage → bimanual
  - Uterotonics → oxytocin, ergonovine, carboprost
  - Uterine tamponade → Bakri balloon

Amniotic Embolism

Amniotic fluid embolism (AFE) is rare but life-threatening. Some sources state mortality as high as 80% in cases. This emergency is caused when amniotic fluid enters the bloodstream and travels to various organs, most commonly the lungs. With the parallels to general pulmonary embolism, you likely have good understanding already.

- Cardiopulmonary collapse
  - Respiratory distress (most common) → oxygen → potential intubation
  - Sudden hypotension → immediate resuscitation and inotropes
  - Push fetus to left side → follow ACLS
  - Emergency C-section
- Coagulopathy and massive bleeding (DIC) → blood and blood products

Sleep Disruption

The necessity of sleep is oftentimes disregarded by ICU staff given the critical nature of the patients. An intubated and sedated patient with 20 care actions to do in 1 hour leaves little consideration for quality of sleep. Nonetheless, physical and mental health of the critically ill is shown in a great deal of research to be very important. *Sensory overload* is the leading cause of sleep disruption in the ICU.

Etiologies and Interventions

- Alarms (monitors, ventilators, IV pumps)
  - Safely alter alarm parameters *if possible*
  - Promptly address and silence alarms
  - Monitor speaking volume and overall traffic
- Clinical care interrupting sleep (med administration, assessments)
  - Cluster care and schedule procedures
  - Remove unnecessary or superfluous care activities during sleep
- Light—day/night routine
  - Expose patient to natural light → encourage daytime activities (sitting in chair, ambulation)
  - Regulate ambient light or unnatural light to reflect normal day hours
  - Melatonin often used to aid in this; however, the use of hypnotics or sedatives is found to worsen the body's ability to self-regulate

Consequences of Sleep Disruption

- Cognitive and physiological negative effects → lengthened ICU stay
- Respiratory → decreased ventilatory response and strength
- Cardiovascular → sympathetic stimulation leads to hypertension and tachycardia
- Immune → decreased function

> **CCRN Tip**
>
> Sleep disruption and deprivation is long thought to be a contributing factor to delirium in the critically ill.

Toxic Ingestions/Inhalations

Regardless of the toxin ingested, a general trauma approach is always utilized; the ABCs (airway, breathing, circulation). Some substances and toxins affect these three issues much more than others. While knowledge of every toxin possibly ingested is not required, the most common are included below with prospective antidotes, if available, and treatments.

Drug/Alcohol Overdose

Alcohol, benzodiazepine, and illicit substances with overdose and withdrawal are covered in detail in Chapter 11, "Behavioral/Psychosocial."

> **CCRN Tip**
>
> Thiamine may be administered in certain overdoses (ethylene glycol), not just in alcohol cases.

Priority Management

- ABCs
  - Airway → aspiration or loss of airway (no gag or cough)
  - Breathing → bradypnea and/or hypoxia (monitor lactate levels)
  - Circulation → hypotension, dysrhythmias, urine output
- Gastric lavage and activated charcoal → within 1 hour of ingestion
  - May be given oral, NG, or OG
  - Intact and peristaltic GI tract necessary for use
  - Activated charcoal may be given up to 4 hours after ingestion
  - Airway necessary before use due to aspiration risk
- Immediate antidote or reversal administration
- Manage metabolic abnormalities
  - Acidosis (watch anion gap) → sodium bicarb
  - Hypoglycemia → dextrose IV
- Manage changes in temperature
  - Hyperthermia → ice packs and cooling blankets
    - Dantrolene and paralytics may be utilized in certain cases. Muscle rigidity worsens hyperthermia, these medications relax or paralyze the muscles.
  - Hypothermia → forced air rewarming (Bear Hugger) and blankets

Toxic Ingestions and Treatments

- **Salicylates (aspirin)** → fluid resuscitation, serum alkalization (aids in elimination) → hemodialysis (severe overdose)
  - Assess for metabolic acidosis and respiratory alkalosis
- **Acetaminophen** → N-acetylcysteine
- **Tricyclic antidepressants (TCAs)** → fluid resuscitation → telemetry
- **Beta blockers/calcium-channel blockers** → insulin/D50
  - Manage hemodynamic instability → inotropes/chronotropes → extracorporeal support
- **Cholinergic agonists** → anticholinergics (atropine)
- **Ethylene glycol (antifreeze, methanol)** → sodium bicarb → ethanol/fomepizole → hemodialysis
- **Heavy metals (iron, arsenic, mercury)** → chelation therapy

Acid–Base Imbalances

Arterial blood gas (ABG) analysis is another section that doubles up in the CCRN blueprint. Acid–base as a whole is covered in detail in Chapter 3, "Respiratory." ABGs remain one of the absolute "must knows" for the CCRN exam.

Review Questions

1. A 65-year-old male was recently admitted to the emergency department after a two-story fall off of his roof. The trauma team assessed and found no issues with the airway. Utilizing the primary survey, which of the following actions are most appropriate for next steps?

   A. Assess pulse ox and lung function followed by establishing IV access

   B. Obtain an ECG followed by administering oxygen

   C. Assess skin color followed by hypoglycemia assessment

   D. Begin neuro assessment followed by immediate FAST ultrasound exam

2. During the compensatory stage of shock, which of the following body homeostatic mechanisms begin in efforts to maintain blood pressure and cellular perfusion?

   A. Increase in bicarbonate production in kidneys, increased perfusion to kidneys

   B. Increase in cardiac output, increase in anaerobic respiration

   C. Tunnel vision, dilated pupils, dry mouth

   D. Adrenocorticotropic hormone (ACTH) release, aldosterone release

3. During septic shock there is an increase in the risk for microclots and fibrin formation. If this response is not stopped or corrected, it may lead to which primary complication?

   A. Pulmonary embolism

   B. Cerebrovascular accident

   C. Septic arthritis

   D. Disseminated intravascular coagulation (DIC)

4. Which of the following signs and symptoms are NOT present in neurogenic shock?

   A. Bradycardia, hyperthermia, oliguria

   B. Tachycardia, hypothermia, normal lactate levels

   C. Tachycardia, hypotension, decreased preload

   D. Reduced vascular tone, decreased SVR

5. Which of the following are examples of required criteria for a systemic inflammatory response syndrome (SIRS) diagnosis?

   A. Hypotension, normal SvO_2, tachycardia

   B. Hyperthermia, hypotension, tachycardia

   C. Hyperthermia, leukocytosis, tachycardia

   D. Hypotension, bradycardia, tachypnea

6. Which of the following is TRUE regarding septic shock?

    A. There is an increase in oxygen consumption

    B. Lactic acidosis would be seen in advancing severe sepsis

    C. Norepinephrine is often avoided due to existing increased SVR

    D. Oxygen delivery (DO_2) is adequate, expected SvO_2 between 60% and 75%

7. A patient with an unknown hypersensitivity is admitted to the emergency room with classic symptoms of anaphylaxis—orbital and tongue swelling. While the admission was serious, intubation was not necessary and the patient improved with treatment. Hours later upon discharge, the nurse is educating the patient on recurrence of hypersensitivity. Which of the following statements is TRUE regarding anaphylaxis for this patient?

    A. Anaphylaxis is typically rapid occurring within minutes

    B. Urticaria is one of the earliest signs of anaphylaxis

    C. Rebound anaphylaxis is less severe than the first reaction

    D. Respiratory distress is caused by rapid buildup of fluid in the lungs

8. An 80 kg woman was recently admitted to the ICU due to hypovolemic shock secondary to large burns. Fluid resuscitation and norepinephrine were implemented immediately. Which of the following outcomes best displays improvement in fluid volume status?

    A. Blood pressure 90/65 mmHg

    B. Urine output 30 mL per hour

    C. CVP 6 mmHg

    D. Heart rate 95 BPM

9. Which of the following interventions is avoided in hypovolemic shock except in extreme cases of hypotension?

    A. Norepinephrine IV titration

    B. Rapid IV boluses of isotonic crystalloids

    C. Place the patient in a recumbent position

    D. Albumin IV infusion

10. Which of the following signs and symptoms is indicative of respiratory failure in multiple organ dysfunction syndrome (MODS)?

    A. PaO_2/FiO_2 ratio greater than 300

    B. Hypercapnia

    C. Increased pH

    D. Bradypnea

11. A patient recently arrived at the emergency department after being shot in the abdomen at close range. The patient is somnolent and very difficult to arouse. Current vital signs are BP 78/55 mmHg, HR 145 BPM, and RR 35. Urine output for the last hour is scant. Which class of hemorrhagic shock is this patient experiencing?

    A. Class IV
    B. Class III
    C. Class II
    D. Class I

12. An 86-year-old patient is in hospice due to terminal pancreatic cancer. The nurse is called to the room with the family disturbed by a loud rattling sound when the patient breathes. Which of the following interventions may help with this situation?

    A. Scopolamine
    B. Reduce oral swabbing
    C. Place the patient supine
    D. Lorazepam IV

13. A patient is suspected of overdosing on aspirin or acetaminophen. For the time being, the patient is conscious and able to ask questions. Which of the following early signs would be suspect for aspirin poisoning NOT acetaminophen?

    A. Tinnitus
    B. Vomiting with metabolic acidosis
    C. Pinpoint pupils and confusion
    D. Hypothermia

14. A patient who fell from a two-story building is in critical condition after losing a significant amount of blood. Which of the following would best explain azotemia and low urine output in this patient?

    A. Intrarenal acute kidney injury secondary to tubular necrosis
    B. Prerenal acute kidney injury secondary to hypoperfusion
    C. Rhabdomyolysis secondary to crush injuries
    D. Post-renal acute kidney injury secondary to urinary tract trauma

15. All of the following represent a high-risk group for healthcare-associated infections EXCEPT?

    A. A patient in the ICU with an internal jugular central line
    B. A patient on beclomethasone for asthma
    C. A patient with end-stage chronic kidney disease
    D. A pregnant patient in triage with three peripheral IVs

16. Which of the following is an important consideration to avoid aspiration and ventilator-associated pneumonia (VAP)?

    A. VAP occurs most often with parenteral nutrition; especially combined with lipids

    B. Pantoprazole is often used to increase gastric motility and decrease aspiration risk

    C. Patients with a history of smoking are at increased risk due to increased cilia motility in the lungs

    D. Abdominal distention may be a sign of enteral feeding intolerance; gastric residual may be assessed

17. All of the following are physiological responses to severe hypothermia EXCEPT?

    A. Vasoconstriction, shivering

    B. Tachycardia, hypotension

    C. Muscle contraction, dysrhythmias

    D. Hyperkalemia, hypoglycemia

18. A 150 kg male patient has been in the ICU for 9 days. The nurse is performing a spontaneous awakening trial. Propofol and midazolam have been held for 2 hours. The patient remains unresponsive. Which of the following should be considered appropriate at this time?

    A. Allow the awakening trial to continue, the medication is taking longer to leave the system

    B. Reverse the effects of midazolam with flumazenil

    C. Consider adding dexmedetomidine (Precedex) to prevent sudden agitation

    D. Notify the physician of the results, expect an order for head CT

19. An alcoholic patient is admitted to the ICU with a diagnosis of ethylene glycol (methanol) intoxication. Which of the following findings would the nurse expect with this patient?

    A. Respiratory acidosis; hypocapnia

    B. Metabolic acidosis; creatinine 1.1 mg/dL

    C. Metabolic acidosis; anion gap 18 mEq/L

    D. Metabolic acidosis; anion gap 6 mEq/L

20. A patient with known depression is brought to the emergency department by EMS. The paramedics state a 60-second episode of ventricular tachycardia occurred during the trip to the ED, then the patient reverted to sinus tachycardia, 120 BPM. The patient was found with multiple bottles of medications. Which of the following medication toxicities would explain the ventricular arrhythmia?

   A. Amitriptyline
   B. Paroxetine
   C. Oxycodone/acetaminophen
   D. Lorazepam

Answer Key

Question 1

Answer: A

Rationale: The primary survey for trauma, ABCDE, states airway always comes first followed by breathing. Breathing assessment may include assessing pulse ox and lung auscultation. Circulation would come next, which includes the placement of the IVs. An ECG would be included in the circulatory part of the survey; however, administering oxygen would come before the ECG, not after. A breathing assessment would also come before skin assessment and hypoglycemia. The same rule applies for the neuro exam; neuro would fall under the "D" in the survey for disability.

Question 2

Answer: D

Rationale: During the compensatory phase of shock, the sympathetic nervous system is activated along with the RAAS system. The sympathetic (fight or flight) response would include symptoms such as tachycardia, increased cardiac output, reduced GI motility. Activation of RAAS would see release of ACTH and aldosterone. The effects will cause retention of sodium and water. An increase in bicarbonate release does not occur and would also not aid in maintenance of blood pressure. An increase in anaerobic respiration is a RESULT of poor cellular perfusion. Tunnel vision, dilated pupils, and dry mouth occur with a sympathetic response, but they do not contribute to maintenance of blood pressure.

Question 3

Answer: D

Rationale: Most commonly associated with septic shock, DIC occurs in sepsis due to activation of coagulation. This causes fibrin to be activated and deposited causing microvascular thrombosis. The activation also decreases the clotting factors leading to bleeding. Pulmonary embolism and CVA would be complications secondary to the DIC itself. Septic arthritis is not a complication of DIC.

Question 4

Answer: B

Rationale: Bradycardia, NOT tachycardia, occurs in neurogenic shock. Widespread vasodilation leads to distributive shock and a lack of perfusion to organs. This would cause an elevation of lactate levels. Hyperthermia is typically seen in neurogenic shock due to autonomic dysfunction. The other answers would be seen in neurogenic shock—reduced vascular tone, oliguria, etc.

Question 5

Answer: C

Rationale: Hyperthermia, tachycardia, tachypnea, and leukocytosis make up the four symptoms of SIRS. Two of the four symptoms need to be present for a SIRS diagnosis. Hypotension is not seen until severe sepsis.

Question 6

Answer: B

Rationale: In severe sepsis, anaerobic respiration begins causing a release in lactic acid. This is due to hypotension and decreased cellular perfusion. While oxygen delivery (DO_2) is adequate in septic shock, oxygen utilization (VO_2) is decreased causing an elevated SvO_2; 60–75% is considered normal. Norepinephrine is commonly used to maintain vascular tone; sepsis causes vasodilation and reduced SVR.

Question 7

Answer: A

Rationale: Anaphylaxis is fairly rapid, typically occurring within minutes, but it may start up to 20 minutes after the initial insult. Urticaria is more delayed than other classic symptoms of anaphylaxis like bronchospasms and angioedema. Rebound anaphylaxis (biphasic) may be less severe or more severe than the first episode. This must be instructed to patients so they may be aware when to come back to the emergency department. Respiratory distress is caused by bronchospasms or laryngeal edema, NOT pulmonary edema.

Question 8

Answer: D

Rationale: Normalization of the heart rate is a good indicator of proper fluid resuscitation. A rate of 95 BPM may be on the high side of normal, but consider that a hypovolemic patient likely was tachycardic into the 120s or higher—95 BPM is an improvement. Urine output should equal 0.5 mL/kg/hr; 30 mL for a 60 kg patient is low. Urine output is $0.5 \times 80 = 40$ mL urine per hour. Blood pressure is NOT the best indicator for fluid volume status, largely due to sympathetic compensation and especially here with the use or norepinephrine. CVP is not a good indicator for fluid volume status. It may be used as an accessory tool, however.

Question 9

Answer: A

Rationale: In hypovolemic shock, the SVR is already elevated. The use of vasopressors is not completely contraindicated, but it is reserved for cases where everything else did not work—a final resort. The other answers are common interventions for hypovolemic shock.

Question 10

Answer: B

Rationale: Hypercapnia and hypoxemia would indicate respiratory distress. The other answers show an opposite of what would be seen. The ratio is less than 300; tachypnea, not bradypnea; and acidosis, not alkalosis.

Question 11

Answer: A

Rationale: It is slightly difficult to memorize the benchmark for the four classes of hemorrhagic shock. One note that makes it slightly easier is to focus on the heart rate. The heart rate in this question is 145, very tachycardic. Greater than 140 is Class IV, between 120 and 140 is Class III. Between 100 and 120 BPM is Class II. A heart rate less than 100 BPM is Class I.

Question 12

Answer: A

Rationale: Anticholinergics or antimuscarinics may be used in cases of death rattle. That may include scopolamine, atropine, and glycopyrrolate, among others. Oral swabbing is palliative for comfort in dry mouth; it is not wise to discontinue palliative treatments as this defeats the purpose of palliative care. Repositioning may aid in minimizing death rattle, but not a supine position. Turning the head or patient's body may reduce the noise. Lorazepam would not help in reducing death rattle.

Question 13

Answer: A

Rationale: Tinnitus is one of the early signs of potential salicylate poisoning. Hyperventilation and respiratory alkalosis are others. Vomiting may be seen early; however, metabolic acidosis would come after. Pinpoint pupils would be seen in opioid use and overdose. Salicylate poisoning results in hyperthermia not hypothermia.

Question 14

Answer: B

Rationale: The most likely explanation for these symptoms is an acute kidney injury caused by hypoperfusion—prerenal AKI. Intrarenal injury is unlikely here without direct damage to the organ itself. Rhabdomyolysis is a type of intrarenal injury. Post-renal AKI is highly unlikely without direct trauma to the urinary tract.

Question 15

Answer: D

Rationale: Pregnancy does not increase the risk of infection by itself. Peripheral IVs, if managed, do not pose a large risk for infection. An internal jugular or femoral central line, immunosuppressed patients (steroid administration), and CKD patients are all high risk for infections.

Question 16

Answer: D

Rationale: Any sign of enteral feeding intolerance should be assessed. Abdominal (stomach) distention, vomiting, diarrhea (especially after immediately starting feedings), and diaphoresis are all symptoms of intolerance. The risk for aspiration is great if vomiting occurs. Parenteral nutrition is not a risk factor for aspiration. PPIs such as pantoprazole decrease the amount of acid produced in the stomach. A common gastric motility medication would be metoclopramide. Smoking causes dysfunction of cilia and poor motility, not increased function; this is certainly a risk factor for VAP.

Question 17

Answer: D

Rationale: Hypothermia causes hypokalemia and hyperglycemia. Patients often require potassium replacement and insulin drips during long courses of hypothermia, whether accidental or induced. The other answers reflect physiological responses to hypothermia.

Question 18

Answer: A

Rationale: Heavier patients (greater amounts of adipose tissue) often require more time to fully come out of sedation. This is due to the lipophilicity of certain medications, especially benzodiazepines. Administering flumazenil in a situation such as this with goals to extubate may cause severe agitation. It is safer to allow more time for the patient to metabolize the medications naturally. Precedex is often used in agitated patients or those expected to be agitated, such as alcoholics or drug users; the patient here does not apply. If after an extended period of time the patient continues to remain unconscious, a neuro consult is likely.

Question 19

Answer: C

Rationale: Ethylene glycol, also methanol or "antifreeze," intoxication leads to metabolic acidosis with an open anion gap. The most common cause is ingestion of antifreeze in a suicide attempt. Intoxication of this substance leads to renal failure, therefore a creatinine would be elevated not normal.

Question 20

Answer: A

Rationale: Tricyclic antidepressant toxicity (amitriptyline) may lead to cardiovascular dysfunctions such as severe dysrhythmias and blood pressure issues. Opioids like oxycodone and benzodiazepines like lorazepam may lead to a bradyarrhythmia but not ventricular tachycardia. SSRIs like paroxetine are not known to cause dysrhythmias in toxicities. While serotonin syndrome is a risk factor for tachycardia, the clinical picture makes more sense with TCA toxicity.

CHAPTER 13

Professional Caring and Ethical Practice

The professional caring & ethical practice section makes up roughly 25 questions on your CCRN exam—or approximately 20%—making it one of the larger sections. AACN defines their "Synergy Model for Patient Care" as a conceptual framework that seeks to align patient needs with nurse competencies. Before the Synergy Model existed, a great deal of nursing care revolved solely around the physiology and medical needs of a patient. The goal of the Synergy Model, and the importance of this chapter, is to look at the patient as a whole and drive nursing competencies by patient needs.

Because this chapter is less to do with specific memorization and more to do with an application of an idea of nursing, this chapter can be difficult to study. A good starting point is to understand the message AACN implies by "synergy." Many of the following concepts may feel natural to you, but others may not. Keep an open mind.

- The *AACN Synergy Model for Patient Care* may be found on the AACN website (www.aacn.org)

Nurse Competencies

Under the Synergy Model, nursing competencies reflect the knowledge, skills, attitudes, and experience needed to meet the needs of patients and their families. The model includes the following competency areas.

Clinical Judgment

The competency of clinical judgment includes treating the patient and communicating with the family about the entire picture. This involves taking into account the complexities of the patient condition, analyzing all data and information, and applying all of these in a critical-thinking manner.

Competency Characteristics
- Formulates solutions based on incomplete information
- Prepares for potential problems ahead of time
- Teaches and communicates with the family about the entire picture of care

Advocacy/Moral Agency

Advocacy includes supporting others and advocating for patients unable to advocate for themselves; representing others' concerns, including patient, family, and nursing staff; serving as a moral broker; and identifying and assisting with resolution of ethical and clinical concerns.

Competency Characteristics
- Understand ethical principles in nursing
  - Autonomy, nonmaleficence, beneficence, justice, veracity, fidelity
- Advocacy
  - Be aware of personal values and feelings → explore personal feelings when placed in uncomfortable or foreign situations
  - Advocate on behalf of the patient, family, and community; most important, advocate for the above regardless of personal views
    - Respect values and personal beliefs
    - Assist, and intervene if necessary, for patients unable to speak for themselves
  - The patient and the family drive moral decision-making; rules or protocol may need to be suspended
- **Moral agency** implies the ability for nurses to act as a moral representative for patients and family. This may include acting as the intersection between patient, family, and the healthcare team.

Caring Practices

Caring nursing practices include maintaining awareness and responsiveness of the care environment; creating a compassionate, supportive, and therapeutic environment; and preventing unnecessary suffering. Nurses engage with vigilant behavior for the patient, family, and other healthcare workers.

Competency Characteristics
- Anticipating patient or family needs and delivering them when needed
  - Includes anticipation of hazards of care and adapting to avoid them → nursing *vigilance*
- Coordinates care and communication across the healthcare needs of the patient as needed
- Explains and ensures patient and family needs through the dying process
  - May include encouraging communication, education about processes, pain management, cultural needs, and others

- Visitation times personalized to the patient and family
  - AACN Practice Alert: *Family Visitation in the Adult Intensive Care Unit*
    - Explains that unrestricted family presence improves recovery and satisfaction
  - AACN Practice Alert: *Family Presence During Resuscitation and Invasive Procedures*
    - Policies should allow for family to choose whether to be bedside or not

Response to Diversity

The nurse must have the awareness and ability to accept views different from their own, including sensitivity across a wide spectrum of differences—cultural, gender, race, lifestyle, age, religion, socioeconomic, disability, sexual orientation, gender identity, among many others—as well as the ability to incorporate these differences into the plan of care.

Competency Characteristics

- Tailoring or creating individualized care to the patient regardless of diversity
  - May include alternative or complementary therapies
- Maintain cultural sensitivity and competence
  - Pain may present differently across cultures
  - Attitude toward death is often different among cultures
  - Understand differences between spirituality and religions
- Care should be provided without bias or stereotyping
  - Be aware of body language, tone of voice, and words chosen

Facilitation of Learning

The nurse must understand and utilize both formal and informal methods of learning to facilitate patient, family, and nursing staff education. This may include other members of the healthcare team.

Competency Characteristics

- Utilize and encourage alternate methods of communication when appropriate
  - Standard practice is "teach, teach-back"
- Individualize teachings to patient and family needs
  - Unique considerations include sensory deficits, learning style, and education aptitude
  - Observe not just verbal understanding, but body language and behavioral cues as well for understanding
  - Goals include improving health, minimizing anxiety, and promoting medication adherence
- Remember that discharge teaching and planning begins upon admission

Collaboration

This entails the ability to work in collaboration with patients, families, and healthcare professionals, including working within the community, in a manner that promotes optimal and realistic goals.

Competency Characteristics

- Beginning nurses may collaborate by seeking out learning for themselves; expert nurses involve themselves in teaching
- Listens to team members and encourage discussions regarding patient care and workplace issues
- Respect and understand the multiples roles in the hospital, not simply medicine and nursing
- Establish multidisciplinary committees or activities such as rounding, committee meetings, quality improvement, etc.
- Use SBAR for communication between team members
- Be a responsible delegator
  - "Five rights of delegation": right task, right circumstance, right person, right supervision, right direction, and communication

Systems Thinking

Systems thinking—the body of knowledge and tools nurses utilize to maintain a multitude of environments both healthcare and nonhealthcare systems—provides nurses with the mental tools to look at the "bigger picture."

Competency Characteristics

- Understands and effectively operates within the healthcare team and institution
  - Shared governance is an organizational structure that gives nurses a seat at the table; governance is shared
  - Patient care delivery models include functional nursing, team nursing, and primary nursing
- Anticipate the needs of patients and families and works within the system to achieve goals
- Understands safety components of the system and utilizes appropriate mechanisms when error (incident reports, hierarchy of nursing, improvement committees)

Clinical Inquiry

The continuous process of questioning and evaluating current practice, including innovating in research and learning, helps lead to new and improved practices and protocols that better align with patient needs.

Competency Characteristics

- Utilizes evidence-based practice and implements changes as appropriate
  - Proficient in learning qualitative and quantitative research models
  - *ACE Star Model of Knowledge Transformation*
    - Discovery research → evidence summary → translation into guidelines → practice integration → process, outcome evaluation
- Individualizes research to specific patient care situations
- Evaluate EBP as it is applied
  - Trend patient outcomes
  - Patient satisfaction
- Follows strict guidelines in relation to patient safety
  - High-risk medications (vasopressors, heparin drip, insulin drip, etc.)
  - Medication errors and reporting
  - Hospital-acquired infection trending

Review Questions

1. A patient in the intensive care unit has remained intubated for the past 7 days and his overall condition continues to deteriorate. The patient does not have a healthcare power of attorney. Family members are unable to agree on what the next steps should be. Which of the following is the best course of action?

   A. Speak with the nurse manager about notifying the ethics committee

   B. Encourage the family to appoint a primary decision-maker

   C. Convince the family to allow their loved one to pass naturally

   D. Arrange for an interdisciplinary conference that includes family members

2. A patient in the intensive care unit was admitted due to an acute exacerbation of COPD. The patient was having difficulty breathing and BiPAP was initiated to avoid intubation. The patient is complaining of discomfort and inability to sleep with the mask on. They continually attempt to take the BiPAP off. Which of the following interventions is most appropriate?

   A. Take the BiPAP off and place the patient on a venturi mask for comfort

   B. Explain to the patient the purpose of the BiPAP

   C. Restrain the patient to ensure adequate oxygenation

   D. Teach the repercussions if they take the mask off and that intubation will be inevitable

3. After a conference with family, the healthcare team believes that end-of-life care is the best option for the patient. The family is hesitant but not unreceptive to this idea. What intervention is best at this time?

   A. Speak with the family about the benefits of palliative care and answer questions asked

   B. Advocate for second opinions and potential alternate options to care

   C. Refer family problems and concerns to the physicians

   D. Restrict family visits to avoid overwhelming the patient

4. The nurse walks in to find the wife of a patient sneaking him a pill from her purse. What would be the best action of the nurse at this time?

   A. Explain outside medications are not allowed and notify the physician

   B. Ask the wife about the pill and its purpose

   C. Confiscate the bottle of pills and coordinate with pharmacy regarding its use

   D. Leave the room and call the physician regarding the improper administration

5. A 65-year-old woman is being discharged home after a series of traumas to her body. The care required at home is complex, but the husband feels he can handle the required tasks. He wants to remain the primary caregiver. Which of the following best evaluates if the husband will be able to manage his wife's care?

   A. He will learn best using handwritten materials with education by the nurse
   B. Begin by asking about the husband's knowledge of his wife's condition
   C. Observe the husband mimicking nurse behavior and skills
   D. Assess the husband's schedule at home

6. A patient with a large family continues to be a challenge for the nursing staff. Multiple demands and many actions deemed "inappropriate" by the nursing staff have made nearly all nurses on the unit request not to be assigned to the patient. Which of the following would be the best decision?

   A. Assign the patient to nursing staff willing to handle the workload
   B. Minimize how many family members may be in the patient's room
   C. Ensure a different nurse is assigned to the patient day to day
   D. Bring the nursing staff into a conference to review the issue

7. A patient is preoperative on the unit for a coronary artery bypass surgery. The patient is visibly anxious. Which of the following interventions is NOT appropriate at this time?

   A. Dim the lights and close the door if able
   B. Administer prescribed lorazepam as needed
   C. Explain interventions to avoid future coronary disease
   D. Encourage family presence in the room

8. The day-nurse received hand-off 15 minutes ago. Upon entry into the patient room for the 8 A.M. assessment, the nurse notices the infusion pump running at an incorrect rate. How should the nurse proceed?

   A. Notify the charge nurse and fill out an incident report
   B. Attempt to contact the night shift nurse to question the infusion pump rate
   C. Determine any harm to the patient and contact the physician
   D. Withhold the error to the patient, but cautiously assess for adverse effects

9. A patient in the intensive care unit was recently admitted due to traumatic brain injury. The neurosurgeon has ordered a repeat CT scan of the patient's head. The nurse contacts transporters to assist in the transfer of the patient to CT. The nurse also calls radiology to coordinate receiving the patient. Which of the following competencies from the Synergy Model is the nurse following?

   A. Systems thinking
   B. Collaboration
   C. Clinical inquiry
   D. Caring practices

10. The nurse suspects that an oncoming nurse is under the influence of alcohol. What should be done at this time?

   A. Speak with the nurse about going home to avoid harming patients
   B. Speak with the nurse manager regarding suspicions
   C. Contact security and bar the nurse from caring for patients
   D. Do not assume suspicions, but monitor closely the nurse's actions

Answer Key

Question 1

Answer: D

Rationale: In situations where the patient has not made their wishes explicitly clear, caring practices include encouraging communication between family and healthcare staff. If the patient has made their wishes known, those wishes should be followed and advocated for. In this case, the family is in disagreement and the healthcare staff sees a deteriorating patient. If the family continues to disagree and a decision-maker is not appointed, reaching out to an ethics committee may be needed down the line. If the family is unable to agree on care, it is unlikely they will agree on who to appoint as a primary decision-maker and the first opportunity should be for a conference; this will allow all of these conversations. It is not the job of a healthcare professional to convince, judge, patronize, or condescend patient or family decisions.

Question 2

Answer: B

Rationale: The primary goal is to avoid intubation of the patient. The patient requires the BiPAP machine, but it would be considered rude or crass to threaten intubation; it's also likely illegal. The best thing for the nurse to do is follow the nursing process (ADPIE) and assess the situation and educate the importance of the current plan. We understand discomfort is a leading factor here. Teaching the necessity of the BiPAP is a good starting point to ensuring adherence. If the patient continues to remove the mask, it would be important to assess for deliriousness or if the patient truly does not want care. Restraints would be considered a last resort if other interventions fail.

Question 3

Answer: A

Rationale: It is important that every patient and every family understands that palliative care is an option for them. The nurse should encourage communication and education about the dying process. The AACN has a practice alert for visitation of family; restricting family visitation is not appropriate. While the physician is an important part of the healthcare team, the nurse is knowledgeable and able to answer family questions. Specific medical questions may require a referral to a physician. The important thing is to manage and utilize your scope of practice. If the healthcare team in conference believes end-of-life is near, it would be inappropriate for the nurse to encourage second opinions unless the family specifically asks for it.

Question 4

Answer: B

Rationale: Institutions do not allow outside medication unless it is previously cleared with the physician and the pharmacist. The wife would need to be told this, BUT the first thing to do is to ask. The nurse may not understand a cultural implication in what the wife is trying to do. The best course is to listen, educate, and then coordinate in a safe way if the pill is possible for the patient to take. Confiscating the bottle is inappropriate at this time.

Question 5

Answer: B

Rationale: As you may begin to see in many questions, the nursing process (ADPIE) comes into play quite a bit. Appropriate interventions by the nurse require an understanding of the problem before acting—hence assessing first. The same applies in this question. To facilitate learning, assessing the level of readiness and education level assists the nurse in tailoring a specific plan for the patient and husband. The other answers would come after this primary assessment. The nurse cannot know the best method of teaching until assessing.

Question 6

Answer: D

Rationale: Again, there is a bit of the nursing process here. By assessing the problem first, the nursing staff can come to the best solution for the family and the unit. They may indeed be formulating a set of rules. By utilizing this process, the unit ensures the highest opportunity for agreement and solidarity among the staff.

Question 7

Answer: C

Rationale: Discharge teaching certainly begins upon admission, but it would be inappropriate to educate or teach a patient in a setting such as this—preop. The patient is also visibility anxious, so it is highly unlikely they will retain any of the information given. The other answers are appropriate interventions for this patient.

Question 8

Answer: C

Rationale: The primary concern is harm to the patient; this should be assessed. Once determined, the physician is contacted, followed by completion of a report. It is not appropriate to notify the charge nurse or attempt to contact the night shift nurse. Withholding an error to the patient goes against nursing ethics; the patient has a right to know.

Question 9

Answer: A

Rationale: Systems thinking involves understanding and facilitating care for the patient. This may involve a multitude of departments and professionals to achieve the desired outcome—in this case, a CT of the head.

Question 10

Answer: B

Rationale: When the nurse suspects another team member is under the influence of a substance, the appropriate action is to notify the nursing manager or supervisor. It is not the staff nurse's position to get involved, and oftentimes doing so can lead to unnecessary conflict. All actions should be taken by the nursing manager or supervisor. It is appropriate to prevent harm to a patient, so allowing the nurse to continue while monitoring may result in harm.

Practice Test 1

Congratulations for making it through the entire book and reading up on the CCRN blueprint. You are ready to tackle the practice exams. Each test contains 125 questions, the same as the CCRN exam. Questions are modeled after the blueprint in type and amount. For this first practice exam, the questions follow topic by topic in order so you may practice each section one by one. All practice exams after this will be mixed. A passing grade on the CCRN exam is 87 questions out of 125 questions. This should be your benchmark for success. Good luck!

1. A 45-year-old patient was admitted to the ICU with a diagnosis of pneumonia. The critical care admission was warranted given increasing oxygen demands. Current oxygen supplementation therapy: high-flow nasal cannula with 40 L of flow and 60% FiO_2. Patient SpO_2 is 90%. Which of the following clinical manifestations would the nurse expect in this patient?

   A. PaO_2 60 mmHg, P/F ratio 200 mmHg
   B. PaO_2 70 mmHg, P/F ratio 117 mmHg
   C. PaO_2 60 mmHg, pleuritic chest pain, dyspnea
   D. PaO_2 80 mmHg, pleuritic chest pain, dyspnea

2. A patient with pneumonia is describing the pleuritic chest pain they experience when breathing and coughing. Which of the following best describes the patient's reports of pleuritic chest pain?

   A. Sharp or burning
   B. Aching or throbbing
   C. Pulsating and severe
   D. Tearing and radiating

GO ON TO NEXT PAGE ➤

3. A 35-year-old male is admitted to the ICU after heroin overdose. After administration of naloxone by paramedics, the patient vomited and began coughing. Upon arrival at the emergency department, the patient required a second dose of naloxone. Due to sustained respiratory depression the patient was admitted to the ICU on a non-rebreather mask, FiO_2 40%. Recent ABG shows pH 7.30, $PaCO_2$ 50 mmHg, HCO_3 24, PaO_2 70 mmHg. Crackles are heard upon auscultation. The patient remains largely somnolent and unable to follow directions. Which intervention is needed at this time?

   A. Stimulate patient breathing by frequent awakenings
   B. Increase FiO_2 via non-rebreather mask
   C. Intubate the patient and place on mechanical ventilation
   D. Administer bicarbonate

4. A patient is recently admitted to the emergency department with a diagnosis of carbon monoxide poisoning. Current SpO_2 is 85% on 100% oxygen. Which of the following best explains the pathophysiology within this patient?

   A. Increased affinity of oxygen to hemoglobin, right shift in oxyhemoglobin dissociation curve
   B. Increased affinity of carbon monoxide to hemoglobin, left shift in oxyhemoglobin dissociation curve
   C. Decreased affinity of oxygen to hemoglobin, left shift in oxyhemoglobin dissociation curve
   D. Decreased affinity of carbon monoxide to hemoglobin, right shift in oxyhemoglobin dissociation curve

5. A patient is being assessed in the ICU after surgical repair of an open-fractured femur. The patient is currently dyspneic with chest pain and petechiae. What does the nurse suspect as the cause of these symptoms?

   A. Fat embolism
   B. Myocardial infarction
   C. Pneumonia
   D. Pneumothorax

6. Which of the following findings would the nurse note upon the assessment of a patient who developed right-sided tension pneumothorax secondary to rib fractures and motor vehicle accident trauma to the chest?

   A. Decreased chest expansion on the left, jugular venous distention
   B. Decreased chest expansion on the left, tracheal deviation to the right
   C. HR 95, BP 150/90, tracheal deviation to the left
   D. HR 135, BP 85/60, tracheal deviation to the left

7. A 55-year-old male patient is currently on CPAP mode through the ventilator. This mode has been ongoing for 1 hour with anticipation of extubation. Given the below results for vitals and ABG, which action is most appropriate by the nurse?

VITAL SIGNS	ARTERIAL BLOOD GAS
BP = 130/85 mmHg	pH = 7.28
HR = 100 BPM	$PaCO_2$ = 55 mmHg
RR = 26	HCO_3 = 24 mEq/L
SpO_2 = 93%	PaO_2 = 85 mmHg

    A. Perform parameters such as negative inspiratory force (NIF).

    B. Increase the FiO_2 on the ventilator, abandon plans for extubation

    C. Order a chest x-ray to assess the lungs

    D. Place the patient on intermittent mechanical ventilation mode, contact the physician

8. An intubated patient is being turned by two nurses. When questioned if he is comfortable, the patient responds "yes" audibly. Which of the following interventions is indicated at this time?

    A. Order a chest x-ray to confirm placement of the endotracheal tube

    B. Turn the patient on their back and elevate the head of the bed

    C. Follow protocol to remove air from the cuff and reinflate

    D. Inflate the cuff to the needed volume

9. A patient is in the ICU status post left thoracotomy 1 hour ago. The surgeon removed the left middle lobe of the lung. There are two chest tubes in place to –20 mmHg of suction. As the nurse enters the room to assess, it is noted both chest tubes have 15 mL of serosanguinous fluid in each. What is the primary reason for the chest tubes?

    A. To remove pleural fluid from the cavity

    B. To maintain negative pleural pressure

    C. To increase the ventilation of the lung

    D. To increase the regrowth of the pleural cavity

GO ON TO NEXT PAGE ➤

10. A 68-year-old Caucasian female arrives at the emergency department due to a witnessed fall at home by her husband. He states after he called 911 she regained consciousness and was complaining of shortness of breath. Mrs. Avanti is diagnosed with an acute exacerbation of COPD (acute on chronic) and given a bronchodilator. She is transferred to the ICU for close monitoring. Given the above case, which of the following ABGs would be expected?

    A. pH = 7.30, $PaCO_2$ = 30, HCO_3 = 30, PaO_2 = 60
    B. pH = 7.29, $PaCO_2$ = 60, HCO_3 = 32, PaO_2 = 37
    C. pH = 7.55, $PaCO_2$ = 25, HCO_3 = 38, PaO_2 = 50
    D. pH = 7.35, $PaCO_2$ = 40, HCO_3 = 24, PaO_2 = 75

11. A 32-year-old patient with cystic fibrosis is hypoxic and in respiratory distress. The current pulse ox is 78%. Taking the correlation between PaO_2 and SpO_2, at what crucial PaO_2 point does severe desaturation occur?

    A. PaO_2 = 40 mmHg
    B. PaO_2 = 50 mmHg
    C. PaO_2 = 60 mmHg
    D. PaO_2 = 80 mmHg

12. A 40-year-old female was admitted to the ICU from the OR 3 days ago. A hysterectomy was performed after a diagnosis of uterine cancer. The patient remained intubated due to bleeding and difficulty weaning off the ventilator. Monitor alarms go off indicating HR 150, BP 160/80, and SpO_2 88%. As the nurse enters the room, the patient is clearly agitated and dyspneic. The ventilator is showing a high-pressure alarm. What is the likely cause of the patient's current condition?

    A. Pulmonary embolism
    B. Pulmonary edema
    C. Pneumothorax
    D. Uterine rupture with hemorrhage

13. A 55-year-old patient is suspected of having pulmonary embolism. The nurse is bedside assessing the situation. The PE is suspected to be caused by a DVT. Which of the following signs and symptoms correlate to PE injury?

    A. Pulseless electrical activity and/or cardiac arrest
    B. Pulmonary artery pressure 18/8 mmHg, petechiae
    C. Normal V/Q, hypoxemia
    D. Audible S_1 and S_2 heart tones

14. A 65-year-old patient is suspected of having pulmonary embolism. She is dyspneic with hypoxemia; she is 2 hours postoperative. Which of the following diagnostic assessments would confirm PE and which treatment would be ordered?

    A. CT pulmonary angiography: heparin
    B. V/Q scan: tPA
    C. Blood cultures: antibiotics
    D. Chest XR: increase oxygen

15. When a patient is experiencing a pulmonary embolism, what best explains why hypoxia occurs?

    A. The clot blocks air flow through the alveoli decreasing ventilation and oxygenation
    B. The clot blocks blood flow and causes increased pressure on the right side of the heart
    C. The clot blocks air flow through the alveoli causing a V/Q mismatch
    D. The clot blocks blood flow through capillaries creating increased alveolar dead space

16. When administering heparin infusion for a patient with pulmonary embolism, which of the following findings would warrant immediate discontinuation of the infusion?

    A. aPTT of 70 seconds
    B. Development of fever
    C. Platelet count of 55,000
    D. Hemoglobin 8.5 g/dL

17. A 24-year-old male patient is admitted to the emergency room with an asthma exacerbation. He is visibly anxious and in respiratory distress. Which of the following signs and symptoms is not seen in early asthma exacerbations?

    A. $PaCO_2$ 55 mmHg
    B. PaO_2 55%
    C. Audible wheezing
    D. Mental status changes

18. A 55-year-old patient is suspected of having pulmonary edema. The patient is intubated on assist control mode. Increased edema has been noted over the past 24 hours with decreasing urine output. Which of the following would be an early finding of pulmonary edema?

    A. Hypercapnia

    B. Decreased static compliance

    C. Increased dynamic compliance

    D. Right-sided heart failure

19. A patient with an internal jugular central line no longer needs the IV access. There is an order to remove the central line. During removal the patient is placed commonly supine with the head down slightly. What is the most important reason for this position?

    A. Prevention of blood pooling in the neck vessels

    B. Prevention of air rushing into the artery

    C. Prevention of carotid artery damage during removal

    D. Prevention of bacterial exposure to the central line site

20. A 22-year-old patient is admitted to the medical ICU with a diagnosis of DKA. Current serum glucose is 230 mg/dL down from 300 mg/dL 1 hour ago, potassium 4.2 mEq/L, and pH 7.30. Which of the following actions is appropriate at this time?

    A. Administer bicarbonate to achieve a pH above 7.35

    B. Titrate up (increase) on the insulin drip

    C. Switch to dextrose IV infusion with mEQs of potassium

    D. Continue normal saline infusion, add potassium

21. A patient with recent surgery on the brain develops increased urine output from baseline. The previous 2 hours of urine output are 150 mL and 200 mL, respectively. Upon urinalysis testing of the urine, specific gravity is found to be 1.004. Vital signs are stable. When assessing osmolality or the urine and serum, which of the following would the nurse expect?

    A. Increased serum osmolality, increased urine osmolality

    B. Increased serum osmolality, decreased urine osmolality

    C. Decreased serum osmolality, increased urine osmolality

    D. Decreased serum osmolality, decreased urine osmolality

22. Which of the following ABG and anion gap analysis is seen in diabetic ketoacidosis?

    A. pH 7.21, $PaCO_2$ 65, HCO_3 20, anion gap 12
    B. pH 7.30, $PaCO_2$ 45, HCO_3 22, anion gap 8
    C. pH 7.55, $PaCO_2$ 25, HCO_3 24, anion gap 10
    D. pH 7.21, $PaCO_2$ 42, HCO_3 13, anion gap 16

23. A critically ill patient in the ICU has been unable to tolerate enteral feedings, and parenteral nutrition has been ordered with secondary lipid administration. TPN began at 1400 via a subclavian central line. Two hours have passed. Based on the below findings, which of the following is the most appropriate at this time?

1400	1600
HR =110	HR – 115
BP = 95/60 mmHg	BP = 100/55 mmHg
SpO_2 = 94%	SpO_2 = 93%
Urine output = 40 mL/hr	Urine output = 100 mL/hr

    A. Discontinue the TPN, contact the physician
    B. Assess serum glucose
    C. Assess central line insertion site for signs of infection
    D. Assess urinalysis, serum sodium and osmolality

24. A 78-year-old female diabetic (Type 2) patient is admitted to the ICU with a diagnosis of HHS. She has neglected to take her insulin over the past few days due to not feeling well with flu-like symptoms. She is currently stuporous but does respond to pain. Given the current vital signs and laboratory findings below, what is the priority treatment at this time?

VITAL SIGNS	LABORATORY VALUES (SERUM)
HR = 120	Glucose = 410 mg/dL
BP = 90/60 mmHg	pH = 7.20
RR = 30 breaths/min	Potassium = 4.2 mEq/L
SpO_2 = 94%	Osmolality = 340 mOsm/kg
Temp = 100.2°F	

    A. Administer infusion of crystalloids, include potassium mEq/L
    B. Assess anion gap and administer bicarbonate
    C. Prepare to intubate the patient and mechanically ventilate
    D. Begin norepinephrine and maintain MAP greater than 60 mmHg

GO ON TO NEXT PAGE ➤

25. A 22-year-old patient arrives at the trauma bay of the emergency department with multiple traumatic injuries. Paramedics estimate 2–3 L of blood loss in the field and continues to bleed. The physician immediately activates massive transfusion protocol. After administering more than 10 units of PRBCs to the patient, which of the following considerations are appropriate at this time?

    A. Administer platelets and fresh frozen plasma

    B. Assess for loss of deep tendon reflexes and muscle weakness

    C. Consider the effects of a right shift in the oxyhemoglobin dissociation curve

    D. Administer potassium and electrolytes

26. A patient has recently been starting on continuous heparin infusion as treatment for a pulmonary embolism. Which of the following would be early clinical signs of complication due to the infusion?

    A. Bleeding from IV sites

    B. Changes in levels of consciousness

    C. Petechiae or purpura

    D. Bright red stool or melena

27. A 60-year-old male patient was admitted to the ICU 3 days ago with a diagnosis of sepsis. 24 hours after admission, the blood pressure begins to decrease requiring vasopressors. The patient presently is on norepinephrine infusion and vasopressin infusion for blood pressure maintenance. The nurse walks in for morning assessment and notices blood seeping from the IV sites and the patient's nose. The nurse is considering specific laboratory tests to confirm disseminated intravascular coagulation. Which of the following would confirm DIC in this patient?

    A. Decreased fibrinogen, increased fibrinogen split products, increased platelets, increased coagulation times, increased D-dimer

    B. Decreased fibrinogen, decreased fibrinogen split products, decreased platelets, increased coagulation times, decreased D-dimer

    C. Increased fibrinogen, increased fibrinogen split products, decreased platelets, decreased coagulation times, decreased D-dimer

    D. Decreased fibrinogen, increased fibrinogen split products, decreased platelets, increased coagulation times, increased D-dimer

28. A 21-year-old was recently admitted to the emergency room after an injury sustained during football. The patient was hit very hard, landed on his back, and immediately reported pain in his upper left quadrant. Upon assessment in the ER, pain was also noted to the left shoulder, bruising around the umbilicus, and a positive Kehr's sign. Current vital signs include BP 90/60 mmHg, HR 125, RR 25 and shallow. What is the most likely explanation for the current set of signs and symptoms?

    A. Ruptured spleen
    B. Musculoskeletal injury to the shoulder
    C. Retroperitoneal bleeding
    D. Septic shock

29. A 20-year-old female was admitted to the ICU after sustaining a blunt injury to the abdomen. Two hours after admission the patient complains of severe diffuse abdominal pain. She is visibly diaphoretic and pale. Current vital signs include BP 85/60, HR 135, RR 30, and temp 101.3°F. What is the priority action for the nurse at this time?

    A. Contact the physician and prepare for emergency surgery
    B. Administer vasopressors and inotropic agents
    C. Assess urine output and urine characteristics
    D. Order an immediate abdominal CT (KUB)

30. Which of the following positions will assist a patient with appendicitis in decreasing the amount of pain they are experiencing?

    A. Supine with the head slightly elevated
    B. Side lying on the right or flat with legs flexed
    C. Side lying on the left or flat with legs flexed
    D. Prone or sims position

31. While caring for a chronic alcoholic with ulcer rupture and bleeding, the nurse is considering the best intravenous fluid for this patient. Which of the following IV fluids is indicated for this patient at this time?

    A. 5% dextrose
    B. Albumin and other colloids
    C. Normal saline
    D. Hypertonic saline

32. A patient with a history of cholelithiasis is admitted to the emergency department with biliary obstruction. The patient complains of epigastric pain for the past week that worsens upon eating. Which of the following diagnostic or laboratory tests would be performed first to aid in diagnosis?

    A. Colonoscopy
    B. Amylase and lipase levels
    C. Arterial blood gases
    D. Endoscopic retrograde cholangiopancreatography (ERCP)

33. An 18-year-old patient is admitted to the ICU after surgical exploration and removal of two bullets. Two hours after admission the patient begins to actively bleed. Which of the following indicates physiological compensation in response to this shock?

    A. Decreased activation of RAAS system, tachycardia, tachypnea
    B. Vasodilation, third spacing of fluid, increased ventilation
    C. Adrenal suppression, tachycardia, dilated pupils
    D. Increased activation of RAAS system, tachycardia, tachypnea

34. Which of the following is the priority consideration for a patient with portal hypertension secondary to liver cirrhosis?

    A. Hematemesis
    B. Hepatic encephalopathy
    C. Aspiration
    D. Third spacing of fluid

35. A patient is admitted to the ICU with a diagnosis of intestinal obstruction of the small intestine. The patient has been vomiting since admission 2 hours ago. The nurse has administered ondansetron and metoclopramide with no relief. Which of the following treatments should be performed at this time?

    A. IV fluids and electrolyte replacements
    B. Mineral oil enemas
    C. Emergency laparotomy
    D. Broad-spectrum antibiotics

36. A patient with chronic kidney disease develops hyperphosphatemia to 6.8 mg/dL. What is the importance in managing elevated phosphorus in patients with CKD?

    A. Prevention of hypomagnesemia
    B. Prevention of hypocalcemia
    C. Prevention of hypokalemia
    D. Prevention of hyponatremia

37. A 32-year-old patient in the ICU is being treated for septic shock with fluids and vasopressors. The patient is also being treated for a pre-renal acute kidney injury (AKI). What is a known risk factor after prolonged decreased perfusion to the kidneys?

   A. Polycythemia vera
   B. Acute interstitial nephritis
   C. Acute tubular necrosis
   D. Goodpasture syndrome

38. A 32-year-old female patient is receiving magnesium sulfate to prevent the progression of preeclampsia. She develops decreased deep tendon reflexes. What treatment plan is indicated at this time?

   A. Administer furosemide IV
   B. Prepare for emergency dialysis
   C. Administer calcium gluconate IV
   D. Prepare for emergency c-section

39. A 45-year-old chronic kidney disease patient is currently receiving hemodialysis (HD) via a fistula in the arm. Fifteen minutes into the treatment the patient experiences a run of ventricular tachycardia 20 seconds long. Immediate analysis reveals a potassium of 7.5 mEq/L. Which treatment is most appropriate at this time?

   A. Hemodialysis
   B. Regular insulin and D50 intravenous
   C. Sodium polystyrene sulfonate
   D. Furosemide IV

40. A pre-renal AKI patient is undergoing IV fluid hydration. Current labs include creatinine 1.8 mg/dL, BUN 30 mg/dL. What is the best indicator for resolution of the kidney injury?

   A. Increased patient weight
   B. Creatinine 1.6 mg/dL, BUN 28 mg/dL
   C. Urine output 0.5 kg/mL/hr
   D. Potassium 4.5 mEq/L

41. Hematuria is witnessed in a female patient admitted after blunt trauma to the abdomen. The patient complains of lower abdominal pain after voiding. What is the most likely injury she is experiencing?

   A. Bladder
   B. Kidneys
   C. Urethra
   D. Uterus

GO ON TO NEXT PAGE ➤

42. A 78-year-old dementia patient was brought to the emergency room after changes in mental status and levels of consciousness were witnessed by the spouse. It was later determined that the patient has been drinking unusually large amounts of water lately. Based upon the laboratory findings below, what is the best course of treatment at this time?

LABORATORY FINDINGS

Na = 115 mEq/L
Cl = 85 mEq/L
K = 3.6 mEq/L
Creatinine = 1.5 mg/dL
BUN = 20 mg/dL

A. Restrict fluids to 1500 mL per day
B. Administer furosemide IV
C. Administer 0.45 saline
D. Administer 3% saline

43. A cardiac patient is receiving lisinopril for management of hypertension. The physician is considering ordering triamterene to add to current treatment. Which of the following electrolyte imbalances is possible with this combination of medications?

A. Hyperphosphatemia
B. Hypercalcemia
C. Hyponatremia
D. Hyperkalemia

44. A patient with a surgical wound on the left hand has received dressing changes for the past 7 days, but the wound does not appear to be healing. The wound now appears purulent and erythemic. What is a secondary cause for inhibition in the healing of this wound?

A. Poor perfusion to the wound site
B. Poor carbohydrate intake
C. Incorrect dressings being utilized
D. Biofilm has not been removed from the wound

45. An 85-year-old female was admitted to the ICU due to a severely infected pressure ulcer of the coccyx. Upon assessment of the ulcer, the nurse notes the skin is not intact and yellowish tissue is exposed. What stage is this deep tissue injury (DTI)?

    A. Stage 1
    B. Stage 2
    C. Stage 3
    D. Stage 4

46. A patient in shock is receiving dopamine intravenously until central access can be obtained. The nurse suspects the IV has infiltrated. Which of the following would the nurse perform first?

    A. Stop the infusion and apply a warm compress
    B. Stop the infusion and maintain the IV
    C. Flush the IV and assess for signs of infiltration
    D. Obtain phentolamine and administer immediately

47. A 45-year-old patient diagnosed with COVID-19 has been intubated and sedated for 2 weeks. Which of the following functional issues would be found with this long-standing immobility?

    A. Reduced muscle mass, myelopathy
    B. Poor oxygenation and ventilation
    C. Muscle wasting, osteopenia
    D. Hypoglycemia, increased cardiac ejection fraction

48. A 65-year-old male patient was discharged home 5 days ago after a left knee replacement surgery. He arrives back to the emergency department with dull pain of the left knee, erythema, and a fever. Given current immunosuppression of the patient, the orthopedic surgeon is taking the patient back to the operating room to explore the surgical area. What is the main reason for this return to the OR?

    A. Removal of synovial fluid from the joint
    B. Removal and redo of the hardware
    C. Debridement and washout with antibiotics
    D. Removal of necrotic tissue

49. A patient was admitted 3 days ago due to multiple crush injuries incurred from a motor vehicle accident. This morning the patient becomes oliguric with tea-colored urine; the nurse suspects rhabdomyolysis. Which of the following treatments should begin immediately?

    A. Fluid resuscitation, spironolactone, antibiotics

    B. Fluid restriction, furosemide, telemetry

    C. Fluid restriction, calcium gluconate, corticosteroids

    D. Fluid resuscitation, mannitol, telemetry

50. A patient is admitted to the neuro ICU after right-sided ischemic stroke and administration of tPA. What is the best timeframe where tPA may be administered after the onset of symptoms?

    A. 60 minutes

    B. 120 minutes

    C. 3 hours

    D. 5 hours

51. A 74-year-old patient is admitted to the ICU after return of spontaneous circulation (ROSC) 15 minutes into the code. Hours later the patient becomes somnolent and difficult to arouse. The nurse notices the pupils are sluggish and poorly accommodate. They are equal in size at this time. What is the most likely explanation for the current deterioration in the patient?

    A. Vasogenic cerebral edema post cardiac arrest

    B. Cytotoxic cerebral edema post cardiac arrest

    C. Increased permeability of the blood–brain barrier leading to edema

    D. Increased osmosis and movement of water due to abnormal osmotic gradients

52. A 32-year-old male arrives at the emergency department after police were called to a bar fight. The patient was struck on the side of the head with a beer bottle. He fell to the ground and briefly lost consciousness according to bystanders. A half an hour after admission to the ED, the patient began speaking incoherently. The left pupil becomes dilated and nonreactive. What part of the brain is likely injured based on these signs?

    A. Left hemisphere

    B. Right temporal lobe

    C. Occipital lobe

    D. Brain stem

53. The daughter of a loved one admitted for a hemorrhagic stroke has many questions regarding the diagnosis. They approach the nurse and ask why the patient has not received tPA; they remember another family member receiving it 3 years prior. What is the best response to give to the family member regarding the diagnosis?

    A. "Tissue plasminogen activator is administered within 4 hours of the onset of symptoms"

    B. "Your father experienced a hemorrhagic or bleeding stroke; giving tPA would worsen the bleeding"

    C. "Your father had a surgery 2 years ago and is ineligible for tPA"

    D. "The neurologist decided not to administer tPA"

54. A 65-year-old patient is recovering in the ICU after a left-sided stroke. Which of the following cranial nerves is crucial to test before administering food or medications PO to the patient?

    A. IX, X, XII

    B. III, IV, V

    C. I, IV, VI

    D. VII, VIII

55. A 22-year-old patient is admitted to the emergency department with suspicions of bacterial meningitis. The patient has nuchal rigidity, fever, and petechiae. Which of the following tests would best confirm the presence of bacterial meningitis?

    A. Blood cultures

    B. Urinalysis—assess for protein in the urine

    C. Kernig's sign

    D. Lumbar puncture

56. A nurse is caring for a 35-year-old trauma patient who was admitted for close monitoring of neuro status. CT of the head displays a left epidural hematoma. The neurosurgeon placed an ICP monitor upon admission, but the nurse suspects it may be clotted. Which of the following, instead of the ICP monitor, would alert the nurse to possible uncal herniation?

    A. Anisocoria of the left pupil

    B. Hemiplegia of the left lower extremities

    C. Breathing irregularities

    D. Tachycardia with dysrhythmias

GO ON TO NEXT PAGE ➤

57. A patient with a subarachnoid hemorrhage secondary to aneurysm rupture develops new-onset headache, blurred vision, and headache 4 days after the aneurysm rupture. The healthcare team suspects vasospasms. Which of the following diagnostic tests might aid in diagnosis and what treatment should be performed?

    A. Angiography, nicardipine IV

    B. Transcranial Doppler, labetalol IV

    C. Head CT, mannitol IV

    D. Chemistry panel, replete electrolytes

58. When caring for a patient with increased intracranial pressure (ICP), which of the following would not benefit the patient in ICP maintenance?

    A. Performing suctioning PRN instead of every 2 hours

    B. Repositioning and administering medications at the same time

    C. Placing the head to the left with the head of the bed in high-Fowler's

    D. Changing alarm parameters safely to remove incessant noise

59. A patient arrives at the emergency department after closed injury to the head from a motor vehicle accident. The patient is unresponsive, is positioned with extremities extended, and has arms hyperpronated. Which of the following does this patient presentation display?

    A. Seizure activity

    B. Decorticate posturing

    C. Decerebrate posturing

    D. Central brain herniation

60. A patient is visibly agitated and speaking to the light in the ceiling; the nurse suspects auditory hallucinations. Which of the following responses for the nurse to the patient is best?

    A. Explain to the patient the need to ground themselves in reality to prevent working themselves up with agitation

    B. Explain to the patient the nurse understands that they are hearing these things, but the nurse does not

    C. Explain to the patient the need to calm down or the nurse will have to calm them down

    D. Explain to the patient the hallucinations are not helpful and should be ignored

61. A violent patient is threatening the nurse with bodily harm. Which of the following does not help in maintaining the safety of the nurse?

    A. Maintain security presence if touching the patient is necessary
    B. Be aware of the exits and place yourself between the patient and the door
    C. Never provide care alone or without help
    D. De-escalate situations with "yes" or "no" questions

62. An intubated patient is in the ICU due to alcohol overdose and severe concussion. It is now 48 hours after admission and the patient is exhibiting signs of agitation. Which of the following would the nurse perform first?

    A. Initiate CIWA protocol; administer lorazepam
    B. Assess for increased intracranial pressure, notify the physician
    C. Increase the sedation to maintain appropriate RASS score
    D. Assess the patient's respiratory status, consider extubation

63. A 35-year-old patient is admitted to the ICU after ingestion of 45 lorazepam pills. They have a history of manic depression. The family states the patient has become increasingly manic over the past day. Which of the following would the nurse associate with a manic episode?

    A. Low or depressed mood
    B. Anhedonia
    C. Decreased need for sleep
    D. Fatigue and loss of energy

64. A patient newly diagnosed with generalized anxiety disorder complains of chronic dry mouth. What is the best explanation for this symptom?

    A. Sympathetic nervous system stimulation inhibits the release of secretions
    B. Parasympathetic nervous system stimulation results from chronic stress and anxiety; this decreases secretions
    C. Cholinergic agonist effects during states of "fight or flight" cause dry mouth
    D. Xerostomia is the likely side effect of a medication

65. A trauma patient arrives at the emergency department after being struck by a car while riding a bike. The patient has multiple obvious injuries. As the nurse assesses, which of the following requires priority intervention?

    A. Pain during inhalation and exhalation
    B. Nonintact wound on the left lower extremity
    C. Open fracture of the left radius
    D. Stridor and increased heart rate

66. A 56-year-old male patient was admitted to the neuro ICU with a diagnosis of neurogenic shock. The patient received a 1 L bolus of normal saline in the ED. Current vital signs and ABG results are below. The nurse administers atropine and dobutamine as ordered. Which of the following is the best indicator of improvement for this patient?

VITAL SIGNS	ABG RESULTS
HR = 45 beats per minute	pH = 7.30
RR = 30 breaths per minute	$PaCO_2$ = 55 mmHg
BP = 85/50 mmHg	HCO_3 = 22 mEq/L
Temp = 39°C	PaO_2 = 60 mmHg
SpO_2 = 87%	

   A. Increase in cardiac output and cardiac index
   B. Urine output 0.5 mL/kg/hr
   C. Decrease in serum lactate
   D. Increase in PaO_2

67. Blood loss has occurred secondary to trauma of the femoral artery. The bleeding was temporized by the physician on duty. Which of the following signs and symptoms would the nurse not early and is associated with minimal blood loss estimated at 10%?

   A. BP 90/60 mmHg
   B. Narrowing pulse pressure
   C. HR 110
   D. Anxiety or agitation

68. A patient in shock has received more than 4 L NS. Current ABG displays pH 7.28, $PaCO_2$ 40 mmHg, HCO_3 16, PaO_2 88%, anion gap 10. The physician orders a switch to lactated Ringer's if further boluses are required. What is the best explanation for using LR over NS in this case?

   A. Hyperchloremic acidosis has developed due to hyposmolality of the blood from normal saline
   B. Hyperchloremic acidosis has developed due to excessive normal saline administration
   C. Metabolic acidosis may be corrected over time with lactated Ringer's solution
   D. Lactated Ringer's will replete electrolyte imbalances whereas normal saline will not

69. A 68-year-old patient is receiving targeted temperature therapy after cardiac arrest in the emergency department. At 0700 the nurse begins rewarming per protocol. At 0800 and 0900 the nurse assesses progress. Which of the following is the most concerning during rewarming of this patient?

0700	0800	0900
HR = 55	HR = 65	HR = 75
RR = 10	RR = 12	RR = 16
BP = 95/70 mmHg	BP = 100/70 mmHg	BP = 100/80 mmHg
Temp = 33°C	Temp = 34.5°C	Temp = 37°C

    A. Heart rate

    B. Respiratory rate

    C. Blood pressure

    D. Temperature

70. Four hours ago, an unconscious patient was brought into the emergency department with suspected overdose of acetaminophen. An empty bottle was found by the patient at the scene. Which of the following would be immediately indicated?

    A. Insert an NG tube and administer acetylcysteine

    B. Draw blood for serum lab tests

    C. Perform gastric lavage with activated charcoal

    D. Intubate the patient and mechanically ventilate

71. A medical ICU patient was diagnosed with septic shock after positive blood cultures and severe hypotension. Which of the following signs is also present in septic shock?

    A. Cardiac output 4 L/min

    B. Central venous pressure 2 mmHg

    C. 480 dynes/sec/cm^5

    D. SvO_2 55%

72. A 70 kg patient with septic shock received two boluses of isotonic crystalloids (1 liter per bolus). Hypotension continues with increasing serum lactate. Which of the following is the first-line agent for refractory hypotension in this case?

    A. Dobutamine

    B. Norepinephrine

    C. Vasopressin

    D. Phenylephrine

GO ON TO NEXT PAGE ➤

73. A woman with hyperemesis gravidarum is admitted due to severe volume loss. Which of the following diagnostic tests is indicative of hypovolemic shock due to hyperemesis?

    A. Serum osmolality 350 mOsm/kg

    B. SVR 600 dynes/sec/cm^5

    C. Urine specific gravity 1.005

    D. Serum potassium 2.8 mEq/L

74. A patient arrives at the emergency department with swollen lips and eyes. The patient states they got stung by a bee an hour ago and they are severely allergic. The patient's speech is difficult to understand and audibly hoarse. Which medication should be given first in this case?

    A. Epinephrine IV

    B. Diphenhydramine IV

    C. Fexofenadine PO

    D. Epinephrine IM

75. A 32-year-old patient is admitted with a suspected overdose of amitriptyline. What important factor should be assessed frequently in the plan of care for this patient?

    A. Cholinergic agonist symptoms

    B. Telemetry and monitoring of dysrhythmias

    C. Assessment of tachypnea

    D. CNS stimulation

76. The nurse suspects cocaine ingestion by a recently admitted patient with angina. What additional symptom of CNS stimulation would the nurse expect to see with cocaine use?

    A. Diplopia

    B. Irritability

    C. Increased urine output

    D. Excessive sleepiness

77. A 34-year-old female was admitted to the ICU due to postpartum hemorrhage. Which of the following is not a risk factor for postpartum hemorrhage?

    A. Induction of labor with oxytocin

    B. Birth of triplets

    C. Labor lasting 2 hours

    D. Large for gestational age fetus

78. A 200 kg patient is approved for admission to the ICU. They have a number of problems in the ED that will need to be addressed once admitted. Which of the following factors would be most important to prepare for first?

    A. SpO_2 91%
    B. Serum glucose 320 mg/dL
    C. Nausea and gastric reflux
    D. BP 150/90 mmHg, previous history of coronary stents

79. A patient is admitted with carbon monoxide poisoning after attempted suicide. What is the leading cause of death in carbon monoxide poisoning?

    A. Hypocapnia
    B. Shock
    C. Hypoxia
    D. Respiratory acidosis

80. Which of the following hematological dysfunctions is not seen in multiple system organ dysfunction?

    A. Platelet count 100,000
    B. Elevated D-dimer
    C. Decreased serum protein-C
    D. INR 1.2 seconds

81. A patient in shock is admitted to the ICU for close management. Current continuous medications include norepinephrine, vasopressin, and phenylephrine. Which of the following signs and symptoms may indicate a complication of the treatment?

    A. Abdominal angina
    B. Peripheral capillary refill less than 3 seconds
    C. Laryngeal edema
    D. Elevated liver enzymes

82. A patient in the ICU has traumatic brain injury with likely herniation. The physician declares brain death. The patient is not eligible for donation; however, the healthcare team has spoken to the family about withdrawing care. It is important to collaborate with disciplines like social services and pastoral care for what reason?

    A. Support the family through the grieving process
    B. Time is better utilized for the nurse to provide palliative care
    C. Explaining the dying process is important to prioritize
    D. Support the healthcare team in patient care decisions

GO ON TO NEXT PAGE ➤

83. A patient in multiple system organ dysfunction is not expected to survive. Organ donation remains a possibility for some of the organs. When the family arrives, they have multiple questions regarding the care of their loved one. Which of the following is most sympathetic to this situation?

    A. Bring the family into the patient room to explain current care and donation

    B. Page pastoral care to come speak to the family

    C. Assess which organs are still functioning and eligible for donation

    D. Guide the family to a private meeting area to speak with the healthcare team

84. Prior to taking a person to a preoperative area, they express some uncertainty about the surgery itself. They appear uncertain about what is going to be done in the operating room. What action should be performed by the nurse at this time?

    A. Contact the charge nurse and express the need to keep the patient on the unit

    B. Contact the physician to come provide additional explanation

    C. Continue to process moving the patient to pre-op and explain any worries the patient may have

    D. Keep the patient on the unit and notify the operating room of the delay

85. A 65-year-old patient is in the ICU when alarms sound; the patient is in ventricular fibrillation. As the nurse walks into the room to begin CPR, the wife is bedside and asks what is going on. What is the best intervention at this time?

    A. Begin CPR and instruct a fellow nurse to explain the situation to the wife

    B. Insist the wife leave the room and speak to someone at the nurses' station

    C. Contact pastoral services to come speak to the wife

    D. Leave the room to locate the physician

86. A sentinel event occurred that resulted in serious patient harm and disability. Which of the following mistakes at the time may open up the nurse to potential lawsuits and litigation?

    A. Failure to anticipate the problem ahead of time

    B. Failure to notify the nurse manager after the incident

    C. Failure to accurately document the situation

    D. Failure to call the family after the incident

87. A 26-year-old patient is in the ICU after a ruptured appendix. The nurse is assessing current pain level. The patient states their pain as 0/10. The face, however, is grimacing. What is an appropriate action by the nurse at this time?

A. Leave the room and reassess the pain in 2 hours

B. Provide privacy to the patient and document pain 0/10

C. Ask the patient to describe what they are feeling reflected in the grimacing

D. Administer pain medications as ordered for moderate pain

88. A patient in the emergency room has a cardiac arrest. Return of spontaneous circulation is achieved after 15 minutes. The patient requires emergency surgery. There is no family at the hospital at this time. How should the nurse proceed in this situation?

A. Contact the family, explain the situation, and request their presence at the hospital

B. Have the physician sign the consent given the emergent nature, contact the family after

C. Wait on the surgery until the family arrives to the hospital

D. Have another nurse contact the family while the primary nurse prepares for surgery

89. The nurse is caring for a patient of foreign descent. Upon assessing, the nurse notes a lack of eye contact when explaining a simple procedure. The patient also recoils when touched to obtain a blood pressure. It states in the chart the patient speaks English. What is an appropriate action by this nurse when interacting with the patient?

A. Ask the patient to confirm understanding with eye contact, document understanding with a nod

B. Have another nurse or nursing assistant obtain the vital signs, ask if the patient responded to English

C. Continue to explain actions in English allowing for no eye contact, ask the patient permission before placing the BP cuff

D. Ask the patient about their heritage and how they would like you to proceed

GO ON TO NEXT PAGE ➤

90. A patient with a severe respiratory infection does not want to be intubated. They sign a DNI order to this effect. The family later finds out and pleads with the healthcare team to intubate the patient and save her life. What is an appropriate intervention at this time?

    A. Revoke the do not intubate order and proceed to follow family wishes

    B. Collaborate with the healthcare team to provide a conference with the family

    C. Contact the physician about intubating the patient

    D. Explain to the family the patient will not be intubated under any circumstance

91. A patient is discussing with the nurse feelings of inadequacy with sex after recovery from a heart attack. The patient describes difficulty managing slight chest pain during sex. What advice would the nurse provide to this patient?

    A. Explain that a nitroglycerin patch may be applied before sex to minimize angina

    B. Instruct the patient to avoid sex and contact his physician

    C. Ask the patient to bring his wife in to discuss his feelings of inadequacy

    D. Tell the patient he should get used to the problem as it likely will not go away

92. A patient in the ICU has recently passed. The family is bedside crying. Which action by the nurse aids in the families coping of the loss?

    A. Speak with the family about the causes of death

    B. Ask the family if they desire the chaplain at this time

    C. Encourage the family to leave the room so the nurse may prepare the body

    D. Allow the family to participate in post-mortem care of the patient

93. An 18-year-old male arrives at the trauma bay of the emergency room with multiple visible traumas. The patient is unconscious. His mother arrives at the ER visibly distraught. Which of the following is not an appropriate intervention in caring for the mother?

    A. Require a registered nurse to speak with the mother for a quick update on the situation

    B. Escort the mother to a private room by the primary nurse, provide an update

    C. Have the physician take the mother aside for privacy and explain the situation

    D. Have the nursing assistant take the mother to a private room and explain the nurse will be with them shortly

94. When caring for a brain-dead patient eligible for organ donation, which of the following statements is true regarding appropriate interventions?

    A. Allow the organ transplant coordinator to speak with the family regarding donation
    B. The nurse should speak with the family regarding patient wishes
    C. Allow the situation to progress naturally, do not influence
    D. Contact the legal power of attorney to make a decision about organ donation

95. A patient is expressing aggravation at the constant alarms and interruptions of patient care activities in the ICU. How would the nurse best rectify these issues for the patient?

    A. Turn off the offending alarms and cancel inappropriate orders
    B. Analyze the specific alarms and care activities to see what can be changed or clustered
    C. Wait until the patient is agreeable to perform patient care activities
    D. Place a sign on the door to stop alternate healthcare workers from entering

96. The husband of a terminally ill patient is providing some water orally. The nurse notices the patient's inability to swallow as water is dribbling out of the mouth. The husband insists that his spouse is thirsty. Which action by the nurse is appropriate?

    A. Offer the husband sponges that may be used to administer water to the mouth
    B. Tell the husband the patient is unable to drink at this time
    C. Remove the water from the room and switch to intravenous hydration
    D. Continue to allow the husband to give water

97. A nurse is caring for a critical patient with a same-sex partner. There are healthcare workers on the unit who are refusing to acknowledge the partner and vocalize their preference to care for other patients. Which of the following actions of caring is appropriate?

    A. Apologize to the patient and partner for the behavior of the healthcare workers
    B. Speak with the nurse manager about forming a conference between healthcare workers
    C. Instruct the charge nurse to avoid assigning the patient to other nurses who voiced disapproval
    D. Take responsibility and care for the patient yourself whenever possible

98. A patient admitted to the ICU for meningitis disclosed to the nurse he is HIV positive. Several family members call inquiring about the patient's personal lifestyle and behavior. How does the nurse proceed?

    A. Speak with the family about risk factors that may have led to contraction of meningitis

    B. Instruct the family to obtain meningitis vaccines

    C. Disclose the diagnosis of the patient and comorbidity of HIV

    D. Do not disclose personal information about the patient to the family

99. Over the period of the previous 2 weeks, the nurse has noted a deterioration of teamwork among the healthcare workers. It is unknown what has led to this issue. What is the most appropriate intervention at this time?

    A. Speak with the nurse manager about forming rounding on the patients with all specialties present

    B. Instruct the ancillary services (social services, dietary) to bring the information directly to the nurses

    C. Ask the physicians to speak with all disciplines about the issues with teamwork

    D. File a complaint with the nursing supervisor, express concern for patient safety

100. A patient was recently admitted to the hospital. They are fearful of the prognosis. Which of the following is an example of nursing veracity?

    A. Allowing the patient to guide care decisions

    B. Collaborating with the physician to bring all the facts to the patient

    C. Providing care in a manner that will not harm the patient

    D. Researching a care activity to administer it to the best of one's ability

101. A 23-year-old male Jehovah's witness is critically ill in the ICU. The physicians have repeatedly explained the dire need of blood to the patient, but the patient and parents refuse. It has been instructed to give blood the moment the patient loses consciousness. What action by the nurse provides the most culturally competent care?

    A. Explain to the healthcare staff that the family understands the severity of the illness, but they remain against blood transfusion

    B. Obtain the supplies and allow for the transfusion of blood when the patient loses consciousness

    C. Contact the ethics committee to become involved

    D. Ask the parents about the reasoning behind the refusal for blood

102. A 75-year-old female patient with a do-not-resuscitate order goes into cardiac arrest with the family bedside. They order you to begin CPR and save their mother. What is the appropriate action?

    A. Initiate CPR as wished by the family
    B. Do not perform CPR
    C. Call the physician and inquire on what to do
    D. Revoke the DNR order in the medical record

103. A patient with mental illness is frequently admitted to the hospital due to lack of medication adherence. The patient is receptive to speaking about the issue. What is the best action for the nurse to proceed?

    A. Explain what happens to the patient when they do not take the medication
    B. Coordinate with the patient, pharmacy, and healthcare staff on creating a system of accountability in taking the medication
    C. Call the case manager assigned to the patient on how they would like to proceed
    D. Contact the patient's friends and family to inquire the reasons for nonadherence

104. An 85-year-old patient with sepsis is on norepinephrine for blood pressure maintenance. Twenty-four hours after initiation of the therapy, the patient wishes to discontinue all life-saving interventions. The nurse explains that turning off the medications will likely lead to death. The patient verbally recognizes this understanding. The physicians do not want the nurse to discontinue the norepinephrine as they believe the patient will recover. What is the most appropriate action by the nurse at this time?

    A. Discontinue the norepinephrine immediately and provide comfort care
    B. Consult with palliative care and contact the family
    C. Speak with the nurse manager about establishing a meeting with physicians, ethics, and the healthcare team
    D. Address the physician concerns directly that the patient does not wish to live

105. A 65-year-old African American male comes into the emergency room due to persistent chest pain lasting longer than 2 hours. He states he has felt unwell for the past 3 days but thought nothing of it. He was walking his dog at the onset of chest pain. While myocardial infarction is most likely, the physician would like to rule out pulmonary embolism. Which of the following orders would be done first to rule out PE?

    A. D-dimer
    B. V/Q scan
    C. Fibrinolytic therapy
    D. Echocardiogram

106. An ECG is ordered immediately upon admission of a patient with chest pain to the ED. The ECG shows ST elevation in leads II, III, and aVF. Based upon these findings what is the location of the MI and the likely coronary artery affected?

    A. Anterior MI—LAD
    B. Lateral MI—circumflex
    C. Inferior MI—RCA
    D. Posterior MI—RCA

107. Which of the following is not indicated in a suspected myocardial infarction induced by cocaine abuse?

    A. Metoprolol
    B. Nitroglycerin
    C. ECG within 10 minutes
    D. Opioid narcotics

108. A patient recently arrived at the emergency department after calling 911 due to chest pain. Arrival to the ED was within 1 hour of onset of pain. ECT shows ST elevations in leads V1, V2, V3, and V4. Troponin was drawn and found to be 2.5 ng/mL. After receiving morphine and nitroglycerin sublingual, the patient continues to complain of severe chest pain. Which of the following is immediately indicated at this time?

    A. Emergency surgery
    B. Emergent PCI
    C. Admission to CCU
    D. Nitroglycerin IV drip

109. A patient recovering from an inferior MI is in the cardiac care unit and is 1 hour post-PCI. A drug-eluting stent was placed in the right coronary artery. The patient was started on GP IIb/IIIa inhibitors immediately upon arrival to the unit. He is resting comfortably in bed when the nurse hears an alarm on the monitor. The following rhythm is shown. Current blood pressure is 90/50 mmHg; the patient is dizzy and nauseous. Which of the following regarding the current situation is true?

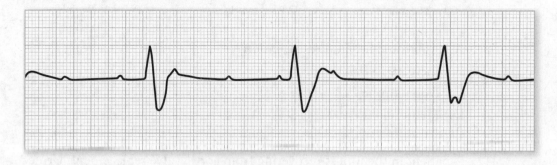

    A. The patient will require coronary bypass surgery

    B. The patient will require transcutaneous pacing

    C. The patient will require atropine

    D. The patient will require epinephrine

110. A 65 year-old Caucasian female has been in the hospital due to aortic stenosis. Aortic valve replacement (mechanical) was performed 2 days ago, but her condition continues to deteriorate. Echocardiogram performed this morning reveals severe left ventricular dysfunction with an ejection fraction (EF) of 20%. Pre-op echo showed EF of 45%. The monitor alarm sounds and the nurse enters the room to the findings below. Which of the following is the patient likely experiencing?

BP = 88/45 mmHg (A-line) MAP = 59	HR = 120 Sinus tachycardia	R = 30
SpO$_2$ = 88% on 40% FiO$_2$ Intubated	T = 98.5°F (37°C)	Pain = 0/10 Sedated
CO = 2.5 L/min	CVP = 5 mmHg	PAP = 20/9 mmHg
PCWP = 20 mmHg	SVR = 1500 dynes	

    A. Diastolic heart failure worsening to cardiogenic shock

    B. Systolic heart failure worsening to cardiogenic shock

    C. Hypertrophic cardiomyopathy

    D. Ventilator associated pneumonia (VAP) worsening to sepsis

111. A patient in the ICU post coronary bypass has the below vital signs and hemodynamics. Which of the following is not indicated at this time?

BP = 85/45 mmHg (A-line) MAP = 58	HR = 130 Sinus tachycardia	R = 22
SpO_2 = 90% on 50% FiO_2 Intubated	T = 98.5°F (37°C)	Pain = 0/10 Sedated
CO = 3.0 L/min	CVP = 3 mmHg	PAP = 16/9 mmHg

   A. Albumin and fluid resuscitation
   B. Increase in FiO_2
   C. Dobutamine IV
   D. Metoprolol IV push

112. A patient in the unit is recovering from aortic valve replacement. Urine output is 35 mL/hr and current SpO_2 shows 94% on 60% FiO_2. BP and CO/CI are low on 12 mcg/kg/min of dobutamine. It is currently being titrated up. Current SVR is 1100 dynes; CVP displays normovolemia. Changes in medications and IV titrations do not improve the patient's condition. What is the next step in care for this patient?

   A. Transplant
   B. Aggressive fluid resuscitation
   C. ICD placement
   D. IABP

113. A patient in the ICU has a blood pressure of 100/72 mmHg. There is an order for an echocardiogram to assess current cardiac output and ejection fraction. X-ray reveals unremarkable lungs but an enlarged cardiac silhouette. With suspected dilated cardiomyopathy, what medications would be ordered to optimize cardiac output in this patient?

   A. Nifedipine
   B. Docusate
   C. Furosemide
   D. Norepinephrine

114. A patient with an aneurysm undergoes graft repair. What location of aneurysm and repair is most commonly associated with the potential complication of a pre-renal acute kidney injury?

   A. Suprarenal abdominal
   B. Infrarenal abdominal
   C. Thoracic
   D. Mesenteric

115. A patient is admitted to the ICU due to dysrhythmias associated with cocaine use. An hour after admission, the telemetry monitor shows a tachyarrhythmia, potentially supraventricular tachycardia. What will dictate the need for electric cardioversion for this patient?

   A. The speed of the heart rate

   B. Blood pressure and hemodynamics

   C. Availability for immediate surgery

   D. Episodes of adenosine given

116. A patient is post-op 6 hours from a coronary artery bypass graft surgery. The surgery was performed on-pump. Which of the following physiological changes would the nurse expect as a result of the heart–lung bypass?

   A. Vascular vasoconstriction and hypertension

   B. Oliguria with pre-renal acute kidney injury

   C. Increased output into the chest tubes

   D. Low-grade fever and mild leukocytosis

117. A patient in the emergency department is being assessed for heart failure. The patient reports being short of breath while sitting on their couch at home. What class of heart failure according to the New York Heart Association would this patient have?

   A. Class 1

   B. Class 2

   C. Class 3

   D. Class 4

118. After an inferior wall myocardial infarction, the patient develops a papillary muscle rupture. What would lead the healthcare professional to believe this?

   A. Systolic murmur with decreased cardiac output

   B. Diastolic murmur with decreased pulmonary artery pressures

   C. Systolic murmur with increased afterload

   D. Diastolic murmur with decreased cardiac output

119. A patient with severe pericardial effusion is admitted to the ICU for close monitoring. Surgery is expected in the near future. Understanding the potential deterioration to cardiac tamponade, what would the nurse expect to see?

   A. Widening pulse pressure and hypertension

   B. Pulsus paradoxus and distended neck veins

   C. Bounding radial pulse and brisk capillary refill

   D. Bradycardia and decreased cardiac output

120. A patient in cardiogenic shock is admitted to the ICU. The nurse is to immediately begin dobutamine as ordered. Which of the following responses to receptors will be primarily affected by this medication?

   A. Stimulation of β_2 receptors (beta 2)
   B. Stimulation of β_1 receptors (beta 1)
   C. Stimulation of dopaminergic
   D. Stimulation of α receptors (alpha)

121. A patient with a history of hypertension is admitted to the ICU with a current blood pressure of 200/110 mmHg. One hour after admission the patient complains of a "tearing" upper back pain that radiates to the shoulders. Which of the following is contraindicated for this patient?

   A. Fibrinolytic therapy
   B. Emergency surgery
   C. Nitroglycerin IV
   D. Hydromorphone IV

122. A patient is in the ICU after a valve replacement. A pacemaker is in place with epicardial wires. Current settings on the pacemaker are DDD. What is the best explanation for this current setting?

   A. Atrial chamber paced, sensed, and inhibited
   B. Ventricular chamber paced, sensed, and inhibited
   C. Atrial and ventricular chambers paced, sensed, and inhibited
   D. Demand ventricular setting, not inhibited

123. A patient arrives via EMS to the trauma bay of the emergency department. A stab wound is present with a knife in the abdomen. The patient is stable at this time. A nurse in the trauma bay expresses the need to remove the knife and assess the wound. What is appropriate at this time?

   A. Remove the knife and assess the wound
   B. Leave the knife and stabilize the entry wound
   C. Transfer the patient to the OR in anticipation of emergency surgery
   D. Apply pressure surrounding the wound to slowly remove the knife

124. A patient is currently being paced via a transfemoral catheter with the goal of 100% ventricular pacing. Upon moving the patient in bed, the nurse notes incorrect pacing on the monitor with 50% capture. The patient complains of dizziness and the blood pressure decreases as witnessed by the radial arterial line. What is the appropriate action by the nurse at this time?

A. Increase the sensitivity on the pacemaker

B. Increase the electrical output on the pacemaker

C. Turn the pacemaker off and assess

D. Decrease the sensitivity on the pacemaker

125. Three days after a myocardial infarction a patient develops pericarditis. Which of the following signs and symptoms would the nurse expect to see in this patient?

A. New-onset S3 murmur

B. Shortness of breath and hypoxia

C. Increased SVR and cardiac output

D. Pericardial friction rub

STOP. You have completed the practice test. Complete your answers before moving forward with the review and rationales.

Answer Key

Question 1

Answer: C

Rationale: Approaching a question like this can be difficult given the specificity of the information provided. Remember that a PaO_2 of 60 mmHg generally correlates to a SpO_2 of 90%. This allows the removal of answers B and D. To choose between the remaining two, perform a calculation for P/F ratio—PaO_2 divided by FiO_2; remember to use the decimal presentation as 0.60%. The current P/F ratio is 100 mmHg indicating potential movement into ARDS or at minimum ALI.

Question 2

Answer: A

Rationale: Pleuritic chest pain occurs upon breathing or coughing. It is typically described as sharp or burning, sudden and intense. There are components in some of the answers that correlate to pleuritic chest pain. The pain can be severe. The pain can radiate, typically to the neck or shoulders. The pain, however, is not pulsating, as is typically associated with an aneurysm, or tearing, which may be associated with dissection or an aortic tear.

Question 3

Answer: C

Rationale: The patient continues to experience the effects of the heroin overdose even after two doses of naloxone. The patient is hypercapnic and acidotic due to inhibited ventilation and oxygenation. To improve these factors, the patient requires mechanical ventilation. Increasing the oxygen will not correct the underlying breathing. The patient remains somnolent, so stimulation seems unlikely to help the situation. The patient is acidotic due to respiratory compromise, not metabolic; the bicarb is also normal and not appropriate for administration at this time.

Question 4

Answer: B

Rationale: Carbon monoxide poisoning results in a left shift in the oxyhemoglobin dissociation curve. This left shift favors oxygen clinging to hemoglobin; unfortunately, carbon monoxide has a 240-fold greater affinity to hemoglobin than oxygen causing this potential fatal displacement.

Question 5

Answer: A

Rationale: The clinical picture here is of a fat embolism caused by the open fracture of the femur. This is a known risk factor for fractures of the long bones such as the femur. Chest pain can be an enigmatic symptom as it is associated with many potential problems; most notably a myocardial infarction. Fat embolism, as in other pulmonary embolisms, may cause chest pain; however, the added symptom of petechiae is not typical in MI. The same rule applies for pneumothorax or pneumonia; chest pain may be found. Remember to look at the full clinical picture to find the correct answer; there is no half-correct answer.

Question 6

Answer: D

Rationale: Tension pneumothorax causes a contralateral deviation of the trachea—in this case, to the left. Hypotension and tachycardia are also expected due to compression of the great vessels resulting in poor cardiac output. This compression may be seen by distended jugular and neck veins. Chest expansion would be decreased on the affected side.

Question 7

Answer: D

Rationale: The patient is showing signs of respiratory distress—hypercapnia and tachypnea. With no added symptoms noted in the question like dyspnea or accessory muscle use, extrapolate the information that is given. CPAP mode requires patient strength to breath, something that is likely lacking here. Extubation is not appropriate at this time, and the patient requires added support through the ventilator; placing them on IMV mode is the best way to temporize this situation while following up with the physician. The patient is not hypoxic at this time so increasing the oxygen is not needed. An x-ray is not needed without additional information that would warrant it.

Question 8

Answer: C

Rationale: If the patient is able to speak while intubated, the cuff is not occlusive to the trachea. Protocol should be followed to minimize the risk of tracheal damage and necrosis due to overinflation. There is no "needed" volume; the volume should be minimally occlusive. A chest x-ray is not indicated, as the issue is with the cuff itself, not the position. Turning the patient on their back with the head elevated is certainly appropriate if there was distress; however, at the moment the concern is the cuff pressure.

Question 9

Answer: B

Rationale: It is common for patients to come out of surgery with chest tubes after a thoracotomy. Due to the breach in the pleural cavity from the surgery itself, the post-op risk of pneumothorax exists. By placing chest tubes, this ensures negative pressure in the pleural cavity. A chest tube also drains fluid, whether it be blood, pus, but preferably not pleural fluid. This is an inevitable result of the chest tube. It is also not the primary reason for the chest tubes in this case. Ventilation, or breathing, is a combination of mechanisms that involve the lungs, diaphragm, and airways. Chest tubes do not assist directly in ventilation, granted they reduce the risk of complications that would hinder ventilation. Growth of the pleural cavity would occur much later and is not the purpose of the chest tubes.

Question 10

Answer: B

Rationale: Given the current state of respiratory distress, a severely acidotic patient is expected. It is also common for COPD patients to be chronically acidotic to begin with. COPD patients also tend to show partial compensation at baseline. The bicarb of this patient is 32 mEq/L, which shows us there is compensation occurring; however, given the abnormal pH of 7.29, this is partially not fully compensated.

Question 11

Answer: C

Rationale: Using the oxyhemoglobin dissociation curve, you can see the correlation between PaO_2 and SpO_2—60 mmHg is the standard tipping point where both numbers begin to decrease much faster. Keep in mind the curve can shift to the right or left given certain circumstances. In this case, a decrease in pH would cause the curve to shift right. Even with this potential shift, 60 mmHg is the most accurate answer.

Question 12

Answer: A

Rationale: The most likely explanation for the clinical signs and symptoms is pulmonary embolism. Given the history of cancer and surgery, this diagnosis correlates. The high-pressure alarm along with hypoxia and tachycardia also correlate to PE. Pulmonary edema would explain many of these symptoms, but the history does not match a typical patient with pulmonary edema. The same rationale applies to pneumothorax; it is not as likely as a PE. Uterine hemorrhage would not explain the respiratory symptoms; not until there was massive blood loss. This patient is also hypertensive, not hypotensive.

Question 13

Answer: A

Rationale: A massive pulmonary embolism may result in pulseless electrical activity (PEA) or other forms of cardiac arrest. The full clinical picture of PE is large; make sure to study in the respiratory chapter. A pulmonary pressure of 18/8 mmHg is normal. Petechiae is indicative of a fat embolism, not PE secondary to DVT. PE causes a V/Q mismatch and would cause hypoxemia. Hopeful an S_1 and S_2 heart sound can be heard; this indicates your patient is alive and has a heartbeat; these are normal heart tones.

Question 14

Answer: A

Rationale: CT pulmonary angiography is the gold standard for diagnosing PE. If angiography is nonconclusive, a V/Q scan may be performed. A venous Doppler may be performed to find the cause of the PE (DVT in the legs). A chest x-ray is not a good conclusive diagnostic tool for a PE. Sepsis is unlikely, so blood cultures at this time are not needed. The primary intervention is to reestablish blood flow through the pulmonary bed; however, the recent surgery places the patient at high risk for bleeding if tPA is administered. At this juncture, heparin would be the treatment of choice to prevent further growth of the clot. The physician will decide if more aggressive therapy is needed at this time. Treatment is typically followed up with coumadin to prevent worsening PE.

Question 15

Answer: D

Rationale: When thinking of pulmonary embolism, remember that the problem is perfusion in nature, not an alveolar problem. The lack of blood flow increases the dead space in the lung not being utilized for gas exchange. PE may cause increased right-sided heart pressure and eventually right-sided heart failure. This is not the cause of hypoxia, however.

Question 16

Answer: C

Rationale: Heparin-induced thrombocytopenia (HIT) is covered in more detail in the hematology chapter. Patients who develop HIT need to have the heparin drip immediately discontinued and be transferred to alternative anticoagulation therapy such as argabatran. Increased aPTT would be expected with heparin infusion. A therapeutic aPTT level is 40–60 seconds, so 70 is slightly high, but it does not warrant immediate discontinuation; the infusion would be slowed down. Fever and anemia are not related to heparin infusion; those would require alternate assessments.

Question 17

Answer: A

Rationale: Hypercapnia is seen in late asthma exacerbations, not early. The body is able to compensate earlier on with tachypnea. Eventually the body tires and is unable to compensate fully causing hypercapnia. This explains why hypoxia is seen before hypercapnia. Wheezing and mental status changes are common in early exacerbation.

Question 18

Answer: B

Rationale: The most common cause of pulmonary edema is left-sided heart failure. Fluid volume excess leading to pulmonary edema affects the compliance of the lungs. Static compliance indicates compatibility at rest, whereas dynamic compliance is during the work of breathing. Pulmonary edema decreases both, but more so static compliance. Hypercapnia would be seen if the pulmonary edema progresses to a severe level.

Question 19

Answer: B

Rationale: The largest and most immediate risk factor during removal of a central line is air embolism. For this reason, the head of the bed is typically slightly lowered to prevent this. This is also the position to place a patient if they actively have an air embolism; lowered head (Trendelenburg) and to the left. The other answers are not an immediate risk during removal of a catheter.

Question 20

Answer: C

Rationale: When serum glucose reaches 250 mg/dL or lower, continuous infusion should be switched to dextrose. In this case, remember that insulin causes potassium to be shifted out of the intravascular space and into the cells, so the serum potassium level will continue to fall. Adding potassium to the continuous infusion is appropriate. Close monitoring of potassium with piggy-back or general replacement would also be appropriate. As the DKA is corrected, the acidosis will correct naturally, there is no need to administer bicarb. The glucose is trending downward, increasing the insulin infusion is not warranted.

Question 21

Answer: B

Rationale: Osmolality is a representation of concentration. As the patient loses more and more volume through *dilute* urine (hypoosmolar—decreased), the serum will become *concentrated* (hyperosmolar—increased).

Question 22

Answer: D

Rationale: In DKA, ABG displays metabolic acidosis with an open anion gap (greater than 12). The others do not reflect this. To review ABG analysis, refer to Chapter 3.

Question 23

Answer: B

Rationale: When patients are initiated on enteral or parenteral nutrition, it is not uncommon for patients to become hyperglycemia. The most appropriate thing to do is to assess for this elevated serum glucose. Remember the 3 P's of hyperglycemia (polyuria, polydipsia, polyphagia). The TPN does not need to be discontinued at this time; if deemed appropriate, a sliding scale insulin order may be ordered. The vital signs provided do not indicate infection at this time. Assessing a urinalysis, serum sodium and osmolality may be appropriate down the line, but at this point the most likely cause is hyperglycemia. This should be assessed first.

Question 24

Answer: A

Rationale: As a prioritization, ABCs should be considered. In this case, the airway is clear and the patient is ventilating adequately as displayed in the pulse ox. What is of concern, however, is the current blood pressure and rebound tachycardia. Given the case study and the vital signs, this patient is showing signs and symptoms of dehydration. The priority is to replace fluids and electrolytes, such as potassium. HHS correlates better in this case than DKA, assessing an anion gap and administering bicarb is not needed at this time. Remember that HHS is "hot and dry" and more commonly associated with Type 2 DM, whereas DKA is more commonly associated with Type 1 DM. Intubation is not needed at this time since the patient is ventilating well. Preload (fluids) should be the priority treatment. If fluids do not correct the problem, and MAP becomes an issue, norepinephrine may be considered by the healthcare team.

Question 25

Answer: A

Rationale: When multiple units of PRBCs are given, remember that this is NOT whole blood. Platelets and FFP will be needed to replace the lost coagulation factors. Due to citrate bindings to calcium and magnesium, patients will become hypocalcemic and hypomagnesemic, requiring replacement of those two electrolytes. Loss of DTR and muscle weakness are symptoms of **hyper**calcemia and **hyper**magnesemia. Potassium may be released by RBCs during transfusion, replacement of potassium will not be needed. There is a left shift in the oxyhemoglobin dissociation curve with large amounts of transfusions leading to 2,3-DPG deficiency in the blood.

Question 26

Answer: C

Rationale: An important consideration in many styles of questions is to immediately notice the word "early." This often changes the nature of the question and answers, as it does here. What are early S&S of bleeding versus late? Petechiae and purpura are oftentimes the first noticeable manifestations of thrombocytopenia and bleeding. The main concern here being heparin-induced thrombocytopenia (HIT) due to the infusion. The other answers would be late manifestations of complications such as intracranial bleeding, GI bleeding, or bleeding from IV sites or wounds.

Question 27

Answer: D

Rationale: The laboratory data during DIC includes decreased fibrinogen and increased fibrinogen split times. This is the cause of the abnormal bleeding. As a result, coagulation times increase. D-dimer increases due to microclots. Platelets are consumed leading to thrombocytopenia and more abnormal diffuse bleeding.

Question 28

Answer: A

Rationale: The clinical picture in this case reflects that of a ruptured spleen. Ecchymosis around the umbilicus (Cullen's sign) and referred left shoulder pain (Kehr's sign) are indicative of a ruptured spleen. The pain is also in the left upper quadrant, which correlates to splenic location. This patient is displaying signs of shock associated with a rupture; the BP is low, with rebound tachycardia and tachypnea.

Question 29

Answer: A

Rationale: This patient is in hypovolemic shock and requires immediate surgery. They are likely internally bleeding due to the blunt trauma as also indicated by the increased temperature. Rupture is possible. Vasopressors may be required after administration of IV fluids, but given the severity of the signs and symptoms, surgery is required right now. Inotropic agents would not help here as the problem is not cardiac in nature. Assessing urine output does not serve much purpose when hypovolemic shock is obvious. The patient will be oliguric. A KUB takes time; this is an emergency situation.

Question 30

Answer: B

Rationale: Peritoneal irritation typically causes patients to maintain a position with the knees flexed; this decreases the irritation. Lying still will also lessen the pain, although not an option here. A test to elicit pain in appendicitis, the psoas sign, has the practitioner place the patient in a left lying position and straighten the right leg and hip; this would elicit pain in appendicitis. The other positions listed in this question would not aid in relieving pain for this patient.

Question 31

Answer: C

Rationale: This patient will be losing volume while actively bleeding. To "fill up the tank" the best option is an isotonic solution like normal saline. Blood may be administered as well if deemed necessary. Lactated Ringer's is an isotonic solution, but it is often not considered safe in liver failure because most lactate is metabolized in the liver. A solution of 5% dextrose is a hypotonic solution and will worsen the hypovolemia. A hypertonic solution is also not indicated as it will cause cellular dehydration and possible organ dysfunction.

Question 32

Answer: B

Rationale: The clinical picture presents like pancreatitis. It is possible this may also correlate to other organs in the area like the liver. A history of gallstones is a risk factor for pancreatitis due to biliary obstruction, a stated point in the question. Cholangitis or choledocholangitis would lead to a rapid onset jaundice, whereas pancreatitis presents differently. Pancreatitis enzymes will be elevated. A colonoscopy will not help identify issues in the upper abdomen. ABG is not warranted, as the question does not state any respiratory issues. An ERCP may be performed but will not be performed first. Be careful with wording; "first" implies just that, a primary test or treatment.

Question 33

Answer: D

Rationale: The sympathetic nervous system, or "fight or flight" response, is activated in situations of bodily threat—in this case, shock. There is a fairly large clinical picture of this activation, but it includes release of adrenaline (tachycardia), release of cortisol, and release of renin as part of the RAAS system. Vasoconstriction occurs, not vasodilation. This thought confuses at times, but do not confuse it with bronchodilation, which is a response to fight or flight.

Question 34

Answer: A

Rationale: Out of the four options, the immediate and priority concern for a patient with portal hypertension is a rupture of esophageal or gastric varices. This manifests with hematemesis or the vomiting of blood. Encephalopathy, while concerning, will not kill the patient at this moment. Focus on ABC issues and emergencies with priority issues. Aspiration is a concern if the person begins to vomit blood, but remember that in the context of a case study, if the question does not say they are vomiting blood yet, it is a concern or risk, not an active problem. Our goal is to prevent these problems. The third spacing of fluid is common in liver cirrhosis as seen in ascites. This may lead to hypovolemia, but again, there are no symptoms of that yet.

Question 35

Answer: A

Rationale: Due to the relentless vomiting, the patient is very likely dehydrated and hypovolemic. Fluids also shift in states of obstruction from intravascular space to other areas further exacerbating the hypovolemia. The immediate concern is loss of circulating volume; this is replaced with IV fluids. When patients vomit, they also lose potassium, this will be replaced. A mineral oil enema may be useful in large bowel obstructions if the obstruction is closer to the rectum. This aids in passage of the hard stool. Emergency laparotomy and broad-spectrum antibiotics would be indicated in cases of bowel perforation. There is no indication of that emergency in this question.

Question 36

Answer: B

Rationale: Remember that phosphorus and calcium have an inverse relationship. When one goes up, the other goes down, and vice versa. This relationship is seen throughout a few disorders, such as CKD, parathyroid issues, and metabolic issues. The other answers do not reflect this relationship.

Question 37

Answer: C

Rationale: Prolonged renal ischemia (pre-renal AKI) may lead to secondary intrarenal AKI—specifically, acute tubular necrosis. Polycythemia vera, or elevated RBCs, is the wrong direction of response. Decreased erythropoietin due to renal failure leads to anemia. Acute interstitial nephritis is another type of intrarenal AKI, but it is not the result of renal ischemia. Goodpasture syndrome is a type of intrarenal AKI, an autoimmune disorder, but it is not the result of renal ischemia either.

Question 38

Answer: C

Rationale: The antidote or antagonist for hypermagnesemia is calcium. This may be given as calcium chloride or calcium gluconate. Furosemide and dialysis would lower the magnesemia in this patient, but the process would take too long. The goal here is to prevent an arrest or further problems right now. A C-section is not indicated unless the patient progresses to eclampsia.

Question 39

Answer: B

Rationale: The goal of immediate treatment is to correct the problem right now before further issues develop. In this case, the patient is in danger of experiencing a code blue or fatal dysrhythmia. Insulin followed by D50 will force potassium out of the blood and into the surrounding tissues and cells. It is a temporizing solution. The patient was already receiving HD; the patient is too unstable to continue treatment at a speed that would correct the potassium fast enough. Insulin/D50 and consideration for CVVH may be warranted depending on blood pressure. Sodium polystyrene sulfonate and furosemide will take too long to work.

Question 40

Answer: C

Rationale: Urine output is almost exclusively the best indicator of overall fluid volume status when resuscitating. This could be with a case like this, pre-renal AKI, a hypovolemic patient, and a severe burn case. Pre-renal AKIs result in oliguria. Correct of this oliguria indicates successful fluid resuscitation. The minimum output generally considered is 0.5 mL/kg/hr. For a 60 kg patient, this comes to 30 mL/hr. Increased weight displays a retention of water. While the creatinine and BUN are slightly improved, they are not the best indicators of fluid resuscitation success. The potassium here is normal; it is also not a good indicator of fluid resuscitation.

Question 41

Answer: A

Rationale: Hematuria is the most common symptom seen after trauma to genitourinary structures. Because the pain is in the lower abdomen, this correlates closest to injury to the bladder. Pain in the flank would indicate kidneys. Suprapubic pain would indicate urethra. While damage to the uterus is possible, there is a difference between hematuria and vaginal discharge. Hematuria specifically describes bloody output upon urinating.

Question 42

Answer: D

Rationale: The patient is experiencing water intoxication. When serum sodium falls below 120 mEq/L, there is a high risk of cerebral edema and seizures. This should be corrected in an expeditious manner; therefore, answers should indicate the speed a necessity needed. Hypertonic solutions like 3% saline are the primary indication here. While furosemide and restricting fluids would work, they would take too long. Hypotonic solutions, 0.45% saline, will make the problem worse and likely kill your patient.

Question 43

Answer: D

Rationale: Triamterene is a potassium-sparing diuretic, same class as spironolactone, its more known sister. ACE inhibitors and ARBs also carry a risk for hyperkalemia. The combination of these two drugs together should be approached with caution. The other electrolyte imbalances are not caused by the combination of these medications.

Question 44

Answer: A

Rationale: A point to note here is the difference between a primary and secondary problem. This question is asking about underlying secondary problems such as poor perfusion, which may be seen in DM 2. Another cause may be poor protein intake, not carbohydrates. Primary causes would be directly on the wound itself like poor dressing changes or removal of healthy granulation tissue or biofilm, which may be linked to infection.

Question 45

Answer: C

Rationale: Yellowish tissue describes adipose (fat) tissue associated with a stage 3 pressure ulcer. If muscle, bone, or tendons were exposed, that would describe a stage 4. All stages may be briefly reviewed in Chapter 7.

Question 46

Answer: B

Rationale: Vasoactive medications like dopamine, epinephrine, norepinephrine, and phenylephrine all cause damage to tissue if infiltration of the IV occurs. This is extravasation. The first thing to always do is stop the infusion. The IV line is maintained to potentially aspirate out as much of the causative agent as possible. It is also maintained in anticipation of administering an antidote, such as phentolamine. Do not use warm compresses in extravasation; it will cause vasodilation and further damage.

Question 47

Answer: C

Rationale: When mechanical stress is not placed on the muscles or bones, they begin to degenerate. Muscles begin to waste and atrophy. Bone begins to demineralize, increasing the risk of osteopenia/porosis. This demineralization potentiates fractures. Myelopathy is injury to the spinal cord, which does not correlate here. Poor oxygenation and ventilation are due to the coronavirus infection itself, not from functional issues. Prolonged bed rest does increase the risk of atelectasis and pneumonia, however. Prolonged immobilization leads to hyperglycemia and decreased cardiac ejection fraction, not increased.

Question 48

Answer: C

Rationale: The clinical symptoms are that of osteomyelitis and infection. After the total knee replacement or other surgeries, the risk for this type of infection increases, especially in an immunosuppressed patient. The surgeon will begin with debridement of the infected tissue and cleans the implant. Removal of the hardware itself would be the next step if deemed necessary by the surgeon. Removal of synovial fluid for diagnostic purposes or treatment is typically performed by needle aspiration, not open surgery. Necrotic or dead tissue would be a much more serious problem and likely to manifest with more severe symptoms like septic shock.

Question 49

Answer: D

Rationale: The first and most important treatment is aggressive fluid resuscitation. This is performed to maintain output of 300 mL/hr or more. Remember that rhabdomyolysis causes intrarenal AKI (tubular necrosis). Flushing out the kidneys will aid in preventing this. Treatment also includes diuretics such as mannitol and furosemide, but not spironolactone due to potassium-sparing. Hyperkalemia is a risk with rhabdomyolysis due to the crush injuries and destruction of muscle. This is also the reason for telemetry—to monitor for dysrhythmias. Calcium and steroids are not indicated at this time; however, if the patient develops dysrhythmias, calcium gluconate may be ordered to protect myocardium.

Question 50

Answer: C

Rationale: Tissue plasminogen activator (tPA) is best administered within 3 hours of the onset of symptoms. Some patients may be considered for tPA up to 4.5 hours after, but 3 hours or less is best, and 5 hours may be close to the "Golden Window"; however, it still falls outside this time. Be a stickler when it comes to these numbers on the CCRN exam. Same for thoughts on "time is muscle," "time is brain," and so on.

Question 51

Answer: B

Rationale: The two main types of cerebral edema are cytotoxic and vasogenic. Hypoosmolar issues and ischemia result in the swelling of "cells" and cytotoxic cerebral edema. In this case, the patient experienced a cardiac arrest and the cessation of blood flow to the brain. This hypoxia leads to ischemia and the death of neurons (cytotoxic). Increased permeability of the blood–brain barrier describes vasogenic cerebral edema. Increased osmosis would be seen in cases of increased fluid retention in the brain such as SIADH, water intoxication, and inappropriate use of certain IV fluids (hypotonic).

Question 52

Answer: A

Rationale: In cases of cerebral edema and increased ICP, ipsilateral pupillary changes and contralateral motor changes. With the pupillary dilation of the left eye, this suggests injury to the left part of the brain. Remember that cranial nerve III (oculomotor) is affected by this increased pressure. Occipital lobe damage would result in vision changes. Do not confuse vision with the eyeball itself or its movement. Brain stem injury or herniation would affect core body functions like breathing and heart rate.

Question 53

Answer: B

Rationale: The main note of this question is hemorrhagic versus ischemic CVA. This patient experienced a hemorrhagic stroke and is ineligible for tPA. This is the best, correct, and most direct response. Whether the symptoms began 4 hours ago or less is moot—tPA is not indicated. Recent surgery is a contraindication to tPA use; 2 years is not recent, and, again, tPA is not indicated anyway. Stating the neurologist decided against is not helpful or informative. Think direct but compassionate.

Question 54

Answer: A

Rationale: Cranial nerves responsible for swallowing and gag will be the most important to assess since these will affect the ability to swallow. The other cranial nerves listed involve other functions.

Question 55

Answer: D

Rationale: There are two decent answers here. A lumbar puncture will definitely elicit bacteria in the cerebrospinal fluid and confirm the presence of bacterial meningitis. A positive Kernig's sign may increase the suspicion of meningitis, but it does not confirm or diagnose the disease. Blood cultures and urinalysis will not show infectious disease in the part of the body of concern, the meninges.

Question 56

Answer: A

Rationale: Anisocoria, or pupillary dilation, occurs on the ipsilateral side of injury, the left in this case. Motor weakness, or hemiplegia, occurs contralateral to the side of injury. Remember to understand the differences between uncal and central herniation. Central herniation would illicit changes in the vital signs due to pressure on the brain stem, e.g., breathing.

Question 57

Answer: A

Rationale: Cerebral vasospasm typically occurs anywhere between 3 and 14 days after SAH. It can be potentially devastating if not caught early. Direct visualization via radiograph or angiography is often preferred to diagnose. Transcranial Doppler may also be used to assess cerebral blood flow and velocity. Vasospasms are treated with calcium channel blockers such as nicardipine and nimodipine.

Question 58

Answer: C

Rationale: A patient with increased ICP should have their head placed midline and in a semi-Fowler's position; 30-45 degrees is typically used. This aids in venous drainage and the lowering of the ICP. Suctioning raises the ICP and should be performed as needed. Auscultate the lungs and suction if appropriate. The clustering of care reduces stimuli and is appropriate in these cases. Changing alarms safely is appropriate here—the main word being safely. As nurses, we can change the alarm parameters to reflect the patient status if it is done within reason.

Question 59

Answer: C

Rationale: Decerebrate posturing is the abnormal extension of the extremities with hyperpronation of the arms. Decorticate posturing is the abnormal flexion with the arms flexed against the chest. The patient is not showing signs of spasticity or seizure. Central brain herniation begins with brain stem compression and vital signs changes eventually leading to flaccidity.

Question 60

Answer: B

Rationale: The best thing for the nurse to do in situations like this is acknowledge that the reality for the patient is "their" reality but not yours. It is not helpful to dismiss or ignore the hallucinations since they are real for the patient. Situations like this may also warrant asking the patient what the voices or auditory hallucinations are saying as they may be violent or commanding in nature. It is inappropriate to threaten a patient with repercussions like forcing them to calm down, likely with medication. This would be borderline assault if not assault already.

Question 61

Answer: D

Rationale: Open-ended questions are best at this time; it allows the patient to express their feelings. It provides therapeutic communication with attempts to de-escalate the situation. The other answers are all good ideas in maintaining nurse safety.

Question 62

Answer: A

Rationale: Given the case study of alcohol abuse, withdrawal is the most likely explanation for the agitation. Agitation may be caused by other factors such as hypoxia or pain, but this question is asking where to begin—what to do first. Increasing the sedation is not appropriate without first assessing the situation (remember nursing process). ICP related issues result in alternate signs and symptoms such as a decreasing level of consciousness.

Question 63

Answer: C

Rationale: A manic episode is characterized by delusions and euphoria. This typically manifests with a decreased need for sleep (insomnia). The other answers are symptoms of hypomania or depression. Not all bipolar patients have to exhibit signs of both cycles.

Question 64

Answer: A

Rationale: The "fight or flight" response, triggered by the sympathetic nervous system, results in anticholinergic type signs and symptoms. This includes dry mouth. Remember the acronym SLUDD for ease of memory (salivation, lacrimation, urination, digestion, defecation). Xerostomia may be caused by medication but is not the likely explanation here given the case of anxiety. The question also makes no mention of medications.

Question 65

Answer: D

Rationale: The primary survey for trauma patients (ABCDE) begins with airway. No matter the presenting factors of a patient, the airway always takes precedence. In this case, stridor is a symptom of airway compromise and should be assessed immediately. The next more important answer would be the pain upon breathing; this may be due to a multitude of reasons such as rib fractures. Both the open fracture and open wound would come later, likely with "exposure" unless indicated otherwise by active bleeding.

Question 66

Answer: C

Rationale: As with shock in general, tissue hypoxia leads to anaerobic respiration and the production of lactic acid. This increases serum lactate. The best indication of resolution of shock is the cessation of anaerobic respiration, aka the decreasing lactate. Dobutamine will increase the cardiac output and index in the efforts to increase oxygen delivery, but it does not tell us if the tissues are utilizing that oxygen. The same reasoning applies to increased PaO_2; the oxygen is available, but is it being used. Oftentimes, a SvO_2 is drawn to assess this oxygen use in the body. Urine output also does not exclusively tell us tissues are utilizing oxygen; it does show, however, adequate perfusion to the kidneys.

Question 67

Answer: C

Rationale: One of the earliest signs of blood loss is tachycardia. In class I hemorrhagic shock, a slight elevation in heart rate and respiratory rate is expected. This indicates minimal blood loss of 10%. Severe hypotension, a narrowed pulse pressure, and changes in mental status indicate a more severe loss of blood.

Question 68

Answer: B

Rationale: Normal saline if administered in large amounts leads to hyperchloremic acidosis. This is also witnessed by an increased chloride amount in the serum. It is associated with a normal anion gap. The acidosis is not the result of hypo-osmolality, but rather the product itself. Lactated Ringer's is given for states of acidosis and does help correct this issue over time; however, it is not the primary reason for switching off of normal saline. LR also contains electrolytes, but it does not correlate to the main concern in this question.

Question 69

Answer: D

Rationale: The patient is being rewarmed too quickly. Remember to move no quicker than 0.5°C to 1°C per hour. Rapid rewarming may lead to a sudden drop in blood pressure due to vasodilation and abnormal shunting. The vital signs are all within normal limits for hypothermia and rewarming.

Question 70

Answer: A

Rationale: Because it has been at least 4 hours since the ingestion, gastric lavage is not indicated. It is unlikely the medication is still in the stomach. What can be done is NG tube placement with administration of the antidote, acetylcysteine. Lab results will be performed, including a liver panel to assess damage, but it is not the most important thing at this time. It would be an expected adverse effect of the toxic ingestion. Airway protection with intubation is a priority when indicated. The case here states nothing of airway loss or difficulty breathing.

Question 71

Answer: C

Rationale: Septic shock, in addition to hypotension, fever, and positive blood cultures, is characterized by a severe reduction in vascular tone. This is displayed with a large decrease in SVR. Remember that a normal SVR is 800–1200 dynes/sec/cm^5. Septic shock would result in an increased cardiac output to compensate. Central venous pressure or right atrial pressure correlates to fluid volume status. This would be more crucial in hypovolemic shocks rather than distributive shocks. SvO$_2$ would be elevated in septic shock as the tissues have difficulty extracting the oxygen from RBCs.

Question 72

Answer: B

Rationale: Refractory hypotension in septic shock is treated first with norepinephrine. If unsuccessful, treatment may add epinephrine or vasopressin followed by inotropes if hypotension is unabating. Alternative agents like phenylephrine and dopamine are reserved for special circumstances of septic shock.

Question 73

Answer: A

Rationale: With states of hypovolemia or severe dehydration, expect concentration of the blood. This may be reflected by a hyperosmolar state and/or elevated hematocrit. The urine specific gravity would also be concentrated. SVR in hypovolemic shock is elevated. Hyperemesis would lead to hypokalemia due to electrolyte losses from vomiting; however, it is not a symptom of the hypovolemic shock itself.

Question 74

Answer: D

Rationale: Epinephrine IM is indicated in states of anaphylaxis. Intravenous epinephrine is reserved for cases of cardiac arrest or cardiovascular collapse. Secondary medications may include antihistamines like diphenhydramine and fexofenadine and steroids.

Question 75

Answer: B

Rationale: Toxicity of TCAs can lead to QRS prolongation and dysrhythmias. This is a priority of care along with any severe vital signs changes. The other answers reflect the opposite direction typically seen. Anticholinergic symptoms, bradypnea, and CNS depression are all seen in TCA toxicity.

Question 76

Answer: B

Rationale: CNS stimulants like cocaine and amphetamines will "increase" what is seen—tachycardia, tachypnea, anxiety or irritability, etc. Diplopia and vision changes are seen in alcohol use. Increased urine output and sleepiness are associated with the parasympathetic nervous system.

Question 77

Answer: C

Rationale: Expeditious labor is not a known risk factor for postpartum hemorrhage. Prolonged labor, however, is. Multiples, use of oxytocin, and an LGA (large for gestational age) fetus are all risk factors. In theory, anything that would tire out the muscle of the uterus could potentially lead to postpartum hemorrhage.

Question 78

Answer: A

Rationale: All of the answers reflect a known risk factor with obesity, but the most important consideration at this time is the hypoxia. This is a priority question— ABCs. If the patient would require intubation, that as well is known to be difficult in obese patients. The other issues can take secondary precedence.

Question 79

Answer: C

Rationale: Hemoglobin has a higher affinity to carbon monoxide than oxygen, displacing the RBCs ability to transmit oxygen to tissues. This results in hypoxia and tissue death.

Question 80

Answer: D

Rationale: Coagulation factors are expectedly increased during MODS. As the body fails to produce clotting factors and platelets, increased bleeding times ensue. The other answers are all seen in MODS.

Question 81

Answer: A

Rationale: Remember that medications that act upon alpha receptors affect vasoconstriction and dilation, whereas medications that act upon beta receptors affect heart rate and heart contraction. With the use of multiple agents simultaneously, it is possible these medications may cause excessive vasoconstriction resulting in ischemia of the heart or mesentery. In this case, the correct answer is displaying mesenteric ischemia. The other answers are not complications of these therapies. The capillary refill of 3 seconds or less is normal. Laryngeal edema would be more associated with an allergic reaction and elevated liver enzymes that of liver failure.

Question 82

Answer: A

Rationale: The priority at this time is to support the family in the needs they may have. That may include a wide variety from education to grieving, to cultural needs. By involving multiple disciplines, including social services and pastoral care, this goal may be achieved.

Question 83

Answer: D

Rationale: Difficult situations like this are best done with privacy and the ability for open dialogue with multiple specialties. The nurse taking direct care is rarely responsible for discussion of donation. The nurse may answer questions regarding patient condition if asked, but at this time, the most important intervention is private conversation with the family regarding their loved one.

Question 84

Answer: B

Rationale: Informed consent is obtained by the physician, with the emphasis on "informed." In this situation there are multiple avenues that may arise whether it is cancellation of the surgery, delay, or continued movement to pre-op; however, none of this can be planned until the physician has had a chance to speak to the patient.

Question 85

Answer: A

Rationale: It is important to allow family to remain bedside if they wish and it is safe to do so. This is an AACN Practice Alert. Because this is a code blue situation, it is also important to immediately begin CPR. A fellow nurse will explain the situation to the wife. Given the emergency nature, it is inappropriate to leave the room.

Question 86

Answer: C

Rationale: Accurate documentation and filing of incident reports is crucial in situations of near-miss or sentinel events. The medical record is a legal document. It is unlikely a nurse would remember every single action they took at the time.

Question 87

Answer: C

Rationale: Given the mismatch between the stated pain and the facial grimace, it is best to further assess the situation. There may be a cultural reason for the withholding of information about pain. It is also important to treat pain as it comes and not allow it to get to a crisis stage. Pain is easier to treat when it is lower.

Question 88

Answer: A

Rationale: It is best to contact the family and provide them with a brief update on the current situation. This way they are aware and able to come into the hospital. It is probable that the physician will sign the consent if the family is unable to be reached or the situation progresses to critical and life-threatening.

Question 89

Answer: C

Rationale: It states in the chart the patient speaks English, so it is unlikely it was placed in error. The nurse should, however, continue to evaluate understanding if the patient is nonvocal. Lack of eye contact may be cultural and should be respected, as well as physical touch. It is best to ask permission before making personal contact or performing procedures. A discussion about heritage and cultural practices may be appropriate at a certain point, but the primary goal is the situation at hand—obtaining vitals. If the patient is open to cultural discussion, the nurse may proceed; otherwise, it may be best to do private research on the side.

Question 90

Answer: B

Rationale: Patient wishes should be followed, especially when a legal document is involved, such as a DNR. Family disagreement with patient wishes is common and is best resolved by sitting everyone down and having a discussion with the healthcare team. The nurse should also be polite and avoid being crass or dismissive. The issue should be resolved if at all possible.

Question 91

Answer: A

Rationale: This is a private matter that should be addressed at such, at least in the beginning. If the patient wishes to have the discussion with his wife present that would be at the patient's direction. Otherwise, the best course of action is to assist the patient with the problem. In this case, nitro may be taken ahead of time. If it is a patch or ointment, it needs to be taken in advance, whereas a pill may be taken at the time of pain. Slight angina is expected in this situation, so sex does not need to be avoided.

Question 92

Answer: D

Rationale: It is helpful in the process of grieving to allow the family to say good-bye by helping with post-mortem care such as bathing. Give the family time to grieve regardless of the specific action.

Question 93

Answer: D

Rationale: The situation should be managed by a nurse or physician given the critical circumstances. A nursing assistant would not have the required information to provide a brief update. The mother will also likely have questions regarding her son.

Question 94

Answer: A

Rationale: The primary responsibility of the nurse is to facilitate the needs of the family in this difficult time. It is not to educate or push any one way. Organ donation assessment and education are performed by the transplant coordinator. They are trained to deal with these difficult conversations.

Question 95

Answer: B

Rationale: Questions like this, while not physiological in nature, do benefit from the nursing process. To fix a problem, one must assess it. It is inappropriate simply to turn off alarms or cancel orders; they are required for patient safety. However, there are possibly certain aspects that could be changed, such as the parameters to safely match patient status. Orders could also be reviewed to cluster care as appropriate.

Question 96

Answer: A

Rationale: The husband is finding comfort by helping his spouse during this period of end-of-life. If the patient can no longer swallow or tolerate large amounts of water, allowing sponges may prevent the dry mouth associated with the dying process. IV hydration is inappropriate, as the patient is end-of-life and curative interventions are not warranted.

Question 97

Answer: B

Rationale: The most appropriate thing to do is sit everyone down to discuss any issues. Whether it being cultural, spiritual, socioeconomic, demographical, or racial, behavior such as this is not welcome in a hospital. Nurses care for a wide variety of patients and must be compassionate to all. Do not ignore or apologize; address the issue head on.

Question 98

Answer: D

Rationale: Confidentiality is key and the law of HIPAA. HIV is a sensitive subject to many and still carries a large stigma within families and society. It is up to the patient on how they would like to disclose this information. Meningitis is a possible co-infection with HIV, but the family is not at any risk of contraction.

Question 99

Answer: A

Rationale: By advocating for patient rounding, this brings all disciplines together and focuses on the patient and care issues. Advocate for these issues yourself without pushing responsibility to others, whether social services or physicians. It is also inappropriate to jump to the nursing supervisor. Follow nursing hierarchy: charge nurse, nurse manager, and so on.

Question 100

Answer: B

Rationale: Veracity means the truthfulness and honesty between the patient and the nurse. The other answers reflect alternate nursing ethics—autonomy, nonmaleficence, and fidelity respectfully.

Question 101

Answer: A

Rationale: The right for patients to dictate their care and decisions is sacred and ethical. Moral agency implies the nurse will advocate and strive to fulfill patient and family wishes, even if they may not personally agree. This is obviously difficult at times when we may feel we know how to help, but again, it is not our judgment call to make.

Question 102

Answer: B

Rationale: Patient wishes must be followed when made clear. In this case, they are in the DNR order. The only person who can revoke the order is the patient. It is a difficult situation to be in, but when patients make their wishes explicitly clear, they should be followed.

Question 103

Answer: B

Rationale: To best facilitate learning, the nature of the problem should be assessed and then a plan engaged. Any plan should involve the patient and all disciplines involved in the patient's case. It is not appropriate to berate the patient at this time about what happens when they don't take the medication.

Question 104

Answer: C

Rationale: It is best to understand the situation fully before moving forward. Patient wishes should be followed, but it is also important that the patient understand the full picture of their care. It is possible the patient does not understand the prognosis and the likelihood of survival.

Question 105

Answer: A

Rationale: The most efficient, least invasive, and least costly method of ruling out a PE is through a serum D-dimer test. Elevated D-dimer indicates there may be thrombus formation and breakdown. A V/Q scan may assist in a PE rule out but is costly and time consuming. Echocardiogram would show right-sided failure secondary to PE, but not likely the PE itself. Fibrinolytic therapy is curative, not diagnostic.

Question 106

Answer: C

Rationale: ST elevation in leads II, III, and aVF displays an inferior STEMI. The right coronary artery is likely affected. Refer to the cardiovascular chapter for a helpful image on how to observe and analyze changes in a 12-lead ECG.

Question 107

Answer: A

Rationale: Beta blockers are contraindicated in variant angina (Prinzmetal's) secondary to cocaine or stimulant abuse. It may block vasodilation and worsen vasospasms. The other answers are indications for all MIs.

Question 108

Answer: B

Rationale: There are a few things happening here that makes an emergent PCI (<90 minutes) necessary. Nitroglycerin and morphine have not abated the pain. The pain is also of new onset (<12 hours). ST elevations are shown in multiple leads defining a STEMI. These are all indications for PCI. Emergency surgery is not necessary at this point, as the problem could potentially be fixed with PCI. Observation on a CCU is likely in the event of an NSTEMI. A nitroglycerin drip is not indicated at this time; a blood pressure is also not provided if considering treatment for severe hypertension.

Question 109

Answer: B

Rationale: Problems with AV node conduction is associated with an inferior MI. This may include heart blocks and bradyarrhythmias. The rhythm above is showing a third-degree heart block. This rhythm in association with the symptoms and blood pressure indicates an immediate intervention is necessary— transcutaneous pacing. There is no need for a CAB at this juncture. Right coronary artery disease may result in these rhythm changes; it is not a re-occlusion or perfusion issue; it is impaired innervation to the conductive system. Positive chronotropes, such as atropine, epinephrine, and others, can certainly be used for heart blocks. They are, however, not often effective in complete heart block. Positive chronotropes would be a better decision if the patient were stable.

Question 110

Answer: B

Rationale: With the systolic BP less than 90 mmHg and an ejection fraction of 20%, this is systolic dysfunction leading to cardiogenic shock. Diastolic dysfunction results in normal ejection fraction but a hypertrophied ventricle. There is no fever, no indication of an infection in this patient, so VAP is unlikely.

Question 111

Answer: D

Rationale: Metoprolol is contraindicated in acute systolic dysfunction. Reflex tachycardia may be assisting the patient with blood pressure and cardiac output. Administration of a beta blocker will decrease the BP. Calcium channel blockers, like nicardipine, are also contraindicated. They will decrease the contractility and worsen blood pressure. The other answers are indicated at this time.

Question 112

Answer: D

Rationale: With continued low BP and CO despite inotropic medications, the next step is IABP. A balloon pump will assist in cardiac output and reduce afterload as indicated by an elevated SVR. On occasion, vasodilators may be used, such as nitroglycerin, in attempts to also reduce afterload. Norepinephrine may also be discontinued depending on the clinic picture since it would be "clamping down" the patient—vasoconstriction. Transplant would be the last resource if the heart is beyond repair and does not improve on IABP. Fluid resuscitation will worsen the condition, especially "aggressive" fluid resuscitation. Preload should be fine tuned; through monitoring of CVP and urine output, both of which at this moment are normal. ICD placement may be likely in dilated cardiomyopathy. The risk being cardiac arrest. This is not the immediate concern here.

Question 113

Answer: C

Rationale: The primary goal in dilated cardiomyopathy is to optimize preload, afterload, and contractility. Furosemide will optimize volume (preload, afterload), whereas positive inotropes will optimize contractility. Negative inotropes are contraindicated (nifedipine). Drugs causing vasoconstriction (norepinephrine) will worsen afterload. Stool softeners like docusate are indicated to prevent constipation and a Valsalva maneuver but do not help in the primary goals in optimization.

Question 114

Answer: A

Rationale: Suprarenal arteries, such as a AAA, most commonly are associated with a post-op complication of pre-renal AKI due to poor perfusion to the kidneys or graft failure. The mesenteric arteries feed the bowel. Infrarenal repairs are below the perfusion of the kidneys and therefore pose little risk. Thoracic repairs may affect renal flow, but AAA locations are the most common.

Question 115

Answer: B

Rationale: The biggest indicator for correction of dysrhythmias in general is the relative stability of the patient (in many cases). The same holds true for SVT and tachyarrhythmias. If the patient is stable in this case, cardioversion is not immediately indicated. The rate is not a factor. Surgery is not necessary for tachyarrhythmias caused by cocaine abuse. Medications like adenosine may be given for tachyarrhythmias, typically before electric cardioversion, but are not a direct reason to cardiovert, nor the rounds of medication given.

Question 116

Answer: D

Rationale: Several physiological changes may be seen by the use of heart–lung bypass during surgery. An inflammatory response is expected due to on-pump usage; this includes low-grade fever and mild leukocytosis. It is worth noting the words "low-grade and mild" for the purposes here. Severe elevation would indicate potential complication. The other answers are not seen directly related to on-pump versus off-pump usage.

Question 117

Answer: D

Rationale: The classes of heart failure progress from best to worst: class 1 to class 4, respectively. This patient reports dyspnea at rest while sitting on the couch. This correlates to class 4, heart failure.

Question 118

Answer: A

Rationale: Mitral regurgitation, a systolic murmur, is often the first signs of a papillary muscle rupture. It can be potentially fatal if not caught early, as cardiogenic shock may be rapid in onset.

Question 119

Answer: B

Rationale: Cardiac tamponade is most associated with muffled heart tones, JVD, narrowed pulse pressure, and pulsus paradoxus. The other answers do not reflect this complication. Tachycardia would be seen, not bradycardia. Peripheral pulses would be weak and thready, not bounding.

Question 120

Answer: B

Rationale: Stimulation of β_1 receptors is the primary response to dobutamine. This results in increased heart rate and contractility. Stimulation of β_2 receptors results in vasodilation and bronchodilation. Stimulation of dopaminergic receptors results in vasodilation of the renal and mesenteric arteries. Stimulation of α receptors results in vasoconstriction as seen in norepinephrine.

Question 121

Answer: A

Rationale: The patient is exhibiting signs of aortic dissection. Fibrinolytic therapy would likely kill the patient and is contraindicated. Emergency surgery is indicated as is management of blood pressure with nitroglycerin IV. Pain management will help manage blood pressure.

Question 122

Answer: C

Rationale: The first letter displays chamber paced, the second letter chamber senses, and third letter chamber inhibited. DDD shows dual-chambers on all three. Pacemakers are a common question on the CCRN exam; study this.

Question 123

Answer: B

Rationale: Any penetrating object should be left until fully assessed by a physician. The nurse should never remove a penetrating object. Stabilize the area until further assessment. The patient is stable at this time, so no emergency or immediate action needs to be taken.

Question 124

Answer: B

Rationale: The current situation is describing a failure to capture the pacemaker. To correct the immediate situation, the electrical output should be increased. Sensitivity will not correct the current issue. Stopping the pacemaker may result in a complete loss of rhythm. Decreasing sensitivity or electrical output would also make the issue worse.

Question 125

Answer: D

Rationale: Symptoms of pericarditis may include a pericardial friction rub and chest pain. Cardiac output may be decreased, not increased. A new S3 murmur would indicate left-sided heart failure.

Practice Test 2

This is the second full practice exam included in this book. The test contains 125 questions, the same as the CCRN exam. Questions are modeled after the blueprint in type and amount. All questions are mixed and random in order. A passing grade on the CCRN exam is 87 questions out of 125 questions. This is your benchmark for success.

1. A physician is explaining the differences between a mechanical or biological valve to a patient in the ICU needing a valve replacement surgery. The patient decides to move forward with a mechanical valve. Which of the following is most important for this patient after the procedure?

    A. Prevention of valve infection

    B. Monitoring of dysrhythmias

    C. Managing hypertension

    D. Adherence to anticoagulation therapy

2. An 86-year-old female patient is in the ICU post fracture of the right arm and subsequent need for anticoagulation and monitoring. X-rays show old fractures as well as previously unknown rib fractures. The nurse is unsure about the findings, but the patient states they are clumsy. The home caregiver will not leave the bedside. Which action by the nurse is best to adequately address this situation?

    A. Contact security and have them escort the caregiver off hospital property

    B. State to the patient and caregiver the unexplained findings on the x-rays

    C. Contact the appropriate authorities to report elder abuse

    D. Consult with a social worker to meet with the patient privately

GO ON TO NEXT PAGE ➤

3. A patient post mitral valve repair develops a complete heart block. Current blood pressure is 85/60 mmHg. Which of the following actions does the nurse perform at this time?

   A. Override the intrinsic heart rhythm and pace the patient via epicardial wires

   B. Attach the patient to pads and pace via transcutaneous pacing

   C. Administer albumin and increase fluid resuscitation

   D. Contact the physician and anticipate administration of dobutamine

4. A 32-year-old male patient is recovering in the ICU after multiple lower extremity open fractures. They were repaired in the operating room by external fixation. A recently drawn arterial blood gas reveals pH 7.50, PCO_2 26, HCO_2 22, PaO_2 72. Which intervention is most appropriate at this time?

   A. Recommend intubation and mechanical ventilation with high PEEP

   B. Assess pain, apply nasal cannula with oxygen

   C. Obtain an order for a V/Q scan STAT

   D. Administer lorazepam PRN for anxiety

5. A patient in the ICU with multiple traumas begins to experience symptoms of delirium tremens. The nurse administers lorazepam IV per CIWA protocol; however, the patient continues to worsen. Which of the following is most likely to aid in this current situation?

   A. Phenobarbital

   B. IV hydration with thiamine

   C. Assess and prevent Korsakoff syndrome

   D. Midazolam

6. A patient with a severe infection develops hyperthermia. Which of the following is true when the oxyhemoglobin dissociation curve shifts to the right as in the case of elevated temperature?

   A. Increased release of oxygen from hemoglobin

   B. Increased SaO_2

   C. Increase in serum 2, 3-DPG

   D. Increased SpO_2

7. A Type 1 diabetic is admitted to the ICU with a serum glucose of 480 mEq/dL and ketonuria. The patient was recently diagnosed with gastroenteritis and has been too nauseous to cat. Which of the following is likely the cause of the current situation?

   A. Decreased caloric intake

   B. Infection resulting in cortisol release

   C. Inadequate insulin administration

   D. Delay in seeking medical attention

8. A patient admitted with multiple traumas has remained intubated for 10 days. The healthcare team believes the patient needs a tracheostomy for continued mechanical ventilation. What is the primary benefit of tracheostomy over an endotracheal tube?

   A. Decreased need to suction/pulmonary hygiene

   B. Decreased need for sedation/analgesia

   C. Decreased cost/level of care

   D. Improved air flow/oxygenation

9. A patient was admitted to the ICU due to esophageal varices rupture with gross hematemesis. A Sengstaken–Blakemore tube was inserted in the emergency department to stop the bleeding. Two hours after the patient arrives in the ICU, alarm monitors alert a SpO_2 of 86% and the patient exhibits signs of shortness of breath. Which intervention is necessary at this time?

   A. Place the patient on a venturi mask at 40% FiO_2

   B. Draw an arterial blood gas STAT

   C. Cut the gastric balloon port with bedside scissors

   D. Pull on the tube gently and pull back 10 cm

10. A patient is admitted to the emergency department with suspected myocardial infarction. Chest pain is reported by the patient at rest. ST elevations exist on the ECG. Which of the following would lead the nurse to believe this was variant angina?

    A. Chest pain is relieved by nitroglycerin

    B. Chest pain is relieved by rest

    C. ST elevations normalize with rest

    D. T-wave inversion is seen on the ECG

11. A patient with a history of alcohol abuse is admitted to the hospital with signs and symptoms of severe dehydration, nausea, and vomiting. Which of the following ABGs would be expected for this patient with chronic alcoholism?

    A. pH 7.26, pCO_2 35, HCO_3 18
    B. pH 7.35, pCO_2 55, HCO_3 34
    C. pH 7.22, pCO_2 50, HCO_3 24
    D. pH 7.55, pCO_2 30, HCO_3 30

12. A patient is admitted to the emergency room with a head trauma. The CT scan shows a skull fracture. In what circumstances would the nurse expect the neurosurgeon to recommend surgery?

    A. The skull fracture is basilar in location
    B. The skull fracture accompanies a concussion
    C. The skull fracture is depressed 6 mm in depth
    D. The skull fracture is linear the full thickness of the skull

13. A patient with COPD exacerbation is currently on a 4 L venturi mask. The patient is exhibiting signs of respiratory distress with intercostal retractions. The physician decides to implement BiPAP in the hopes of avoiding intubation. After the patient is placed on BiPAP, what finding would best indicate to the nurse an improvement in the patient condition?

    A. Patient is anxious stating the mask is uncomfortable
    B. Decrease in arterial $PaCO_2$
    C. Patient states an improvement
    D. SpO_2 currently 84%

14. In the ICU, a unit maintenance item cannot be agreed upon between day shift and night shift nurses. The discourse is causing difficulty in the unit and is resulting in poor teamwork. What is an important first step to resolving this issue?

    A. Have the nurse manager meet with the staff nurses one by one
    B. Include both day shift and night shift nurses in a committee meeting
    C. Instruct two or three senior nurses to make a decision
    D. Implement different protocols for the day shift and night shift

15. Which of the following signs and symptoms is not associated with delirium in the ICU?

    A. Delirium only occurs in people with previously normal baselines (alert and oriented)
    B. Delirium may affect thought processes and attention
    C. Delirium may cause psychomotor slowing
    D. Delirium is typically acute and reversible

16. A patient with bowel obstruction is suspected of perforation. Which of the following signs or symptoms would suggest perforation if assessed by the nurse?

    A. Recent blood work showing a WBC of 5,000
    B. Pain that is lessened by lying flat or supine
    C. Stiff abdomen upon palpation with guarding
    D. Complaints of radiating lower back pain

17. The nurse caring for a patient with a low hemoglobin recently began a unit of packed red blood cells. The initial infusion rate was 100 mL/hr. Fifteen minutes after initiation, the patient is reporting difficulty breathing and urticaria present on the torso, neck, and face. Given the vital signs below, what is the most appropriate intervention by the nurse?

BP – 80/35	HR – 135	RR = 32	SpO$_2$ = 93%

    A. Slow down the blood transfusion, contact the HCP
    B. Norepinephrine, rapid fluid resuscitation
    C. Oxygen via non-rebreather mask, diphenhydramine
    D. Intramuscular epinephrine, intravenous steroids

18. A patient with pulmonary hypertension is admitted to the cardiac ICU due to worsening right-sided heart failure. A Swan-Ganz catheter is inserted for close monitoring. The patient has jugular venous distention and generalized edema. Current CVP is 14 mmHg, and PAP 32/14 mmHg. Given these findings, which of the following treatments is best?

    A. Initiate a dobutamine infusion
    B. Administer 500 mL bolus normal saline
    C. Initiate a milrinone infusion
    D. Administer sildenafil or epoprostenol

19. A patient was immediately taken to the operating room upon arrival due to suspected aortic dissection. The surgery was successful and the patient is due to arrive to the ICU momentarily. Which of the following should the nurse consider in the immediate postoperative hours?

    A. Rewarming the patient may result in a drop in blood pressure
    B. MAP below 60 mmHg is a target goal
    C. Maintain blood sugar below 120 mg/dL
    D. Strip chest tubes to maintain outward blood flow

GO ON TO NEXT PAGE ➤

20. A nurse is assisting with the turning of a patient when they notice the infusion pump for heparin is running at an abnormally high rate. The primary nurse is not present. The patient was admitted to the ICU with a deep vein thrombosis. Which of the following actions is most appropriate at this time?

    A. Contact the physician about the rate of infusion

    B. Change the rate on the infusion and notify the charge nurse

    C. Stop the infusion and fill out an incident report

    D. Speak to the primary nurse about the infusion drip and rate

21. A patient in the cardiac care unit has diastolic heart failure. The patient is currently on a beta blocker and ACE inhibitor. The ejection fraction remains low. Which of the following medications may improve the patient condition?

    A. Amlodipine

    B. Digoxin

    C. Dopamine

    D. Losartan

22. A patient in hemorrhagic shock is to receive blood transfusions. Which of the below blood reactions is the most dangerous and potentially fatal?

    A. Non-immune-mediated reaction

    B. Transfusion-associated circulatory overload

    C. Immune-mediated reaction (mismatched blood)

    D. Allergic reaction with urticaria and pruritus

23. A 65-year-old patient with acute on chronic kidney injury is admitted to the ICU for treatment. Which of the following electrolyte imbalances would the nurse expect?

    A. Hypokalemia, hypercalcemia, hyperphosphatemia

    B. Hyperkalemia, hypocalcemia, hyperphosphatemia

    C. Hyperkalemia, hyponatremia, hypomagnesemia

    D. Hypokalemia, hypernatremia, hypercalcemia

24. A 45-year-old patient has been admitted to the ICU for close monitoring. Chart reviews show this is the second admission by this patient in the last three months for this reason. The patient is stable and relaxing in bed. Which of the following statements by the nurse would inquire into potential reasons for the frequent admissions?

    A. Is your medication too expensive?

    B. Do you need help at home?

    C. Why do you think you are in the hospital?

    D. Do you use the hospital for your primary care?

25. A patient with chronic kidney disease is admitted to the critical care unit with a potassium of 7.0 mEq/L, hypotension, and an audible S_3. Oxygen is being administered by a venturi mask. Immediate intervention would be most effective by which of the following?

    A. Diuretics

    B. ACE inhibitors

    C. Norepinephrine

    D. Dialysis

26. A 63-year-old female patient is admitted for a hip fracture requiring surgical repair. This is her second major fracture within a 12-month period. She has experienced fatigue and weight loss in the previous 6 months. What problem is this patient likely experiencing?

    A. Osteogenesis imperfecta

    B. Calcium and vitamin D deficiency

    C. Hyperphosphatemia

    D. Vitamin C deficiency

27. A 75-year-old male patient is admitted from a nursing home for failure to thrive and multiple pressure ulcers. Which of the following is not a consideration for increased risk of pressure ulcers according to the Braden scale?

    A. Nutrition lacking adequate protein

    B. Peripheral neuropathy

    C. Autonomic neuropathy

    D. Urinary and fecal incontinence

28. During placement of a pulmonary artery catheter (Swan-Ganz), the nurse is assisting by inflating and deflating the balloon as ordered by the physician. As the catheter is threaded through the right-sided chambers of the heart, the nurse suspects the balloon is now wedged in the pulmonary artery. What is the next step?

    A. Note the pressure and deflate the balloon

    B. Instill 5 mL of air into the balloon catheter and advance

    C. Maintain the inflated balloon for 60 seconds and read the pressure

    D. Withdraw the catheter back to prevent wedging

29. A patient is admitted to the ICU from the floor due to sustained hypotension due to hypovolemia. Which of the following would the nurse see in the early stages of shock?

    A. Decreased urine output
    B. Increased work of breathing
    C. Increased cardiac output
    D. Decreased blood pressure

30. An hour into the administration of a potassium infusion to a patient, the nurse notices the bag hung includes 40 mEq of potassium instead of the ordered 20 mEq. What is the first step in correcting this error?

    A. Fill out an incident report and notify the nurse manager
    B. Assess infusion pump rate and obtain the correct bag
    C. Notify the physician immediately
    D. Change the volume to be infused to only 20 mEq

31. When administering an insulin drip to a patient in diabetic ketoacidosis, when does the nurse begin to administer dextrose infusion instead of normal saline infusion?

    A. When the anion gap is closed
    B. When metabolic acidosis is corrected
    C. When serum potassium normalizes
    D. When the serum glucose reaches 250 mg/dL

32. A 24-year-old asthmatic patient is admitted to the ICU with status asthmaticus. Which of the following is a true statement regarding the current condition of this patient?

    A. This condition is often exacerbated by upper respiratory tract infections
    B. This condition typically responds well to albuterol
    C. This condition results in increased forced expiratory volume
    D. This condition automatically requires intubation and mechanical ventilation

33. A 55-year-old patient is admitted to the ICU with multiple traumas. Pain management has been difficult for this patient; multiple opioid narcotics have not been helpful. The nurse would like to incorporate nonpharmacological therapies—specifically, guided imagery that may be played on a nearby computer. What would be the most appropriate first intervention by the nurse?

A. Assess previous research on effectiveness of guided imagery

B. Set up the computer and search for appropriate guided imagery

C. Call the family to ask for permission to use guided imagery

D. Ask the patient if guided imagery would be something of interest to them

34. A 45-year-old patient has complaints of dull abdominal pain and recent nausea and vomiting. The patient describes the vomiting as "forceful." Further assessment by the nurse reveals high-pitched bowel sounds. What condition does this patient most likely have?

A. Ruptured appendicitis

B. Small bowel obstruction

C. Acute esophagitis

D. Large bowel obstruction

35. A patient reports chest pain while walking down the sidewalk. When they arrived back home, the patient took a sublingual nitroglycerin and the pain dissipated. Out of fear, the patient arrived at the emergency department. What is the most accurate statement to make to the patient at this time?

A. This was unstable angina and will require admission to the hospital

B. This was not a heart attack; this pain is common in stable angina

C. This will require an immediate cardiac catheterization to rule out a heart attack

D. This situation is benign and will not require follow-up in the future

36. The ICU nurse has received an order to begin a heparin infusion for a patient with an active DVT. Which of the following is most important in reducing an error regarding this medication?

A. Contact the pharmacy for the exact rate of infusion

B. Double check or triple check the work with oneself

C. Obtain a double sign-off with another registered nurse

D. Obtain a coagulation panel 6 hours after initiation

GO ON TO NEXT PAGE ➤

37. A 74-year-old male patient is admitted to the ICU with probable subdural hematoma. There is a previous history of stroke due to atrial fibrillation. A pacemaker was placed to manage tachyarrhythmias. Which of the following diagnostic tests is best for this patient to assess current neurological bleeding?

    A. Computed tomography (CT)
    B. Magnetic resonance imaging
    C. X-ray film
    D. Fluoroscopy

38. A patient in the neuro ICU is recovering post craniotomy for a subarachnoid hemorrhage by ruptured aneurysm. The physician orders control of blood pressure with a nicardipine infusion. Which problem is the healthcare team attempting to prevent by utilizing this infusion?

    A. Vasospasms
    B. Increased intracranial pressure
    C. Cardiac ischemia
    D. Rebleeds

39. A 36-year-old female is in her first trimester of pregnancy when she arrives at the emergency department complaining of a headache. She states the headache does not go away. Which of the following findings is of most concern?

    A. Blood pressure 160/95 mmHg
    B. Lower abdominal pain
    C. Edema around the ankle
    D. Quickening of the fetus

40. A patient is admitted to the emergency department with cocaine intoxication and potential overdose. Which of the following signs and symptoms would be expected in this patient?

    A. Bradycardia
    B. Nystagmus
    C. Anxiety
    D. Abdominal pain

41. A patient in heart failure has a current blood pressure of 90/50 mmHg, cardiac output 2 L/min, and SVR of 1800 dynes/sec/cm⁵. Current treatment with inotropes has failed; the patient is now in cardiogenic shock. The physician decides to begin intra-aortic balloon pump treatment for which purpose?

    A. Decrease preload and cardiac ischemia
    B. Decrease afterload and increase coronary artery perfusion
    C. Decrease afterload and improve cardiac output
    D. Decrease preload and improve right ventricular output

42. A patient with a femur fracture is admitted to the ICU with planned surgery for tomorrow. They have a history of chronic kidney disease. The patient complains of mild pain requiring intervention. Which of the following medications is contraindicated in this patient?

    A. Acetaminophen
    B. Naproxen
    C. Oxycodone
    D. Hydromorphone

43. After a myocardial infarction with intervention, the nurse notes gradual resolution of ST elevations on the ECG. The patient is transferred to a step-down unit the following day for continued monitoring. An ECG taken days after the initial MI may show what changes?

    A. Large-peaked T waves
    B. Q waves
    C. Inverted p waves
    D. Widened "QRS" complex

44. When deciding the best intravenous fluid for infusion, the nurse notes a serum sodium of 115 mEq/L. The patient is suspected of fluid overload. Which of the following intravenous fluids would be contraindicated in this patient?

    A. Normal saline (0.9% NaCl)
    B. Half-normal saline with dextrose 5% (0.45% NaCl with D5%)
    C. 3% saline
    D. Dextrose 5%

45. The nurse is reviewing evidence-based practice for reducing the risk of catheter-associated UTIs. Which of the following correctly identifies how EBP is utilized in practice?

    A. EBP begins with setting guidelines for practice
    B. Clinical guidelines are built off of research
    C. EBP is almost exclusively applied for patient satisfaction
    D. Quantitative research is built off of clinical practice

46. While assessing a number of patients in the ICU, the nurse would note which treatments as being effective control of preload and afterload?

    A. Nitroprusside decreasing afterload in hypertensive crisis
    B. Bumetanide infusion increasing preload in heart failure
    C. Norepinephrine decreasing afterload and SVR in septic shock
    D. Administration of blood decreasing preload in severe anemia

47. A patient with a pacemaker displays a spike before the p wave but no spike before the QRS. As the nurse helps the patient out of bed to the bathroom, the heart rate increases on the monitor. Which of the following settings is this pacemaker?

    A. VVI
    B. AAI
    C. DDD
    D. VOO

48. A patient is admitted with a severe upper respiratory infection and increasing work of breathing with mild intercostal retractions. The patient is visibly anxious. Given the below vital signs and ABG results, which intervention is most appropriate?

VITAL SIGNS	ABG RESULTS
BP = 145/90 mmHg	pH = 7.34
HR = 135/min	$PaCO_2$ = 50
SpO_2 = 90% on 4L nasal cannula	PaO_2 = 62
Temp = 39°C	HCO_3 = 32

    A. Immediate intubation and mechanical ventilation
    B. Increase the nasal cannula to 8 L
    C. Administer lorazepam IV push
    D. Transition the patient to high-flow nasal cannula

49. A patient with suspected meningitis undergoes a lumbar puncture for confirmation. The physician orders supportive treatment with a diagnosis of viral meningitis. Which of the following findings of the lumbar puncture correlate to this diagnosis?

    A. Glucose 75 mg/dL
    B. Elevated WBC
    C. Elevated protein
    D. Cloudy CSF

50. A 55-year-old male patient has had recent problems focusing at work. He states he recently got a divorce. He also has complaints of insomnia and flat affect. The past few days he states he has been unable to remember simple tasks like taking out the trash or paying bills. What is the most likely cause of this patient's memory loss?

    A. Psychotic break
    B. Early-onset dementia
    C. Situational depression
    D. Mild acute delirium

51. A 36-year-old female patient is admitted with an infected wound on the left arm. She has a history of IV drug use and is positive for HIV. Upon admission, the wound is erythematous and painful. When the nurse returns to round on the patient, the wound has spread to the upper arm and now appears purple. The patient complains of excruciating pain on the arm. What is the likely condition this patient is experiencing?

    A. Severe cellulitis complicated with likely sepsis
    B. Localized infiltration of IV drugs
    C. Necrotizing fasciitis
    D. Traumatic wound due to repeated needle penetration

52. A 78-year-old female patient with a history of schizophrenia is admitted to the critical care unit with multiple traumas. She is not oriented at this time but remains calm. There are blood dyscrasias upon laboratory assessment. Which of the following is a priority at this time?

    A. Contact the patient's psychiatrist to confirm current treatment
    B. Perform a medication reconciliation on all home medications
    C. Hold all psychiatric medication
    D. Obtain a consult for inpatient psychiatry

GO ON TO NEXT PAGE ➤

53. A patient is receiving intravenous diltiazem therapy for recent episodes of atrial fibrillation with rapid ventricular rate (RVR). Which of the following is an important assessment while utilizing this infusion?

    A. Close heart rate monitoring

    B. Measuring of QT interval

    C. Assessment of cardiac output

    D. Obtain baseline serum magnesium levels

54. A patient receiving amiodarone, ciprofloxacin, and furosemide is on a cardiac care unit for close monitoring. The monitor alarms and current rhythm is interpreted as torsades de point. After ACLS protocol, the patient is stabilized. What is the priority and quickest assessment the nurse may perform to assess causes of this rhythm?

    A. Draw immediate lab tests for electrolytes

    B. Assess current QT interval

    C. Contact pharmacy to review potential drug interactions

    D. Assess for worsening acute kidney injury

55. A 21-year-old patient arrives at the emergency department after a minor motor vehicle accident. The patient was restrained. Upper left quadrant pain is present that radiates to the left shoulder especially upon exertion. The patient also reports recently being sick of mononucleosis. What is the most likely diagnosis given the clinical findings and history?

    A. Ruptured bowel

    B. Pancreatic laceration

    C. Ruptured aortic arch

    D. Ruptured spleen

56. A 55-year-old patient is admitted with severe constipation and abdominal cramping. The patient does not remember when their last bowel movement was; it is likely a week or more. Large bowel obstruction is suspected. The patient has a BMI of 34, hemoglobin of 8.5, and a history of smoking. What is the most common cause of large bowel obstruction and the likely culprit for this patient?

    A. Crohn's disease

    B. Colorectal cancer

    C. Surgical adhesions

    D. Intussusception

57. A patient with a current BP of 210/90 mmHg is prescribed nitroglycerin IV infusion. The primary goal being to prevent the rupture of a current intracranial aneurysm. Where is the location of the aneurysm if it is located in the most common area?

    A. Circle of Willis
    B. Carotid artery
    C. Intraventricular space
    D. Hypothalamus

58. The increased production of immunoglobulin E results in which type of distributive shock?

    A. Neurogenic shock
    B. Septic shock
    C. Anaphylactic shock
    D. Endocrine shock

59. A 55-year-old patient in the ICU developed ARDS as a complication to septic shock. Which of the following diagnostic findings would not be seen in this patient?

    A. PaO_2/FiO_2 <250
    B. PAWP <16 mmHg
    C. SVR <600 dynes/sec/cm^{-5}
    D. Refractory hypoxia

60. A 55-year-old patient arrives at the emergency department with left-sided hemiparesis and aphasia. Family states the symptoms began 2 hours before bringing him to the hospital. Thrombolytic therapy is indicated. As the nurse briefly reviews history, which of the following would contraindicate the use of tPA?

    A. History of pulmonary embolism
    B. Peripheral arterial disease
    C. Head trauma 6 months ago
    D. Cerebral AV malformation

61. A patient is suspected of having a pulmonary embolism (PE). Which diagnostic test is the best indicator for diagnosis of PE?

    A. Chest x-ray
    B. CT pulmonary angiogram (CTPA)
    C. D-dimer
    D. Ventilation/perfusion scan

GO ON TO NEXT PAGE ➤

62. A 52-year-old female patient is in the ICU with severe respiratory illness. Over the course of the last 2 weeks, the patient has lost 5 kg. Continued severe diarrhea has made tube feedings difficult and the decision to initiate total parenteral nutrition (TPN) is made. When beginning TPN, what adverse effect would be the initial concern?

    A. Hyperglycemia

    B. CLABSI

    C. Infection

    D. Liver dysfunction

63. A female patient is admitted to the ICU with shortness of breath, fever, and tachypnea. She also has complaints of chest pain upon breathing and chills. A diagnosis of pneumonia is made. Ultrasound exam reveals a large pleural effusion of the left lung in addition to bilateral lung infiltrates seen on the chest x-ray. Given the vital signs, lab and ABG analysis, what is the likely condition and expected intervention?

VITAL SIGNS	LABORATORY FINDINGS	ABG ANALYSIS
BP = 135/95 mmHg	RBC = 4.3×10^3/ul	pH = 7.2
HR = 125/min	Hgb = 12.4×10^3/ul	$PaCO_2$ = 58
SpO_2 = 90% on 60% FiO_2 (non-rebreather)	Plt = 135,000/ul	PaO_2 = 65
Temp = 39°C (102.2°F)	WBC = 16,000/ul	HCO_3 = 25

    A. Empyema/chest tube placement

    B. Renal failure/dialysis

    C. Tension pneumothorax/thoracentesis

    D. Septic shock/antibiotics

64. A patient arrives from surgery to the critical care unit. The patient had a kidney transplant performed. The nurse notes a new order for tacrolimus in the chart. Which of the following clinical manifestations should the nurse pay particular attention for?

    A. Decreased muscle tone

    B. Decreased urine output

    C. Increased serum potassium

    D. Increased platelet count

65. A patient with valvular disease is being assessed by the cardiologist. After the physician auscultates, they state the patient has a loud systolic murmur that is associated with systolic dysfunction. It is also noted the murmur is likely from stenosis. Which valves are potentially the culprit of this murmur?

    A. Pulmonic/tricuspid
    B. Aortic/mitral
    C. Mitral/tricuspid
    D. Aortic/pulmonic

66. A patient with terminal cancer decides to enter hospice care. The healthcare team is reviewing palliative care for the patient and items to be included in the plan of care. Which of the following is not an aspect of palliative care?

    A. Coordinating care with multiple disciplines
    B. Respecting patient cultural practices
    C. Expressing the need for curative treatment
    D. Administer pain control methods

67. A diabetic patient is being assessed for peripheral arterial disease (PAD) due to new onset pain in the lower extremities. An ankle–brachial index reveals a ratio of 0.7. How would the nurse interpret these results?

    A. This patient may have venous congestion, the extremities should be elevated above the heart
    B. This patient may have severe stenosis, surgical bypass is likely
    C. This patient likely has PAD, the ankle–brachial index is specific to diagnosis
    D. This patient may have PAD, the extremities should be kept dependent of the heart

68. A patient arrives at the emergency room by ambulance after being picked up in a park by police. The patient was screaming the world was under attack by aliens. Upon arrival, the patient is found to be hypertensive, tachycardic, and hyperthermic with sweating. Which of the following substances has this patient likely ingested?

    A. Marijuana
    B. LSD
    C. Cocaine
    D. Alcohol

GO ON TO NEXT PAGE ➤

69. Which of the following is not a known cause for systolic heart failure?

    A. Myocardial infarction
    B. Hypertension
    C. Atrial fibrillation
    D. Aortic stenosis

70. A 32-year-old male patient arrives at the emergency department with symptoms of the flu. He states the symptoms began last night. How long after exposure would symptoms of the flu typically begin?

    A. 14 days or more
    B. 24 hours or less
    C. 1 to 2 weeks
    D. 1 to 4 days

71. A patient arrives at the critical care unit after a coronary bypass surgery. Which of the following is not an appropriate nursing intervention to prevent complications after the patient is extubated?

    A. Administering a sedative and splinting the chest upon coughing
    B. Overriding a second-degree heart block with a temporary pacemaker
    C. Administering aminocaproic acid to prevent post-op bleeding
    D. Providing a insulin infusion to combat hyperglycemia from catecholamines

72. A nurse is utilizing the nomogram "PQRST" to aid in the pain assessment of a patient. Which of the following findings would reflect the "P" in this assessment?

    A. Increased pain upon coughing
    B. Radiating pain to the umbilicus
    C. Pain 8/10
    D. The pain is worse at night

73. A patient in heart failure develops fluid overload. Which of the following would not be seen in this patient?

    A. Jugular venous distention
    B. Lung crackles upon auscultation
    C. New onset S3 and S4 murmur
    D. Decreased GFR with azotemia

74. A 23-year-old female gymnast was competing when she experienced a sudden and excruciating headache. Upon arrival to the hospital, she was immediately admitted to the neuro ICU. At this time, she had additional complaints of neck stiffness. Which of the following is the likely diagnosis given the symptoms?

    A. Epidural hematoma
    B. Subarachnoid hemorrhage
    C. Intracranial hemorrhage
    D. Coup-contrecoup injury

75. A patient has a current blood pressure of 80/40 mmHg. In which type of shock is intra-aortic balloon pump therapy indicated?

    A. Cardiogenic
    B. Hypovolemic
    C. Anaphylactic
    D. Neurogenic

76. A nurse working on a med-surg floor calls a rapid response on a patient they believe to be in severe sepsis. The patient is immediately transferred to the ICU. All of the following items the nurse should perform within the first hour of admission EXCEPT:

    A. Measure lactate level
    B. Obtain blood cultures
    C. Initiate inotropic therapy for refractory hypotension
    D. Immediate administration of crystalloids

77. A patient is admitted directly to the ICU from a nursing home for an infected pressure ulcer. The wound base is healing with large amounts of exudate coming out of the wound. Which of the following dressings is most appropriate for use in this wound?

    A. Duoderm and tegaderm dressings
    B. Aliginates and hydrogel dressings
    C. Wet-to-dry dressings
    D. Hydrocolloid and silver sulfadiazine dressings

78. A patient with unknown abdominal trauma complains of diffuse pain and difficulty breathing. The abdomen is visually distended. Which position would the nurse place the patient to best assist with improving ventilation?

    A. High-Fowler's
    B. 30–45-degree elevation
    C. Supine
    D. Prone

GO ON TO NEXT PAGE ➤

79. During assessment of a patient with a previous stroke, the nurse notes the left arm has full range of motion against gravity and some resistance. The right arm does not move although the patient states a muscle contraction. How would the nurse grade the movement of the left arm?

    A. Grade 5
    B. Grade 1
    C. Grade 2
    D. Grade 4

80. The family member of a patient on norepinephrine infusion notes discoloration of the patient's toes. What is the most appropriate action by the nurse?

    A. Kindly ask the patient to wait while you notify the physician
    B. Explain the discoloration is normal and will not harm the patient
    C. Assess the discoloration and peripheral pulses
    D. Advocate to the healthcare team switching to an alternate vasopressor

81. A patient is diagnosed with osteomyelitis of the left femur after an open fracture. What is the priority action for this patient?

    A. Administer intravenous antibiotics
    B. Obtain an intraosseous catheter
    C. Notify the orthopedic surgeon
    D. Obtain blood cultures

82. A patient in DKA is receiving a normal saline infusion and insulin infusion for the past 3 hours. Which of the following should the nurse anticipate giving to prevent adverse effects of this treatment?

    A. Administration of magnesium sulfate
    B. Administration of potassium chloride
    C. Administration of calcium gluconate
    D. Administration of vitamin B6 supplements

83. An elderly patient is admitted to the ICU with multiple diagnosis. They are expected to remain on bed rest for an extended period of time. Which of the following would not be helpful in reducing adverse outcomes of prolonged immobility?

    A. Perform active and passive range of motion exercises
    B. Encourage movement within bed and help with turning
    C. Utilizing deep-breathing techniques
    D. Activate bed alarms and round hourly

84. The nurse in the ICU is rounding on a patient with a psych history. The nurse wishes to assess potential changes in mental status. Which of the following is not a part of the mental status examination?

A. Orientation to person, place, situation, and time

B. Ability to concentrate

C. Encouraging nurse–patient rapport

D. Presentation of appearance and affect

85. A patient in the ICU is diagnosed with an acute kidney injury secondary to excessive contrast use. Which of the following characteristics of the patient's urine would be expected?

A. Low urine sodium, high specific gravity

B. High urine sodium, low specific gravity

C. Low urine sodium, low specific gravity

D. High urine sodium, high specific gravity

86. The ICU has recently updated a handful of protocols involving patient care. The majority of staff have enacted the new protocols without issue; however, some staff are complaining that a few staff are incredibly resistant to the changes and have continued to refuse. What is the best action to fix this current problem?

A. Bring the staff refusing to follow protocols into the nurse manager's office

B. Send the staff refusing e-mails educating the new protocols

C. Hold a staff meeting to discuss the new protocols

D. Give the staff more time to adapt to the changes and reevaluate in 3 months

87. A patient arrives at the emergency department after being extracted from a burning building. There is high suspicion of smoke inhalation. The physician believes intubation to be the best course of action. Which arterial blood gas would indicate intubation is likely?

A. pH 7.55, $PaCO_2$ 32 mmHg, PaO_2 79 mmHg

B. pH 7.40, $PaCO_2$ 35 mmHg, PaO_2 85 mmHg

C. pH 7.32, $PaCO_2$ 48 mmHg, PaO_2 64 mmHg

D. pH 7.45, $PaCO_2$ 33 mmHg, PaO_2 64 mmHg

GO ON TO NEXT PAGE ➤

88. Which of the following actions would not safeguard privacy and confidentiality of a patient in regard to the use of electronic medical records (EMR)?

    A. Setting up automatic closure of the EMR after 3 minutes of no activity
    B. Encouraging the use of patient passwords
    C. Auditing chart access by healthcare staff
    D. Withholding information for insurance reimbursement

89. The mother of a gunshot victim is in the waiting area. The patient passed away 5 minutes ago and the nurse is cleaning the body of blood to present to the mother. When bringing the mother into the room, which of the following would aid in the grieving process?

    A. Explain the reasons for the death of her child
    B. Stand quietly with the mother as she holds her child's hand
    C. Leave the room if the mother begins to cry
    D. Call the chaplain to be with the mother

90. A patient diagnosed with ARDS is being mechanically ventilated. The patient is on sedation with propofol and fentanyl. The patient is asynchronous with the ventilator and has a pulse ox of 86%. Increasing the sedation does not fix the problem. The blood pressure is also low. Which of the following is indicated at this time?

    A. Switch the ventilator mode from assist control to SIMV
    B. Consider the use of neuromuscular blocking agents
    C. Consider adding another form of sedation, such as midazolam
    D. Place a bite block in the patient's mouth, assess high pressure

91. A patient in the ICU is critically ill and unable to work. A manager from the patient's work calls to inquire about when they may be able to return to work. How should the nurse respond?

    A. Explain the patient is critically ill and unlikely to return anytime soon
    B. Do not disclose the diagnosis, but explain the patient cannot work right now
    C. Do not disclose any information; suggest they speak to the patient's wife
    D. Explain the manager should call back at a later time when the patient is able to speak

92. A critically ill patient recently had a central line placed for continuous administration of medicine. Which of the following is not helpful in reducing the risk of central line associated bloodstream infection (CLABSI)?

    A. Following appropriate hand hygiene
    B. Utilizing nurse-driven protocol for removal of unnecessary catheters
    C. Encouraging the use of femoral vein catheters
    D. Change the transparent dressing minimum every 7 days

93. The nurse is caring for a number of patients who came into the emergency department with complaints in line with an ongoing respiratory viral pandemic. Which of the following would be most important for the nurse to enact immediately?

    A. Quarantine the patients if possible, have each patient wear a surgical mask
    B. Perform appropriate tests to confirm the presence of infection
    C. Notify respiratory therapy, prepare for impending interventions
    D. Call the state health department, disclose positive cases

94. A 60-year-old patient with advanced pancreatic cancer is told by the healthcare team his prognosis is very poor. He likely does not have much time yet. This morning he is unable to tolerate any PO intake without becoming severely nauseated with dry emesis. He states he no longer wants food or other interventions besides medication for pain. How can the nurse best approach this situation?

    A. Allow the patient to clearly describe his wishes
    B. Leave the room to allow the patient privacy
    C. Encourage intake of food to preserve strength
    D. Sit with the patient and describe hospice care

95. A patient in the ICU is experiencing severe pain requiring q2h IV boluses of morphine. The patient no longer wants morphine as it makes them excessively sleepy and unable to perform even simple tasks. The nurse advocates for a move to a patient-controlled device to avoid overmedication and assures the patient pain control will be adequate. Which two nursing ethics is the nurse following by advocating this move?

    A. Autonomy and nonmaleficence
    B. Nonmaleficence and beneficence
    C. Fidelity and justice
    D. Autonomy and fidelity

GO ON TO NEXT PAGE ➤

96. A patient in the ICU had a transvenous pacemaker placed a short while ago. The current settings on the pacemaker were set by the physician and is reflected on the monitor as 100% pacing at a rate of 90 BPM. The nurse wants to test the capture threshold to minimize battery failure. How would the nurse perform this action?

    A. Decrease the sensitivity

    B. Increase the sensitivity

    C. Decrease the electrical output

    D. Increase the electrical output

97. A large healthcare team is present in a patient room due to instability and potential emergency. While waiting, the alarms begin beeping and ventricular fibrillation is seen on the monitor. After pushing the code blue button, which of the following actions should the bedside nurse perform first?

    A. Leave the room and obtain a crash cart

    B. Initiate cardiopulmonary resuscitation

    C. Assess for a carotid pulse

    D. Obtain 1 mg of epinephrine and administer immediately

98. The nurse witnesses a sentinel event on a patient they are responsible for. What is the obligation of the nurse from the standpoint of documentation?

    A. Omit information regarding the sentinel event from the patient medical record

    B. Document minimal information in the patient chart, use vague language

    C. Document information as witnessed in the patient chart, fill out an incident report

    D. Fill out an incident report and place in the patient's medical record

99. A 23-year-old transgender female patient is admitted to the ICU from the emergency department. The patient has multiple traumas and requires the placement of an indwelling catheter. What is the first step the nurse should take in providing sensitive care?

    A. Speak with the charge nurse about switching assignments if the nurse is uncomfortable

    B. Reflect on personal knowledge and feelings regarding transgendered patients

    C. Assess whether the patient has female or male genitals

    D. Obtain the indwelling catheter and prepare for the procedure

100. A 65-kilogram patient in respiratory distress is intubated to provide adequate ventilation. The settings ordered by the physician are assist control mode 16/min, tidal volume 450 mL, FiO$_2$ 60%, and PEEP 16. Which of the following adverse effects might the nurse see due to the intubation and current settings?

    A. Sudden decrease in cardiac output

    B. Increase in pulmonary artery perfusion

    C. Improvement in ABG results

    D. Barotrauma secondary to excessive tidal volume

101. A patient with hypercalcemia secondary to hyperparathyroidism is in the ICU for close monitoring. Morning labs show a serum phosphorus of 1.6 mg/dL and serum calcium of 12.6 mg/dL. Which of the following complications of hypophosphatemia should the nurse especially monitor for?

    A. New onset Chvostek's sign

    B. Osteoporosis

    C. Excessive diarrhea and vomiting

    D. Respiratory muscle weakness

102. A patient in the ICU with COPD exacerbation is being intubated at the request of the pulmonologist. Which of the following considerations with the ventilator is best for a patient with COPD exacerbation?

    A. Shorten inspiratory time by setting fast respiratory rates

    B. Prolong inspiratory time by setting low respiratory rates

    C. Shorten expiratory time by setting fast respiratory rates

    D. Prolong expiratory time by setting low respiratory rates

103. A patient in septic shock develops petechiae, hematuria, and oozing from the IV sites. The nurse suspects disseminated intravascular coagulation and confirms with a blood draw to test for fibrin split products. The physician orders cryoprecipitate for what reason in this patient?

    A. Increase circulating thrombin

    B. Increase circulating fibrinogen

    C. Increase circulating plasmin

    D. Increase circulating platelets

104. A patient receiving massive transfusion protocol due to multiple traumas will likely develop which problem due to the citrate in the transfused blood?

    A. Hypokalemia

    B. Hyponatremia

    C. Hypermagnesemia

    D. Hypocalcemia

GO ON TO NEXT PAGE ➤

105. A patient arrives to the ICU due to an acute on chronic injury to renal insufficiency. The nurse is reviewing nutritional requirements with the dietician. Which of the following would not be restricted from the diet of this patient?

    A. Potassium
    B. Fluids
    C. Proteins
    D. Carbohydrates

106. A patient with fluid overload arrives at the emergency department with dyspnea and crackles upon auscultation. They state missing three dialysis appointments over the past two weeks. Emergency dialysis is ordered to begin immediately. Which of the following is the best method to gauge successful fluid removal in fluid overload?

    A. Decrease in pulmonary crackles
    B. Trend blood pressure goals
    C. Obtain daily weights
    D. Increase in GFR

107. A patient who sustained multiple abdominal injuries is admitted to the ICU. CT scan shows injury to multiple organs, including the liver, spleen, and stomach. Acute liver failure is suspected when recent lab work shows transaminitis and increased ammonia levels. Due to injury to the stomach, the patient is unable to receive any medication through the NG tube. It remains to low intermittent suction. How would the nurse advocate the immediate removal of ammonia in this patient?

    A. Lactulose enema
    B. Decrease protein in the diet
    C. Peritoneal dialysis
    D. Neomycin

108. An intubated patient is admitted to the neuro ICU after a serious motor vehicle accident. The patient has a critical traumatic brain injury as seen on a head CT. Upon admission, the nurse notes bilateral pupillary size of 8 mm, flaccidity of the body, and a negative corneal reflex. Which of the following actions should the nurse take at this time?

    A. Report the findings to a physician, anticipate the need for an apnea test
    B. Assess for loss of brain-stem reflexes
    C. Call organ procurement services
    D. Document the findings, assess an ABG

109. A patient in the ICU with a psych history reports intense fear with chest tightness, diaphoresis, and visual disturbances. The nurse suspects a panic attack. What physiological changes does the nurse understand to cause panic attacks?

    A. A decrease in gamma-aminobutyric acid
    B. An increase in parasympathetic function
    C. A decrease in amygdala activity
    D. There are no physiological changes as the issue in psychological

110. The nurse is teaching a class about the important pathophysiological changes seen in patients with sepsis. Which of the following is not a main pathophysiological feature of sepsis?

    A. Decreased serum neutrophils
    B. Systemic inflammation
    C. Abnormal coagulation
    D. Disordered fibrinolysis

111. A patient is admitted to the ICU with suspected overdose. The patient is unconscious, bradycardic, and bradypneic. Excessive secretions have required multiple deep suctionings. The patient also has constricted pupils and has urinated and defecated in the bed. Which medication has the patient likely overdosed on?

    A. Anticholinergic agents
    B. Acetaminophen/oxycodone
    C. Beta blockers
    D. Cholinergic agonists

112. A patient in the ICU being treated for new-onset asthma has a history of heart failure and is on captopril, metoprolol, and furosemide. Which of the following considerations should the nurse recommend to the physician?

    A. Increase the dose of furosemide
    B. Stop the captopril
    C. Stop the metoprolol
    D. Hold ordered albuterol

113. A patient with a stab wound to the right leg is hemorrhaging from the site of injury. Current vital signs include blood pressure 75/55 mmHg, heart rate 150 BPM, respiratory rate 35/min, and SpO_2 90% on 15 L mask. What class of hemorrhagic shock is this patient in?

    A. Class IV
    B. Class III
    C. Class II
    D. Class I

114. A nurse is walking down the hall when they see another nurse shove a patient back into bed aggressively. The patient has dementia and has repeatedly been trying to get out of bed throughout the shift as witnessed by the floor staff. How should the nurse respond?

    A. Ask the patient later about the potential abuse
    B. Report the behavior to the nurse manager immediately
    C. Walk away from the situation and file a report
    D. Contact the family to report the behavior

115. A tensilon test is ordered for a patient with suspected myasthenia gravis. An improvement in muscle strength after the injection of edrophonium would suggest what diagnosis?

    A. Myasthenia gravis
    B. Cholinergic crisis
    C. Guillain–Barre
    D. Huntington's disease

116. A patient is intubated in the emergency department after being found unconscious on a sidewalk. The healthcare team suspects the patient is inebriated by alcohol. Upon auscultation the nurse notes crackles. Which of the following is true regarding aspiration in this patient?

    A. Aspiration is most likely to occur in the left lung
    B. Aspiration is likely due to decreased gag reflex
    C. Aspiration will likely result in the need for a bronchoscopy
    D. Aspiration recovery will benefit with antibiotic use

117. ST elevations are seen in leads II, III, aVF, and V2–V5. A friction rub can be heard upon auscultation regardless if the patient holds their breath. The patient complains of chest pain, especially when lying flat in the bed. Which problem is this patient likely experiencing?

   A. Anterior wall STEMI
   B. Inferior wall STEMI
   C. Endocarditis
   D. Pericarditis

118. A patient is critically ill in the ICU. There are multiple avenues for treatment, but the patient is intubated and sedated. The power of attorney lies with a young family member who is a physician. There is discourse because a current girlfriend disagrees with the HPOA on the next course of action. What is the best course of action in dealing with this issue?

   A. Explain to the girlfriend that decision making capacity lies with the HPOA
   B. Follow the wishes of the HPOA and ignore the girlfriend
   C. Hold a meeting with the healthcare team, girlfriend, and HPOA
   D. Have the girlfriend and HPOA speak about these issues bedside

119. After an abdominal aortic aneurysm repair a patient's morning labs display new onset azotemia. What is the likely cause for this change?

   A. Expected outcome—will normalize with time
   B. Intrarenal acute kidney injury
   C. Prerenal acute kidney injury
   D. Postrenal acute kidney injury

120. A 200 kg patient is in the ICU after surgery to remove a lobe of the liver secondary to cirrhosis and cancer. Which of the following is not an inpatient risk factor associated with this patient's weight?

   A. Dysfunctional breathing with possible pneumonia
   B. Difficulties with vascular access
   C. Increased risk of decubitus ulcers
   D. Poor glycemic control

GO ON TO NEXT PAGE ➤

121. A patient with a history of cholelithiasis is admitted to the ICU with anticipated surgery the following day. The next morning the patient exhibits a fever with abdominal pain and new onset jaundice. Which of the following does the nurse suspect?

    A. Acute cholecystitis

    B. Acute cholangitis

    C. Acute pancreatitis

    D. Acute hepatitis

122. A 65-year-old patient is admitted to the ICU due to worsening sepsis. A central line is placed in anticipation of the need for vasoactive agents. When speaking with the family regarding the current condition of the patient, they state the patient has a long history of heroin abuse and is known to be using before admission. Which of the following early symptoms of withdrawal would be important for the nurse to assess?

    A. Piloerection, diarrhea, pupillary dilation

    B. Leukocytosis, chest pain, tachypnea

    C. Pupillary constriction, constipation, muscle weakness

    D. Hypovolemia, hypernatremia

123. Before performing a carotid endarterectomy, the physician is likely to request the administration of which medication?

    A. Magnesium sulfate

    B. Normal saline bolus

    C. Alteplase

    D. Heparin

124. The physician orders a renal dose of dopamine to improve the urine output in a critically ill patient. Which of the following doses reflects a renal dose?

    A. 1–2 mcg/kg/min

    B. 5 mcg/kg/min

    C. 10 mcg/kg/min

    D. Greater than 10 mcg/kg/min

125. Interpret the following ABG: pH 7.45, $PaCO_2$ 28 mmHg, HCO_3 14, PaO_2 82%.

    A. Compensated respiratory acidosis with hypoxemia

    B. Compensate metabolic acidosis without hypoxemia

    C. Partially compensated metabolic acidosis with hypoxemia

    D. Compensated respiratory alkalosis without hypoxemia

STOP. You have completed the practice test. Complete your answers before moving forward with the review and rationales.

Answer Key

Question 1

Answer: D

Rationale: Lifelong anticoagulation therapy is required for those who undergo valve replacement with a mechanical valve. The risk of thrombus formation and stroke is high. The other answers are important for all valve surgeries, but it is not the primary concern with a mechanical valve.

Question 2

Answer: D

Rationale: The situation will be more appropriately assessed by speaking with the patient separately without the caregiver glaring over the shoulder. Provide a safe environment and listen. If the situation warrants it and elder abuse is suspected, the proper authorities should be, as mandated by law, contacted.

Question 3

Answer: A

Rationale: Valves, especially those close to conductive pathways (mitral, aortic, tricuspid), when replaced may lead to dysrhythmias like heart blocks. These patients leave the operating room with epicardial wires for the needs of pacing. The patient is experiencing hemodynamic instability and requires pacing override. Transcutaneous pacing is not needed since epicardial wires are present; it also might not work given the scar tissue of the surgery. Albumin and fluid are not indicated at the time since the problem at hand is the heart rhythm. Dobutamine is not indicated at this time for the same reasons.

Question 4

Answer: B

Rationale: The results of the ABG show respiratory alkalosis. This is likely caused by pain or anxiety. The most accurate answer is to intervene on the current hypoxia and assess for pain. Do not assume the patient is in pain or experiencing anxiety. Simply administering lorazepam without performing an assessment is not appropriate. Pulmonary embolism may result in respiratory alkalosis; however, the initial intervention is not a V/Q scan. CT angiography or D-dimer is more appropriate. Intubation is not needed at this time.

Question 5

Answer: A

Rationale: Benzodiazepines are the first-line medication in CIWA protocol and delirium tremens. If the medication is unsuccessful, phenobarbital is commonly added. IV hydration with thiamine will not assist in this problem, nor will assessing Korsakoff syndrome. Versed (midazolam) is used in some occasions when other benzodiazepines and phenobarbital do not abate the symptoms. This is not the next step in this case.

Question 6

Answer: C

Rationale: A right shift of the oxyhemoglobin dissociation curve causes hemoglobin to more readily release oxygen to tissues. It increases the release of 2,3-DPG. It will decrease both SaO_2 and SpO_2, as these two numbers often correlate. Remember not to confuse PaO_2 with SaO_2.

Question 7

Answer: B

Rationale: Infection causes a release of hormones such as cortisol and catecholamines like adrenalin. This further propagates hyperglycemia and may lead to diabetic ketoacidosis as is evidenced by the symptoms in this case. This is the most likely explanation given the story of current gastroenteritis.

Question 8

Answer: D

Rationale: The main reason to switch a patient from endotracheal tube ventilation to tracheostomy ventilation is the improvement of air flow with a tracheostomy. Consider an ETT like breathing through a straw. There is increased dead space and need for mechanical ventilation assistance. When switching to a tracheostomy, it is typically easier to wean from the ventilator. This decreases ICU stay and length in the hospital. Suctioning and pulmonary hygiene are often required with tracheostomies as well as ETT. The other answers are benefits to a trach, but they are not the primary reason for the switch.

Question 9

Answer: C

Rationale: Respiratory distress may occur due to migration of the balloon and pressure placed on the trachea. If this occurs the tube should be cut to release air and deflate. The other answers do not address the immediate danger and ABC problem here being caused by the balloon itself. Sengstaken–Blakemore tubes, like other NG tubes, are not manipulated by the nurse once placed. Like other NG tubes they are also confirmed by pH aspirate and later by chest x-ray.

Question 10

Answer: A

Rationale: Variant angina, or Printzmetal's angina, is most characterized by the relief of chest pain, signs, and symptoms with treatment of nitroglycerin. A true STEMI or NSTEMI would see symptoms continue, such as ST elevation or elevated troponin. Chest pain at rest does not exclusively describe variant angina, this may also be unstable angina or MI in general. T-wave inversions are very nonspecific, being caused by a wide variety of things, hypokalemia and myocardial ischemia being two.

Question 11

Answer: A

Rationale: Chronic alcoholism is most commonly associated with the ABG abnormality of metabolic acidosis. This is due to liver dysfunction and elevation of lactic acid in the body.

Question 12

Answer: C

Rationale: Depressed skull fractures 5 mm or deeper typically require surgical intervention. A basilar skull fracture does not need surgery unless CSF drainage continues or the patient is at very large risk of meningitis or if meningitis is suspected. A linear skull fracture is defined as the full thickness of the skull. This is expected. A concussion does not determine the need of surgery; however, bleeding such as an epidural bleed would warrant emergency surgery, but this is unrelated to the skull fracture itself.

Question 13

Answer: B

Rationale: The goal of pressure support ventilation whether it be noninvasive or invasive is to improve ventilation. This includes the gas exchange of oxygen and carbon dioxide. A decrease in arterial carbon dioxide shows improved ventilation. Stated feelings expressed by the patient are important; however, an objective finding is better to a subjective interpretation of improvement.

Question 14

Answer: B

Rationale: Bringing the entire team together is the most effective way to resolve disagreements. This will allow everyone to voice their opinions in an open setting.

Question 15

Answer: A

Rationale: A popular misconception is that delirium only occurs in once-healthy people. This is untrue. It may be compounded onto other issues, making it a difficult comorbidity to manage. One such example is delirium in addition to underlying dementia. The other answers are true statements reflecting delirium.

Question 16

Answer: C

Rationale: A rigid, board-like (stiff) abdomen is indicative of peritonitis. In this case, the peritonitis is secondary to the bowel perforation. Blood work would show leukocytosis, not 5000. Pain is improved by positioning with the knees flexed and the pain does not typically radiate to the lower back.

Question 17

Answer: D

Rationale: The vital signs, symptoms, and case story suggest an allergic reaction with anaphylaxis. Epinephrine is immediately needed to stabilize the patient due to the overwhelming histamine response in the body. Steroids will also aid in negating these effects. Vasopressors and fluid resuscitation may be required if epinephrine and steroids do not correct the issue. In distributive shock-like anaphylaxis, vasodilation leads to this severe decrease in BP. Vasopressors may assist in this. The blood would be stopped all together, not slowed.

Question 18

Answer: D

Rationale: The primary problem is pulmonary hypertension (PH). Utilizing phosphodiesterase-5 inhibitors such as sildenafil vasodilate the pulmonary bed. Most people know this medication as Viagra, but remember the drug was originally researched for PH. Prostacyclins like epoprostenol will also help vasodilate the pulmonary arteries. Administering a milrinone infusion may assist with the right-sided heart failure, but it will not correct the underlying problem that is PH.

Question 19

Answer: A

Rationale: For the vast majority of surgeries, especially those expected to be long, most patients arrive at the surgical ICU slightly hypothermic. During rewarming vasodilation may occur and result in a sudden drop in blood pressure. This likely will necessitate in adding preload (volume). MAP goals almost always are 60 mmHg or higher to maintain perfusion to organs. Sugar is typically maintained at 140–180 mg/dL after major surgeries. Do not strip chest tubes unless there is an order. The risk being damaging the suture linings or dislodging a clot that will result in bleeding.

Question 20

Answer: D

Rationale: The best action is to speak with the primary nurse themselves to inquire about what appears to be an abnormal rate. There may be specific reasons for this rate unknown at the time. It is inappropriate to stop an infusion without good reason first. Abnormal does not necessarily mean wrong. The other answers do not give the benefit of the doubt first.

Question 21

Answer: A

Rationale: Calcium channel blockers (amlodipine), or negative inotropes in general, help increase the filling time in diastole. These medications, however, are contraindicated in systolic heart failure. Losartan, an ARB, may be added to therapy for either type of heart failure. Given that an ACE inhibitor is already in use, treatment would move to a different class of medication completely.

Question 22

Answer: C

Rationale: A hemolytic reaction can be potentially fatal if immune-mediated. This occurs due to improper administration of mismatched (wrong type) blood. A non-immune-mediated reaction is less severe. An allergic reaction is not fatal unless anaphylaxis or airway closure is imminent. TACO or TRALI reactions are serious, but with proper interventions manageable.

Question 23

Answer: B

Rationale: Injury to the kidneys disrupts the excretion of water, electrolytes, and waste products. This results in hyperkalemia, hypermagnesemia, hyperphosphatemia, and hypernatremia. Calcium, however, decreases because the active component of vitamin D is not produced—this and the opposing influence of phosphorus.

Question 24

Answer: C

Rationale: Open-ended questions are best when inquiring about patient knowledge or reasoning. The other answers may be factors, but they are yes or no questions.

Question 25

Answer: D

Rationale: The immediate problems are severe hyperkalemia and hypotension. Out of the possible answers, dialysis is the only plausible intervention to correct these issues. If the patient is too unstable for hemodialysis, CRRT may be required. Diuretics do not work without functioning kidneys (CKD). Norepinephrine may correct the hypotension, but it will likely worsen hyperkalemia and certainly not correct it. ACE inhibitors would not be indicated here. They may also worsen the potassium level.

Question 26

Answer: B

Rationale: The most likely explanation for this patient is nutritional and vitamin deficiency in the form of calcium and vitamin D. These deficiencies often lead to osteomalacia, osteopenia, or osteoporosis in older adults, especially post-menopausal women.

Question 27

Answer: C

Rationale: The Braden scale and understanding the components within is important knowledge for pressure ulcer risk. Autonomic neuropathy involves dysfunction of the autonomic nervous system most closely related to heart rate and blood pressure in this sense. This is not a component of the Braden scale. Sensory perception and the ability to feel discomfort, however, is a component. Do not confuse autonomic versus peripheral neuropathy.

Question 28

Answer: A

Rationale: When wedging a pulmonary artery, it is important to not to prolong the length of inflation as this can lead to infarction or the more fatal complication of pulmonary artery rupture. Most PA catheters only require 1.5 mL of air or less to fully inflate the catheter balloon. Instilling more air can lead to pulmonary artery rupture and death.

Question 29

Answer: C

Rationale: Early compensation of hypovolemic or hemorrhagic shock includes activation of the sympathetic nervous system (fight or flight). This would manifest by an increase in heart rate and cardiac output. SVR would increase in attempts to compensate for loss of volume. The other answers display later signs if the volume loss was severe.

Question 30

Answer: B

Rationale: Potassium is infused at 10 mEq/hr regardless of the amount contained within the bag. Only 1 hour has passed, so theoretically only 10 mEq should have been administered by this time. It would be potentially dangerous to keep the original bag hung in case more potassium is administered than ordered; therefore a new bag should be obtained and hung. If excessive potassium was believed to be administered, the first step with errors is to always assess the patient first before any other action.

Question 31

Answer: D

Rationale: DKA protocol involves a switch to dextrose infusion once the serum glucose reaches 250 mg/dL. That number does change slightly depending on institutional policy, but it remains the general rule of thumb. When the anion gap closes and acidosis has resolved, insulin infusion is typically switched to subQ sliding scale. Acidosis may cause hyperkalemia; however, that is a separate problem than the DKA itself.

Question 32

Answer: A

Rationale: The most common cause of status asthmaticus is exacerbation with upper respiratory tract infections. Other causes may include stress or sensitivity to certain particles. Status asthmaticus does not typically respond well to bronchodilators, hence the emergency. It results in a decreased FEV_1 and does not always require intubation; the condition may be managed with positive pressure ventilation such as BiPAP. Decreased LOC or cardiac arrest are two main reasons intubation would become inevitable.

Question 33

Answer: D

Rationale: There are many forms of nonpharmacological interventions for pain, but the most important factor above all else is if the patient even has a desire to try. If the patient is not on board, it is unlikely the intervention will be successful.

Question 34

Answer: B

Rationale: Dull pain typically describes bowel obstructions in general; however, the high-pitched bowel sounds and forceful vomiting specifically point to a small bowel obstruction. Change in bowel habits or bowel movements would point more to a large bowel obstruction. A ruptured appendix would exhibit symptoms of peritonitis among others not listed in this question. Esophagitis manifests with swallowing difficulties and GERD-like symptoms.

Question 35

Answer: B

Rationale: Stable angina is the most common form of angina and is not a heart attack, although it may be a precursor down the line. It will require outpatient monitoring. Stable angina dissipates when exertion is removed and/or nitroglycerin is effective. Unstable angina is present even at rest. Cardiac catheterization is not indicated at this time.

Question 36

Answer: C

Rationale: High-alert medications like a heparin infusion or insulin infusion require a two RN sign-off. This is the most important factor. Whether the nurse double checks their own work or calls the pharmacy, the nurse is still the only person theoretically to hang and program the infusion without a second registered nurse. Coagulation panels are drawn typically every 4 to 6 hours, but this would not help reduce error at the beginning of the infusion.

Question 37

Answer: A

Rationale: The CT scan will provide the best picture for this suspected bleeding. An x-ray does not provide a specific location of the bleeding and is too vague to be useful. An MRI is contraindicated due to the pacemaker. Fluoroscopy is not needed in this case. Most fluoroscopy cases involve the movement of a catheter or object, such as coiling an aneurysm or placement of orthopedic devices.

Question 38

Answer: D

Rationale: Rebleeding is a potential complication of aneurysm repair. Hypertension may lead to the artery rupturing again and causing rebleeds. Calcium channel blockers like nicardipine are useful in preventing vasospasms; however, this question specifically addresses blood pressure management as the current question. Increased ICP and cardiac ischemia are not primary risk factors for the use of this drug.

Question 39

Answer: A

Rationale: A long-standing headache may be a sign of hypertension and potential pre-eclampsia. Blood pressure above 140 mmHg systolic warrants further investigation for pre-eclampsia. Abdominal pain associated with pre-eclampsia is typically in the RUQ or epigastric areas. Ankle edema is expected in many pregnancies. Quickening of a fetus occurs when the baby moves—a good finding.

Question 40

Answer: C

Rationale: Cocaine is a stimulant. Therefore, signs and symptoms will be in line with central nervous system stimulation: tachycardia, tachypnea, hypertension, and anxiety. Nystagmus is seen in alcohol intoxication. Abdominal pain may be expected due to overstimulation, but assessment of the abdominal organs would be warranted in case of ischemia or dysfunction. This would be a complication of the intoxication, however, not a symptom of the intoxication itself.

Question 41

Answer: C

Rationale: IABP treatment's primary goal is to improve left-ventricular function. This is accomplished by counterpulsation of the balloon to reduce afterload thereby increasing cardiac output. Another goal of IABP is to improve perfusion through the coronary arteries. The case presented here is of heart failure and cardiogenic shock. There is no presentation of myocardial infarction being an issue here, although it could be in a different question.

Question 42

Answer: B

Rationale: NSAIDs like naproxen or ibuprofen worsen GFR thereby exacerbating the CKD. These medications are generally contraindicated in CKD for this reason. The other medications are safe for this patient to receive although the dose may need to be reduced in some cases.

Question 43

Answer: B

Rationale: Progression of ECG changes through an MI follows a typical order beginning with large-peaked T waves, ST elevation, T wave inversion, then finally Q waves. Q waves are the result of damaged tissue electricity cannot pass through. It is a sign of previous MI. An inverted p wave is commonly from an ectopic beat. A wide QRS denotes signaling from the ventricles, not the SA or AV nodes.

Question 44

Answer: D

Rationale: Hypotonic solutions are contraindicated in this situation of severe hyponatremia. This will worsen the current sodium level. The other answers are adequate to correct this hyponatremia. An isotonic or hypertonic solution may be used; however, remember changes in sodium must be done slowly over time to prevent a rapid shift of water in brain cells.

Question 45

Answer: B

Rationale: The ACE Star Model of Knowledge Transformation explains the general process of EBP and how it is applied into clinical practice. Similar to the scientific method in general, research or a question is asked, followed by research, and evaluation. In this case, the method is used to apply changes into clinical practice.

Question 46

Answer: A

Rationale: Questions of this nature are not uncommon; however, the larger concept is even more important. Understand common medications used in the ICU and how they affect preload, afterload, and contractility. Nitroprusside is a potent vasodilator and will therefore decrease afterload. The other answers are incorrect.

Question 47

Answer: B

Rationale: In this pacemaker, the atrium is paced, sensed, and inhibited when an atrial event is sensed (inhibited). This allows for intrinsic speed to go above the setting of the pacemaker. The p wave denotes depolarization of the atrium. In a VVI, setting the spike would be seen right before a wide QRS complex. DDD paces both chambers. VOO (asynchronous) ventricular pacing allows for pacing faster or slower than a dysfunctional heart.

Question 48

Answer: D

Rationale: The clinical picture is showing partially compensated respiratory acidosis. The main issue here is poor ventilation. The patient is retaining carbon dioxide and not ventilating enough oxygen. The best treatment for this at this time is a positive pressure ventilation like high-flow nasal cannula or BiPAP. Increasing the oxygen may improve the hypoxia but not the ventilation as a whole. Intubation is not necessary at this time as the problem is still considered relatively mild to moderate. Severe acidosis with changes in LOC would warrant intubation. Administration of a sedative like lorazepam will worsen overall ventilation of carbon dioxide and oxygen. The anxiety will improve if the underlying hypoxia is corrected.

Question 49

Answer: A

Rationale: In viral meningitis, the CSF of a lumbar puncture matches that of the serum glucose or is slightly below. The CSF is clear. Elevated protein and WBCs are found in both viral and bacterial meningitis.

Question 50

Answer: C

Rationale: The patient is exhibiting classic signs of depression. Flat mood, insomnia, difficulty focusing that may in turn lead to difficulty with certain aspects of memory. Given the history with the divorce, the most likely answer is depression. A psychotic break would manifest with some degree of dissociation. A formal dementia diagnosis would require many more tests that span a period of time. Delirium is typically caused by an underlying medical reason.

Question 51

Answer: C

Rationale: The patient is displaying signs of necrotizing fasciitis. The most obvious sign being the color changes (red to purple) over a short period of time and the rapid expansion of the wound bed. Severe pain and erythema also describe NF, but also correlate to cellulitis, granted pain associated with cellulitis is typically not severe. Localized infiltration would not typically spread up the arm unless a vesicant was administered. A traumatic wound does not describe an infected wound as such. It may explain the pain, but not the erythema or expanding color.

Question 52

Answer: B

Rationale: The priority concern at this moment is the potential cause for the blood dyscrasias. These dyscrasias may be caused by a medication the patient is currently taking. If the patient was actively psychotic, violent, or in crisis, priority would shift in addressing that first; however, the patient in this case is calm. This is also why inpatient psychiatry is not a priority at this time; physiological treatment comes first. Holding all psychiatric medication is not appropriate as this could exacerbate a psychotic break; assess first.

Question 53

Answer: A

Rationale: Most calcium channel blockers (CCB) do not cause bradycardia, but diltiazem is a different type of CCB called non-DIIP. These may cause severe sinus bradycardia or sinus arrest. The patient should be monitored closely (telemetry) when receiving this infusion. Most of these patients receive this treatment in the ICU due to this reason. The other answers are not considerations for use of this infusion.

Question 54

Answer: B

Rationale: QT prolongation may occur due to a number of medications—amiodarone, haloperidol, erythromycin, and ondansetron (among others). Two leading factors causing torsades de pointes is QT prolongation and hypomagnesemia. This patient may be hypomagnesemic or hypokalemic given the current use of furosemide. These electrolyte imbalances are known to cause torsades; however, the question is asking for the priority and fastest assessment possible. Assessing a QT prolongation is one, a more common cause of torsades, and two, a rapid assessment off of ECG. Drug interactions are a possibility, but not a priority at this time. The case does not allude to renal issues in this patient, although it would potentially explain electrolyte imbalances and dysrhythmias.

Question 55

Answer: D

Rationale: A ruptured spleen is typically caused by blunt trauma to the left upper quadrant. Previous history of infection like mono may precipitate the rupture given possible splenomegaly. Kehr's sign is present with the radiating left shoulder pain, a common finding in splenic rupture. Ruptured bowel would result in symptoms of peritonitis. Pancreatic laceration is a difficult diagnosis and is often nonspecific. Ruptured aortic arch would inevitably result in loss of consciousness and severe hypotension. This location of aneurysms or dissections typically present with patients describing ripping or tearing back pain or chest pain that may radiate.

Question 56

Answer: B

Rationale: Colorectal cancer is the most common cause of a large bowel obstruction. The patient history of smoking along with obesity points to risk factors of colorectal cancer. Current anemia is also suggestive of cancer itself. Crohn's disease and adhesions are risk factors for a small bowel obstruction. Intussusception may occur in both the small or large bowel, but a common symptom present in this obstruction is a red currant jelly–like stool; this is not present.

Question 57

Answer: A

Rationale: Aneurysms most commonly exist within the Circle of Willis; the leading location being the anterior communicating artery. The carotid artery is a common location of aneurysms, but this is not intracranial. A burst aneurysm may cause dysfunction of the hypothalamus, but the hypothalamus is not the location of the aneurysm itself. Intraventricular aneurysms are rare.

Question 58

Answer: C

Rationale: Immunoglobulin E exists on mast cells and basophils. When they react to antigens, this is an allergic reaction. These antigens may range from medications to foods like peanuts. Mast cell activation can cause a wide array of problems because of their presence in almost all tissues. Activation leads to massive histamine release, vasodilation, with resulting shock among many other problems. The other answers do not reflect this pathophysiology.

Question 59

Answer: B

Rationale: PAWP is typically greater than 18 mmHg in those with ARDS. A reading of 16 mmHg would NOT be found in this patient. All of the other answers are diagnostic findings in ARDS or shock (low SVR).

Question 60

Answer: D

Rationale: There are a number of absolute contraindications to tPA. Some examples to commit to memory: intracranial bleeding including subarachnoid hemorrhage, neurosurgery/head trauma/or stroke within 3 months, known AV malformation or aneurysm, and active internal bleeding. The other examples are not contraindications.

Question 61

Answer: B

Rationale: The gold standard for PE diagnosis is CT pulmonary angiography. Other tests may be performed in the assistance of the diagnosis such as d-dimer and ABG evaluation but this is not definitive for diagnosis as there are many other causes for elevated d-dimer and acidosis. A V/Q scan is helpful but is more common if other tests come back inconclusive.

Question 62

Answer: A

Rationale: Typical TPN bags contain 20–50% dextrose. This amount of glucose causes hyperglycemia. A patient on TPN will have a sliding scale insulin order to manage any hyperglycemia. Infection or CLABSI are risks for TPN as well;

however, this is not the immediate or first concern. Liver dysfunction is also a risk for TPN, but again would take some time to develop.

Question 63

Answer: A

Rationale: The most likely diagnosis with this collection of findings is an empyema. Ultrasound displayed a pleural effusion; however, it is unknown what this material contains. Serous fluid, blood (hemothorax), pus (empyema), or another type of fluid may be the culprit. Until drainage occurs definitive diagnosis is difficult. With the chest tube, fever, leukocytosis, and chills, these symptoms point to an empyema.

Question 64

Answer: B

Rationale: Two main adverse effects of tacrolimus is increased risk for infection (leukopenia) and renal dysfunction. A decrease in urine output would suggest an acute kidney injury due to the medication. The other answers are not associated with tacrolimus use.

Question 65

Answer: D

Rationale: Systolic murmur associated with stenosis are the atrioventricular valves. The semilunar valves are associated with a systolic murmur of insufficiency. The other answers do not reflect a combination. The types (semilunar versus atrioventricular) of valves always open and close together.

Question 66

Answer: C

Rationale: It is inappropriate to inflict patients with one's own personal viewpoints. If the patient is terminal and has made a decision for hospice and palliative care, treatment is no longer curative in nature. The other answers are all included in palliative care.

Question 67

Answer: D

Rationale: The ankle–brachial index is not a sensitive tool for diagnosis, but it may assist in arriving at the bigger picture. A ratio less than 1 may indicate PAD. Remember to dangle the arteries and elevate the veins in reference to a larger diagnosis. Stenosis or atherosclerosis may be likely here, but the index is not specific to any particular diagnosis. A bypass surgery would be warranted when there is severe lack of blood flow distally on the extremity.

Question 68

Answer: B

Rationale: Out of the potential list of substances, LSD is the only one known to cause hallucinations with use. Alcohol is known to cause hallucinosis, but more so with chronic abuse. The vital signs are also more in line with LSD abuse.

Question 69

Answer: C

Rationale: Atrial fibrillation is a complication of systolic heart failure, but not a cause of it. CAD such as an MI can weaken the muscle and cause systolic heart failure. Hypertension and aortic stenosis may both force the heart to pump harder and therefore become dilated and weak.

Question 70

Answer: D

Rationale: Symptoms of flu typically begin 1 to 4 days after exposure, with 2 days being the most common. Symptoms can last up to 1 to 2 weeks.

Question 71

Answer: A

Rationale: Pain control is crucial in post-op thoracotomy surgeries. Cracking the ribs is incredibly painful. A sedative does not offer pain control. This would likely increase the risk of aspiration, atelectasis, and pneumonia. Appropriate pain management would include anti-inflammatory agents and opioid narcotics. The other answers are appropriate interventions.

Question 72

Answer: A

Rationale: The "P" of PQRST reflects palliative or precipitating factors. Q for quality, R for region or radiating, S for subjective descriptions, and T for temporal nature.

Question 73

Answer: D

Rationale: Hypervolemia (fluid overload) may be caused by a multitude of problems. Chronic kidney disease or acute kidney injuries affect the kidneys ability to filter and remove excess fluid. This is a cause of fluid overload, however, not a symptom of it. The other answers reflect commonly seen signs and symptoms of fluid overload.

Question 74

Answer: C

Rationale: An aneurysm rupture is the likely culprit given the case presented. An athlete performing taxing or strenuous exercise may rupture an undiagnosed aneurysm or AV malformation. Patients typically complain of "the worst headache of my life." Neck stiffness is also in line with a SAH. The other answers do not fit the symptomatology as well or etiology.

Question 75

Answer: A

Rationale: The two primary goals of IABP are to decrease the afterload to help the heart pump more effectively, and to increase the perfusion through the coronary arteries. IABP is indicated for cardiogenic shock.

Question 76

Answer: C

Rationale: Initial treatment for refractory hypotension is norepinephrine, followed by vasopressin or epinephrine. Inotropes are reserved as a last line after all else. The bundles have likely changed since the last time you studied this topic. Review the 1-hour and 24-hour bundles. It has since become slightly more simplified but nonetheless very important. The other answers are included in the 1-hour bundle.

Question 77

Answer: B

Rationale: The primary goal of dressing therapy for this patient is to encourage the exudate removal. This is a healthy process of wound healing. Dry dressings are to be avoided as this will pull out healthy granulation tissue and delay wound healing. DuoDERM and Tegaderm encourage autolytic debridement. They are not able to absorb large amounts of fluid. This is not appropriate in this case.

Question 78

Answer: B

Rationale: Whenever increased abdominal fluid is suspected of causing dyspnea, the correct action would be to place the patient in a semi-Fowler's position (30–45 degrees). This allows the fluid to spread out over the largest possible space. This may occur due to an unknown trauma leading to buildup of abdominal fluid (possibly blood) or is also known to be an issue in liver cirrhotic patients with ascites. The fluid pushes up on the diaphragm and causes breathing difficulties.

Question 79

Answer: D

Rationale: A slightly difficult topic to memorize, grading of muscle strength is found in Chapter 9. Grade 0 defines no movement. Grade 5 defines full range of motion against gravity and resistance. The left arm in this case has full range of motion against gravity, but some resistance. This is grade 4 muscle strength.

Question 80

Answer: C

Rationale: Discoloration of the toes is an adverse effect of norepinephrine therapy. Potent vasoconstriction often decreases perfusion potentially causing ischemia and necrosis. Assess the problem so it may be noted and tracked in the case it becomes worse. Norepinephrine therapy is needed to maintain blood pressure so switching medications based upon this finding is not appropriate. The physician should be notified, but that is not the first action.

Question 81

Answer: A

Rationale: Osteomyelitis is a severe infection with a high likelihood of spreading without immediate treatment. IV antibiotics give the best chance to prevent this. Intraosseous access is not needed for the delivery of adequate antibiotics. Without symptoms of sepsis or septic shock, blood cultures are not appropriate. There is also no indication that emergency surgery is needed. If the infection does not subside, this may warrant a surgical consult.

Question 82

Answer: B

Rationale: Insulin causes potassium to leave the intravascular space and move into surrounding cells. This will decrease serum potassium and potentially lead to hypokalemia. It is important to replete this electrolyte in these cases. The other electrolytes and vitamins would be replete as needed, but they are not a direct effect of insulin use.

Question 83

Answer: D

Rationale: Bed alarms and frequent rounding would decrease the risk of falls, but not that of immobility itself. The other answers may all reduce the risks of immobility (muscle atrophy, atelectasis, etc.)

Question 84

Answer: C

Rationale: There are multiple components of a full mental status exam, although orientation (person, place, situation, time) is the most commonly used. A nurse–patient relationship is important to encourage, but it is not part of the formal exam itself. The other answers reflect options within a mental status exam.

Question 85

Answer: A

Rationale: When the kidneys have difficulty filtering water, solutes, and electrolytes, the result is more concentrated urine with decreased sodium. Concentrated urine may be reflected by dark color, a high specific gravity, or elevated urine osmolality.

Question 86

Answer: C

Rationale: When collaborating with a large staff and enacting new policy or protocols, the best way to ensure solidarity and understanding across the board is to hold a staff meeting. Information can be lost in translation if allowed to disseminate slowly or via nonpersonal methods, such as e-mail. Punishing is inappropriate. Waiting and hoping the problem will go away is inappropriate.

Question 87

Answer: C

Rationale: Airway obstruction and respiratory distress is the leading concern among smoke inhalation or facial burns. This would be reflected in an ABG by advancing respiratory acidosis with hypoxemia. In questions like this, it is often easier to search for the answer with the worst results. Two answers show hypoxemia, but only one of those in combination with acidosis.

Question 88

Answer: D

Rationale: There are certain situations where the disclosure of patient information does not require patient consent. The first and most commonly used is for continuity of care. Other examples include information for billing and contagious diseases requiring reporting to health agencies.

Question 89

Answer: B

Rationale: The immediate needs of the mother at this time is support. This does not require explanation unless she specifically asks. The technology and devices surrounding the patient may be frightening to see; pointing them out is not helpful. It is unknown if the patient is religious or spiritual so a chaplain may not be desired. Leaving the room does not offer support.

Question 90

Answer: B

Rationale: Asynchronous ventilation is a potential problem with ARDS among many other intubated patients. If sedation does not correct the problem, paralytics are a common next step (vecuronium, rocuronium). Continued asynchronous ventilation is linked to decreased overall ventilation and increased ICU mortality. Changing the mode or using a bite block will not solve the underlying problem. Adding a third sedative when the blood pressure is low is not appropriate.

Question 91

Answer: C

Rationale: HIPAA dictates no information can be released without patient consent. If the patient is incapacitated, the next of kin would execute this release unless an advance directive with healthcare power of attorney was present.

Question 92

Answer: C

Rationale: Appropriate CLABSI bundles include a variety of tools to reduce the risk of infection. Aside from the other correct answers, utilizing disinfectants prior to engaging the hub (chlorhexidine, alcohol, povidone-iodine), covering open hubs, strict sterile insertion, among many others are included. Using the femoral vein is typically the last resort when other access cannot be obtained or if an emergency dictates the need. The femoral site is dirty and much more difficult to keep clean. Because of this, it is not a preferred site.

Question 93

Answer: A

Rationale: The priority intervention at this time is to contain the potential spread of the pathogen. Regardless of the contagion, quarantining those suspected of infection should be performed first if possible. Patients suspected of being infected should wear appropriate PPE as well as all healthcare professionals in contact with the patients. The general order of operation is first, quarantine; second, protection with PPE; and third, treat the patient.

Question 94

Answer: A

Rationale: When dealing with emotional and stressful situations the patient may experience, it is best to allow open dialogue for questions, but not pressure the topics. Allow the patient to speak their mind while providing emotional support. Follow patient wishes if they are made; in this case, no more food means no more food. It would be inappropriate to push the idea of hospice, however likely it is. The topic will come up in due time.

Question 95

Answer: D

Rationale: The patient no longer wants frequent boluses of morphine, by following those wishes the nurse is adhering to the autonomy of the patient. By suggesting an alternative that will continue to benefit the patient and be competent to the scope of practice, the nurse is adhering to fidelity. Following up on the promise of pain management adheres to fidelity as well.

Question 96

Answer: C

Rationale: By decreasing the electrical output (milliamps), eventually the capture will be lost and the pacer spike will no longer be seen. This action can be dangerous if there is no underlying rhythm (native) to continue a heart rate. For this reason, once the threshold is determined, the output is typically doubled from the threshold. Decreasing the sensitivity would test the sensing threshold not the capture threshold.

Question 97

Answer: B

Rationale: The CCRN exam presents information in a manner where ACLS protocol knowledge is required. In this question, this is even more rudimentary into BLS than necessarily ACLS. Ventricular fibrillation will always result in a pulseless patient. The first and foremost action, proven by research from the American Heart Association, is the immediate need for CPR to reestablish some degree of blood flow and perfusion. The actions of obtaining a crash cart and administration of epinephrine will be performed by a secondary nurse. The primary or bedside nurse's responsibility is to immediately begin CPR until someone else takes over.

Question 98

Answer: C

Rationale: A sentinel event occurs when there is patient harm or death. The event is generally unexpected or avoidable. The primary nurse's responsibility is to document the facts about what happened. The incident report should be filled out and submitted to the appropriate person; oftentimes a committee or manager. The incident report does not go in the patient chart; its use is to prevent similar errors in the future. It is improper and illegal to withhold information from a chart about what happened.

Question 99

Answer: B

Rationale: Certain questions may come up regarding sensitive topics like abortion, LGBT patients, or even a critically ill pedophile. It is important to assess personal beliefs before anything else since it is inappropriate to inflict personal viewpoints or judgments onto the patient regardless of how much one might disagree. Switching assignments is not allowed except in extreme cases. Whether the patient has female- or male-presenting genitals is a moot point; the nurse should understand how to insert a catheter for either. If unaware of the terminology, transgender female means a male-to-female patient. A transgender male means a female-to-male patient.

Question 100

Answer: A

Rationale: PEEP increases intrathoracic pressure. This pressure inhibits venous return or preload back to the right side of the heart. This will decrease cardiac output and decrease blood pressure. This is a known adverse effect to PEEP itself, but especially high PEEP as is this case. An improvement in ABG is a good thing, not an adverse effect; remember to pay attention to wording and semantics. A 6–8 mL/kg tidal volume calculation is average. A tidal volume of 450 mL is adequate for this patient. Barotrauma is possible with excessive PEEP as well as volume, but this answer specifically says volume.

Question 101

Answer: D

Rationale: Hypophosphatemia may result in general muscle weakness. This may include the muscles responsible for breathing like the diaphragm. Respiratory weakness may result in hypoventilation and worsening problems with oxygenation. Chvostek's sign is a result of hypocalcemia. Osteoporosis is a result of hyperparathyroidism itself, not of hypophosphatemia. Constipation, not diarrhea, is a result of hypophosphatemia.

Question 102

Answer: D

Rationale: The primary goal for a patient with COPD exacerbation or asthmaticus is to promote longer expiratory time. Allow the patients to exhale the maximum amount of air (carbon dioxide) to prevent acidosis and air trapping. This is accomplished by slowly respiratory rates and the maximum use of the lung.

Question 103

Answer: B

Rationale: Cryoprecipitate is high in fibrinogen. Decreased fibrinogen exists in DIC, leading to abnormal bleeding. Increasing thrombin, a component of clots, would make the problem worse. Plasmin is an enzyme that breaks down fibrin—most nurses know this as tPA or a fibrinolytic. This is also the cause of DIC itself; to further exacerbate the breakdown of fibrin would worsen the problem. Platelets are often given to patients in DIC but are not the purpose of cryo.

Question 104

Answer: D

Rationale: The citrate in transfused blood binds to calcium leading to hypocalcemia and a decrease in ionized calcium. Hyperkalemia also results from large amounts of transfusion due to increased potassium in the blood itself (RBC lysis releases potassium). The other answers are not common in massive transfusion protocol, nor are a result of citrate.

Question 105

Answer: D

Rationale: A renal diet consists of restricting protein, sodium, potassium, and phosphorus. Because of the difficulty eliminating water, a restriction of fluid is also common in renal diets. Think about what the kidneys are responsible for eliminating and what would typically increase due to this kidney failure. Remember the breakdown of protein leads to increased nitrogen waste (BUN).

Question 106

Answer: C

Rationale: Daily weights remain the best method to gauge successful fluid removal. Blood pressure is managed by a number of physiological methods (sympathetic tone, volume, RAAS, etc.). A decrease in crackles would display success for specifically the likely cause of the patient's dyspnea; however, this is not the best measure of fluid loss. A patient in CKD or ESRD will not see improvement in their GFR. The nature of the disease is reduced GFR; the only true cure is organ transplant.

Question 107

Answer: A

Rationale: Lactulose remains the beginning gold standard for high serum ammonia. It is most commonly given orally, but that is not possible in this patient. Therefore, a lactulose enema is the best option. All of the other answers are methods to treat ammonia as well, but each has drawbacks whether it is adverse effects or time to effectiveness. The question asks for immediate removal, peritoneal dialysis takes time. This patient has no diet at this time, so decreasing a nutrient is not appropriate since they are NPO. Neomycin has many toxic adverse effects on organs.

Question 108

Answer: B

Rationale: The clinical picture is displaying likely brain death. Following with additional assessments like a gag reflex or other brain-stem reflexes would provide additional information on this likely brain death. Once that is complete, the nurse would reach out to the physician for orders. An apnea test is likely if the physician agrees. Organ procurement services would be contacted but is not the next action. An ABG is not necessary at this time.

Question 109

Answer: A

Rationale: A decrease in GABA is one of the understood causes of anxiety and panic attacks. The sympathetic nervous system is stimulated. Amygdala activity is increased. These changes are physiological albeit manifest with psychological features such as fear.

Question 110

Answer: A

Rationale: The clinical pathophysiology of sepsis is often described as a triad—systemic inflammation, coagulopathy, and dysfunctional fibrinolysis. Neutropenia would be a cause of sepsis, but not a feature of it.

Question 111

Answer: D

Rationale: Understanding the mechanisms of cholinergic agents is important. The difference between a cholinergic agonist and anticholinergic luckily is they have opposing signs and symptoms. The acronym SLUDD is typically used to assist with this. Agonist = wet, anti = dry. This patient is exhibiting the wet signs, incontinence and secretions. This toxicity seen here is also in line with a potential cholinergic crisis. Opioid and beta blocker overdose match some of the symptoms, but not as closely as a cholinergic agonist.

Question 112

Answer: C

Rationale: Certain medications are typically contraindicated in asthma. These include beta blockers and NSAIDs, therefore given the new onset asthma, this medication should be switched. The other medications are appropriate to continue for this patient.

Question 113

Answer: A

Rationale: This patient is severely tachycardic and tachypneic. The pulse pressure is narrowed and severely decreased. There is also evidence of hypoxia given the current pulse ox on 15 L. This is most closely aligned with a class IV hemorrhagic shock.

Question 114

Answer: B

Rationale: The immediate concern is patient safety. Even in situations that may be stressful or aggravating, such as constantly reminding patients not to get out of bed, physical or verbal assault is inappropriate and illegal. This behavior should either be immediately dealt with by speaking with the nurse themselves or reported to the nurse manager. Most questions that have illegality point to reporting the behavior immediately to the nurse manager. If the manager is not available, a direct conversation is required.

Question 115

Answer: A

Rationale: When Tensilon (edrophonium) is administered, if the muscle weakness improves the patient likely has myasthenia gravis. If the muscle weakness does not change or becomes worse, a cholinergic crisis is likely. Tensilon is an acetylcholinesterase inhibitor. It prevents the breakdown of acetylcholine within motor neurons. Remember acetylcholine is also responsible for glandular activity, so if the patient exhibits an increase in SLUDD symptoms, this is a cholinergic crisis.

Question 116

Answer: B

Rationale: Alcohol is a sedative that suppresses a number of bodily functions. One of those functions would be the gag reflex and ability for the body to cough strongly to anything that may work its way down into the airways. This is the most likely explanation. Aspiration is most common in the right lung, not left. Bronchoscopy may be ordered if other interventions do not solve the problem. Antibiotics may be ordered if infection ensues, main word "if."

Question 117

Answer: D

Rationale: The symptoms listed are most in line with pericarditis. A pericardial friction rub will be heard regardless of breathing as the heart docs not stop when holding the breath. ST elevations are seen globally across the ECG in pericarditis. The pain is also worse when the inflammation is rubbing against surrounding structures.

Question 118

Answer: C

Rationale: The best form to find solidarity is to hold interdisciplinary conferences. Questions like these may be worded a hundred different ways, but the general idea remains the same. It is not appropriate to ignore or be dismissive to anyone. The HPOA does ultimately have the final say, but to avoid unhappiness or anger, talking it out is best. Speaking about these matters in front of the patient will likely result in anger and yelling. Privacy is needed here.

Question 119

Answer: C

Rationale: AAA repair is typically done with a graft. This graft may occlude the renal arteries and decrease perfusion. This injury may also have occurred during the surgery itself when the physician cross-clamp the aorta. This would result in a prerenal AKI.

Question 120

Answer: D

Rationale: Glycemic control is managed by the healthcare team. Morbid obesity does not affect the team's approach to managing hyperglycemia in this patient. The sliding scale will manage this. The other answers are common difficulties, inpatient, related to morbid obesity.

Question 121

Answer: B

Rationale: Fever, abdominal pain, and new onset jaundice is called Charcot's triad. This is a clinical picture of cholangitis, especially given the history of cholelithiasis. The majority of cholangitis cases are related to biliary obstruction from gallstones.

Question 122

Answer: A

Rationale: Heroin withdrawal is typically believed to be mild and not life-threatening. It can cause death, however, usually from severe fluid losses from vomiting and diarrhea. The clinical picture of heroin withdrawal is rather large, but some common symptoms are yawning, sneezing, diarrhea, vomiting, lacrimation, rhinorrhea, among many others. Piloerection is more commonly known as goosebumps. Remember to pay attention to the words "early" versus "late"; this would dictate correct answer choices.

Question 123

Answer: D

Rationale: Prior to undergoing carotid endarterectomy, the patient should receive anticoagulation unless contraindicated. This is most commonly done by heparin. The main purpose of this administration is to reduce the risk of stroke associated with the procedure itself.

Question 124

Answer: A

Rationale: A renal dose of dopamine is a low dose meant to improve renal perfusion and therefore urine output. The higher doses of dopamine increase blood pressure and cause vasoconstriction.

Question 125

Answer: D

Rationale: First, identify the primary problem. In this case, and with many fully compensated ABGs, this may be difficult since the pH is normal. The trick is to identify at which end of normal the pH lies; in this case, it is on the alkalotic side of normal. This is the primary problem and can be identified by the other information from there.

Practice Test 3

This is the third full practice exam included in this book. The test contains 125 questions, the same as the CCRN exam. Questions are modeled after the blueprint in type and amount. All questions are mixed and random in order. A passing grade on the CCRN exam is 87 questions out of 125 questions. This is your benchmark for success.

1. The nurse is admitting a patient to the ICU directly from a nursing home. The patient has a history of multiple allergic reactions, many of which have resulted in hospitalizations. What is the first action the nurse will take during this admission?
   A. Perform a complete medication reconciliation
   B. Identify previous reactions and the resulting symptoms
   C. Consult immediately with an allergist to perform testing
   D. Avoid the use of latex and latex-containing products

2. A patient admitted with multiple traumas has a history of psychiatric illness. Which of the following interventions is not an appropriate method to de-escalate agitation?
   A. Bilateral soft wrist restraints
   B. Speak with the patient in open-ended questions
   C. Suggest the use of music or alternative therapies
   D. Obtain chaplain assistance when asked by the patient

3. A patient with heart failure is currently on metoprolol and lisinopril but due to worsening ejection fraction must be admitted. Which of the following measurements is commonly used to determine left ventricular end-diastolic pressure?

   A. Systemic blood pressure

   B. Pulmonary artery wedge pressure (PAOP)

   C. Cardiac output/cardiac index

   D. Systemic vascular resistance (SVR)

4. A patient with severe traumatic brain injury has pupillary dilation with bradycardia and abnormal posturing. Aside from bradycardia, what are the other two findings consistent with Cushing's triad?

   A. Hypotension and bradypnea

   B. Decreased cardiac output and increased SVR

   C. Widening pulse pressure and hypoxia

   D. Hypertension and irregular breathing

5. A patient refuses to allow the physician to place a central line catheter for immediate continuous renal replacement therapy (CRRT). The physician educates the need for this treatment as well as the nurse and others. By putting patient autonomy aside, which ethical term is the healthcare team enacting by continuing to advocate for CRRT therapy?

   A. Fidelity

   B. Nonmaleficence

   C. Paternalism

   D. Justice

6. A nurse in the ICU has an order to begin enteral feedings on an intubated patient. Which of the following considerations is most appropriate when beginning enteral tube feedings?

   A. It is not necessary to confirm placement before administration

   B. It is best to start at 50% of the intended goal rate per hour

   C. Ensure the head of the bed is elevated a minimum of 30 degrees

   D. Decompress the stomach with an NG tube before enteral feeding initiation

7. An 86-year-old male patient complains of abdominal pain and diarrhea that comes and goes over the past 3 days. He states the reason he came to the hospital was profound weakness and fatigue this morning. He has visible dry mucous membranes. Urinalysis shows elevated specific gravity that is dark in color. The physician orders a CT scan of the abdomen to rule out internal issues. Which of the following orders would be most appropriate at this time?

    A. Fluid resuscitation with isotonic fluids

    B. Place an NG tube for water flushes and enteral feedings

    C. Obtain a urine culture, anticipate administration of antibiotics

    D. Administration of loperamide

8. A diabetic patient arrives at the emergency department after fainting. A family member acted quickly and administered glucagon for suspected hypoglycemia. The nurse is educating the patient on hypoglycemic unawareness and neuroglycopenia. Which statement best describes the pathophysiology of what this patient is experiencing?

    A. The failure of the parasympathetic response leads to decreased glucose delivery to the brain

    B. Repeated hypoglycemic episodes cause heightened awareness of body responses

    C. The failure of the adrenergic response leads to decreased counterregulatory hormones

    D. Gluconeogenesis in the liver is dysfunctional leading to hypoglycemia

9. A patient with systolic heart failure after a myocardial infarction is experiencing repeated episodes of syncope in the ICU. The patient is unable to ambulate safely. The following assessment from a syncope workup is as follows:

VITAL SIGNS—SUPINE POSITION	VITAL SIGNS—SITTING POSITION
BP = 122/75	BP = 105/80
HR = 110	HR = 130
RR = 28	RR = 32
SpO_2 = 94%	SpO_2 = 93%

Given the above syncope workup, which of the following interventions should be performed first?

    A. Obtain an order for a formal tilt-test

    B. Administer isotonic fluids

    C. Increase the dose of digoxin

    D. Administer beta blockers

GO ON TO NEXT PAGE ➤

10. A patient with suspected heart failure arrives to the ICU with a decreased ejection fraction and cardiac output. Which of the following pathophysiological responses will attempt to compensate for this decrease in EF/CO?

    A. Decreased heart rate

    B. Increased oxygen use

    C. Peripheral vasodilation

    D. Decrease in renin release

11. A 33-year-old patient presents with shortness of breath, tachypnea, and coughing, auscultation reveals wheezing. The patient reports symptoms for the past hour. Suspecting an asthma attack or potentially status asthmaticus, the nurse draws an arterial blood gas. Which of the following ABGs would be expected at this time?

    A. pH 7.28, $PaCO_2$ 52, HCO_3 26, PaO_2 82

    B. pH 7.30, $PaCO_2$ 30, HCO_3 18, PaO_2 90

    C. pH 7.60, $PaCO_2$ 40, HCO_3 35, PaO_2 72

    D. pH 7.50, $PaCO_2$ 32, HCO_3 26, PaO_2 78

12. A postoperative patient is high risk for pulmonary embolism. Which of the following signs and symptoms would alert the nurse to potential PE?

    A. Dyspnea, tachypnea, hypoxemia

    B. Dyspnea, bradypnea, crackles

    C. Hypertension, bradycardia, wheezing

    D. Atrial gallop, bradypnea, hypotension

13. A sedated patient in the medical ICU has the following ABG result: pH 7.50, $PaCO_2$ 30, HCO_3 26, PaO_2 75. Which changes to the ventilator settings does the nurse anticipate?

    A. Increase the tidal volume, increase FiO_2

    B. Increase the respiratory rate, maintain current FiO_2

    C. Decrease the tidal volume, decrease FiO_2

    D. Decrease the respiratory or tidal volume, increase FiO_2

14. Thrombus formation may occur throughout the entire body. Which of the following increases the risk of thrombus rupture resulting in a traveling embolism?

    A. Increased turbulence of blood flow around the thrombus

    B. Decreased macrophages and size of the thrombus

    C. Thrombus covered with stable fibrous caps

    D. Decreased turbulence of blood flow around the thrombus

15. After a CT scan of the head, a patient is admitted to the neuro ICU diagnosed with hemorrhagic stroke. The patient is alert with expressive aphasia and mild hemiparesis of the left lower extremity. Which of the following treatments are indicated for this patient?

    A. Administration of opioids and benzodiazepines
    B. Administration of recombinant tissue plasminogen activator (rtPA)
    C. Administration of FFP and vitamin K
    D. Administration of enoxaparin or clopidogrel

16. A patient in severe respiratory distress undergoes emergency intubation at the bedside. Which of the following interventions would be immediately performed after intubation to confirm proper placement of the endotracheal tube (ETT)?

    A. Call the radiology department for portable chest x-ray
    B. Auscultate for bilateral breath sounds
    C. Document the centimeter at the lip, confirm cuff inflation
    D. Observe color change in the end-tidal carbon dioxide (ETCO$_2$) device

17. A bulimic patient is admitted to the ED after complaints of severe and prolonged vomiting with occasional blood. The patient complains of epigastric pain and weakness. What is the most likely reason for a physician to order an esophagogastroduodenoscopy (EGD) in this patient?

    A. Observation of gastric or duodenal ulcers
    B. Confirmation of Mallory–Weiss tears of the esophagus
    C. Confirmation of gallstone obstruction of the sphincter of Oddi
    D. Observation of gastroesophageal varices

18. Cardiac tamponade may manifest with muffled heart tones and decreased cardiac output. When a pulmonary artery catheter is placed, the nurse may also witness which changes in pressures?

    A. Decrease in CVP, increase in PAD and PAOP
    B. Diastolic pressures within 2 to 3 mmHg of each other
    C. Increase in CVP, decrease in PAD and PAOP
    D. Systolic pressures within 2 to 3 mmHg of each other

GO ON TO NEXT PAGE ➤

19. A patient is stung by a bee and arrives at the ED. Three years prior the patient was stung by a bee and was hospitalized for 5 days due to a severe anaphylactic reaction. Which of the following clinical manifestations of anaphylaxis would be seen in the respiratory system of this patient?

    A. Hypotension and tachycardia

    B. Massive immune-mediated IgE release

    C. Pneumothorax and tachypnea

    D. Stridor and hypoxemia

20. A nurse notes a rise in CAUTIs over the past 2 months. When reviewing protocol surrounding indwelling catheters, which of the following would the nurse address and change due to updated evidence-based practice?

    A. Irrigating the catheter frequently to prevent clots and occlusions

    B. Collecting urine specimens with aseptic technique

    C. Hand-washing before accessing or manipulating a catheter

    D. Removing the catheter as soon as it is no longer indicated

21. A patient in the early stages of chronic kidney disease chooses to begin peritoneal dialysis (PD) instead of fistula placement for hemodialysis. While being monitored in the hospital during the early exchanges of PD, the outflow dialysate starts to be brownish in color. Which of the following complications might the nurse expect?

    A. Peritonitis

    B. Bleeding in the peritoneum

    C. Perforation of the bowel

    D. Clotting of the outflow tubing

22. During a colonoscopy with fentanyl and midazolam the patient becomes unresponsive and the respiratory rate is decreasing. The pupils are slightly dilated. After 60 seconds, the SpO_2 begins to fall below 90%. The nurse anticipates administration of which medication first?

    A. Naloxone

    B. Neostigmine

    C. Flumazenil

    D. Epinephrine

23. Central lines are preferred over peripheral lines for the infusion of vasoactive agents. What is the best explanation for this reasoning?

    A. Central lines are more common in the ICU and easier to manage

    B. Infusion of vasoactive agents peripherally is contraindicated

    C. Vasoactive agents cause tissue injury during extravasation

    D. Norepinephrine and other vasoactive agents hit the heart faster when given centrally

24. A patient is diagnosed with a brain tumor. The location of the tumor is placing pressure on the posterior pituitary gland, causing an increase in hormone secretion. Which of the following diagnostic findings would be expected in this patient?

    A. Serum osmolality 265 mOsm/kg

    B. Urinary output 5 L per 12-hour shift

    C. Urine specific gravity 1.035

    D. Serum sodium 155 mmol/L

25. Acute hypoglycemia crisis may be life-threatening if not corrected. What serum glucose level would the nurse expect if only tachycardia and diaphoresis is present in the patient?

    A. 125 mg/dL

    B. 60 mg/dL

    C. 50 mg/dL

    D. 30 mg/dL

26. A 32-year-old patient arrives in the ICU after severe burns to the lower back, buttocks, and both legs. Fluid resuscitation is currently being administered. Two hours after admission the patient complains of numbness of the left leg. Suspecting the cause is patient position, the nurse shifts the patient in bed. One hour later, the patient complains of severe pain in the same leg. It is difficult to inspect the leg fully given the extent of the burns; however, Doppler reveals a weaker dorsalis pedis pulse in relation to the right leg. What complication is likely in this case?

    A. Hypovolemic shock

    B. Femoral artery perforation

    C. Lumbar nerve damage

    D. Compartment syndrome

27. A 50-year-old patient with a history of alcohol abuse is admitted to the hospital with worsening liver failure. The toxicology report is negative and the blood alcohol concentration (BAC) is zero. The patient is lethargic at this time and is making incomprehensible sounds but not formed words or speech. What is the most likely cause for these symptoms?

    A. Alcohol overdose
    B. Wernicke's encephalopathy
    C. Alcohol withdrawal
    D. Acute hypoglycemia

28. A patient in the hospital inadvertently receives a medication they are allergic to. Anaphylaxis develops and the nurse administers epinephrine. Why is epinephrine a first-line drug in anaphylaxis?

    A. Epinephrine offsets the effects of histamine
    B. Epinephrine is a negative inotrope correcting hypotension and shock
    C. Epinephrine blocks beta receptors aiding in bronchodilation
    D. Epinephrine stimulates the body's parasympathetic system

29. Multiple organ dysfunction syndrome (MODS) devastates the entire body eventually ending in death. Which of the following neurological changes would the nurse see as MODS progresses?

    A. Increasing alertness with anxiety
    B. Decreasing levels of consciousness
    C. Diplopia and nystagmus
    D. Decreased urine output, elevated lactate levels

30. A patient arrived at the critical care unit 30 minutes ago after a small bowel repair. The estimated blood loss during surgery was 250 mL. Current IV infusions include 5 mcg/min of norepinephrine and IV maintenance with plasmalyte. The patient recently received a fluid bolus. Current vital signs upon admission and the present are as follows:

VITAL SIGNS ON ADMISSION	VITAL SIGNS 30 MINUTES LATER (PRESENT)
Temp = 34.5°C	Temp = 35.5°C
BP = 105/85 mmHg	BP = 95/80 mmHg
HR = 85	HR = 95
RR = 16	RR = 18
SpO_2 = 95%	SpO_2 = 94%

What changes does the nurse expect in this patient?

A. Increasing need for norepinephrine

B. Increasing need for oxygen

C. Decreasing need for fluid replacement

D. Switching fluid maintenance to normal saline

31. The family of a critically ill patient insist on remaining in the hospital. It has been days since any of them have been home. The family looks disheveled and tired. How can the nurse address this situation with sensitivity?

A. Instruct the family to go home to clean up and sleep

B. Assist the family with any hygiene or sleep needs in the hospital

C. Remove the family from the hospital, but allow them to come back later

D. Consult with the social worker regarding the situation

32. A patient with advanced liver failure is intubated and unlikely to survive the day. Before he was intubated in the emergency department, he stated he did not wish his brothers to be able to visit him in the hospital. The patient's mother and brothers are at the front desk of the hospital insisting on seeing the patient. What is the most appropriate action by the nurse?

A. Allow all three family members to visit for 10 minutes

B. Tell the family the patient is dying and not likely to survive the day

C. Explain the mother may see the patient, but not the brothers

D. Do not allow the family to visit the patient

GO ON TO NEXT PAGE ➤

33. A 65-year-old female patient with multiple pulmonary embolisms is immediately started on an IV infusion of heparin. She develops heparin-induced thrombocytopenia (HIT) and the heparin is discontinued. She has a planned surgery for removal of multiple DVTs. Preoperative lab results display a platelet count of 30,000. Which action by the nurse is most appropriate?

    A. Call the operating room and cancel the surgery

    B. Monitor the patient for spontaneous bleeding

    C. Obtain an order to transfuse platelets

    D. Contact the surgeon and inform the results

34. A patient in the ICU is in the early stages of septic shock. A pulmonary artery catheter is inserted for close monitoring. Which of the following hemodynamic parameters would be expected for this patient?

    A. SvO_2 85%, cardiac output 7.5 L/min, SVR 1200 dynes/s/cm^{-5}

    B. SvO_2 66%, cardiac output 2.5 L/min, SVR 1600 dynes/s/cm^{-5}

    C. SvO_2 55%, cardiac output 5.5 L/min, SVR 1200 dynes/s/cm^{-5}

    D. SvO_2 79%, cardiac output 7.5 L/min, SVR 600 dynes/s/cm^{-5}

35. After a myocardial infarction a patient experiences sustained left ventricular failure. Echocardiogram shows increased left-sided filling pressures and decreased ejection fraction. Which of the following treatments would be appropriate for this patient?

    A. Calcium channel blockers

    B. Vasodilators

    C. Beta blockers

    D. Fluid resuscitation

36. A 75-year-old Type 2 diabetic patient is admitted to the critical care unit. A bedside fingerstick glucose test is unable to read a specific number due to range. The monitor states greater than 600 mg/dL. The patient is a poor historian and moderately confused. Which of the following findings would be expected in this patient?

    A. Serum osmolality 340 mOsm/kg, potassium 5.8 mEq/L, pH 7.38

    B. Serum osmolality 170 mOsm/kg, BUN 24 mEq/L, pH 7.35

    C. Serum osmolality 310 mOsm/kg, sodium 135 mEq/L, pH 7.28

    D. Serum osmolality 350 mOsm/kg, potassium 3.0 mEq/L, pH 7.55

37. When a patient diagnosed with hypothyroidism develops an infection, a severe decrease in thyroid hormone may develop. What assessment findings would the nurse associate with this dangerous decrease in thyroid hormone?

    A. Heat intolerance, hypotension, anxiety
    B. Fluid overload, hypertension, lethargy
    C. Weak and thready pulses, hypotension, polyuria
    D. Neck swelling, hypotension, stupor

38. After a thoracotomy, an intubated patient is admitted to the surgical critical care unit for close monitoring. The patient has one pleural chest tube to suction. Which of the following actions related to this patient may result in a complication?

    A. Leaving the chest tube unclamped during transport
    B. Keeping the chest tube lower than the level of the chest at all times
    C. Stripping the chest tube when ordered
    D. Increasing the PEEP on the ventilator

39. A nurse in the neuro ICU is entering the room of a ventilated patient to provide a number of care items. The patient requires suctioning and cleaning due to an incontinent episode. The patient recently had a spinal cord injury and remains on norepinephrine to maintain elevated MAPs. Upon turning the patient, the patient becomes hypotensive. Which of the following actions would the nurse perform first?

    A. Notify the physician of the sudden drop in blood pressure
    B. Increase the infusion rate of norepinephrine
    C. Place the patient in a supine position with the head flat
    D. Perform a digital rectal exam for impacted stool

40. The mother of an 18-year-old patient has remained at the bedside and wishes to spend the night. The unit rules do not allow visitation after 8 P.M.; however, the patient appears to have less anxiety when his mother is present. What would be the most appropriate response by the nurse?

    A. Explain to the mother she can stay an hour longer but then must leave
    B. Allow the mother to spend the night with her son
    C. Ask the physician for permission to let the mother stay
    D. Gently explain visitation rules exist for the benefit of the entire unit and patients

GO ON TO NEXT PAGE ➤

41. A patient is expected to be discharged within the next 24 hours. The husband of the patient will be required to provide wound care at home but does not show proficiency to perform the task. Which intervention would be the most appropriate?

    A. Provide bedside teaching with husband and observe him repeating the dressing change

    B. Consult with the wound care specialist to provide teaching

    C. Coordinate with case management to provide home health care

    D. Print out step-by-step instructions for the husband to follow

42. Abdominal assessment of a patient with end-stage liver disease reveals massive ascites. Two weeks earlier the patient had 6 L drained via paracentesis. The patient has decreased cardiac output and rapid shallow breathing. What is the most likely cause of the current patient condition?

    A. Third-spacing of fluid and hypovolemia

    B. Fluid buildup placing pressure on the diaphragm and vena cava

    C. Hyperammonemia and hepatic encephalopathy

    D. Portal hypertension and decreased preload

43. A physician was recently speaking to a patient about their prognosis with and without treatment. As the nurse enters the room, the patient is visibly distraught and crying. The patient does not make eye contact with the nurse but requests to be alone. What is the most appropriate response by the nurse at this time?

    A. Ask the patient questions regarding their feelings around the prognosis

    B. Call the chaplain and request they spend time with the patient

    C. Remain with the patient and sit quietly

    D. Provide the patient with peace and privacy, check back later

44. A patient in the emergency department has an ABG drawn that reveals the following: pH 7.28, $PaCO_2$ 45, HCO_3 16, PaO_2 85. What is the most likely cause for this acid–base imbalance?

    A. Status asthmaticus

    B. Frequent antacid consumption

    C. Hyperventilation

    D. Excessive diarrhea

45. Which of the following statements regarding the initial treatment for myocardial infarction is false?

    A. The primary goal is to reduce ischemia to the myocardium
    B. ECG may oftentimes show no ST elevation
    C. Propranolol is the beta blocker of choice
    D. Oxygen should be administered only when necessary

46. While rounding on the critical care unit the nurse notices a telemetry monitor reading the heart rhythm incorrectly. Upon closer assessment, the electrodes are found to be placed improperly. Which of the following electrode placements found is incorrect?

    A. V_6 at the fifth intercostal space, mid-axillary line
    B. V_1 at the fourth intercostal space, right of the sternum
    C. V_2 at the fifth intercostal space, midclavicular line
    D. White lead at the right arm

47. Certain respiratory conditions may affect either the ventilation or perfusion of oxygen and carbon dioxide. Which of the following conditions inhibits perfusion but not ventilation?

    A. Pulmonary embolism
    B. Pneumonia
    C. COPD/emphysema
    D. Pulmonary edema

48. A patient is admitted to the ICU with a COPD exacerbation. The patient is also diagnosed with pneumonia. Which of the following signs and symptoms are expected with pneumonia but not COPD?

    A. Shortness of breath
    B. Decreased expiratory flow
    C. Fine crackles
    D. Chronic cough

49. Immediately postpartum a young female was admitted to the ICU due to DIC. Prior to confirmation of DIC, there was estimated blood loss of 1L. Which of the following findings would not be expected in this patient at this time?

    A. Petechiae and purpura of the skin
    B. Decreased cardiac output
    C. Serum platelets 50,000
    D. Hemoglobin 8.6 g/dL

50. A patient was admitted to the neuro ICU after being diagnosed with a subarachnoid hemorrhage. MRI shows the cause as an aneurysm rupture likely due to cocaine abuse. Which of the following treatments is included in the management of this patient in the ICU?

    A. Intravenous fluids to maintain hypervolemia
    B. Intravenous fluids to maintain normovolemia
    C. Intravenous fluids to maintain hypovolemia
    D. Intravenous fluids would help in subarachnoid hemorrhage

51. A 78-year-old patient presents to the emergency department due to increasing lethargy. The family states the patient has dementia but has been acting odd lately and reports the patient drinking excessive amounts of water, likely 6 L or more in the past 24 hours. Which of the following lab values should the nurse look to for the cause of these symptoms in the patient?

    A. Potassium
    B. Creatinine/BUN
    C. Ammonia
    D. Sodium

52. A 24-year-old patient is admitted to the ICU postoperatively due to a minor complication. The surgeon requested ICU admission for close 24-hour monitoring. The patient has a history of anxiety and is frightened to be in a critical care setting. Which medication would be a first-line anxiolytic commonly given in the ICU?

    A. Midazolam
    B. Lorazepam
    C. Fentanyl
    D. Phenobarbital

53. A patient in the early stages of chronic kidney disease requires a CT scan with contrast. The benefits of the scan outweigh the risks at this point. What is the most important thing for the nurse to implement after the CT scan?

    A. Administration of continuous hypotonic saline
    B. "Flushing" the kidneys with adequate fluid intake
    C. Obtaining serum creatinine and BUN levels
    D. Discontinuing any medications that are nephrotoxic

54. An obese patient is postoperative in the ICU from a bowel resection. One hour after surgery the patient develops a fever, a tender bowel upon palpation, and absent bowel sounds. Which complication is this patient likely experiencing?

    A. Pancreatic duct leak

    B. Retention of a surgical towel

    C. Anastomotic leak

    D. Adhesion development

55. After discharge home, a patient who had a gastrectomy is called by an ICU nurse for follow-up. The patient describes experiencing palpitations, anxiety, and weakness 2 hours after eating. What is the most likely explanation for the patient's symptoms?

    A. Hyperglycemia secondary to rapid food movement into the duodenum

    B. Hypovolemia secondary to dumping syndrome

    C. Hypokalemia secondary to gastrointestinal losses

    D. Hypoglycemia secondary to rapid insulin response to dumped food

56. A patient in the ICU is high risk for DVT due to immobility and sedation. Which of the following prophylaxis is indicated for this patient?

    A. Sequential compression devices

    B. Scheduled low molecular weight heparin

    C. Heparin infusion to therapeutic effect

    D. Aspirin or clopidogrel

57. Platelet dysfunction affects the coagulation process throughout the body. At which level would thrombocytopenia potentially increase the risk of bleeding?

    A. 50,000

    B. 100,000

    C. 20,000

    D. 5000

58. A patient with ARDS is showing poor lung compliance on the ventilator; a common symptom of ARDS. What is the best definition for lung compliance?

    A. The lungs' ability to ventilate oxygen and carbon dioxide

    B. The lungs' ability to stretch and expand

    C. The lungs' ability to perfuse blood in the alveoli

    D. The lungs' ability to respond to movement of the diaphragm

GO ON TO NEXT PAGE ➤

59. Which of the following correctly compares and contrasts asthma and COPD?

   A. Asthma and COPD are irreversible and chronic

   B. Oxygen assists patient with asthma, but not COPD

   C. Airway obstruction in asthma may improve, whereas COPD does not

   D. Sputum production is less common in COPD than in asthma

60. A 45-year-old patient recently underwent a laparotomy for multiple internal injuries secondary to trauma. The current vital signs are BP 105/80 mmHg, HR 110, RR 18, SpO_2 94% on 40% FiO_2. The patient is currently receiving inotropic therapy to increase cardiac output and remains sedated. Which of the following is not a risk factor for the development of an acute kidney injury?

   A. Hypovolemic shock

   B. Post-operative vancomycin infusions

   C. Naproxen use for pain management

   D. Inotropic therapy

61. A patient in the ICU is receiving hemodialysis due to an acute kidney injury superimposed on top of previous chronic kidney disease. The pre-dialysis lab values show a creatinine of 3.4, a BUN of 24, and a potassium of 6.2 mmol/L. The patient monitor exhibits intermittent PVCs. The goal of treatment is to remove 2 L of fluid and correct the lab values. What consideration is the most important for the nurse to monitor once hemodialysis has completed?

   A. Dysrhythmias

   B. Azotemia

   C. Hypovolemia

   D. Delirium

62. After a near-fatal car accident, a patient is withdrawn and does not speak to the nurse. The patient does not make eye contact and only mumbles toward the window. As the nurse turns to leave the room the patient speaks a name unfamiliar to the nurse. What is an appropriate action at this time?

   A. Give the patient privacy as they likely want to be alone

   B. Inquire about the name spoken by the patient

   C. Encourage the patient to speak with their family about the experience

   D. Ask the patient if they would like an anxiolytic

63. Refractory hypoxemia is present in a patient with a suspected pulmonary shunt. Which of the following is not a likely cause for this shunt?

   A. Pulmonary edema

   B. Pneumonia

   C. Atelectasis

   D. Pulmonary embolism

64. A 65-year-old female patient is admitted with a viral respiratory disease. Her history includes hypertension, osteopenia, and myasthenia gravis. What is the most important assessment for this patient at this time?

   A. Obtain baseline vital capacity

   B. Auscultate the lung sounds

   C. Analysis of spirometry for peak flow

   D. Observe the plethysmograph

65. After 2 days, a patient in the critical care unit begins to develop agitation, yawning, and rhinorrhea. The vital signs are BP 160/80 mmHg, HR 130, RR 22, and SpO$_2$ 95%. Which of the following interventions should the nurse include in the plan of care?

   A. Assess CIWA protocol and administer lorazepam PRN

   B. Administer antihypertensive medications

   C. Administer PRN opioids

   D. Initiate COWS protocol for opioid withdrawal

66. After an inferior wall myocardial infarction, a patient develops large V waves on the pulmonary artery catheter waveform when it is wedged (occluded). What is the likely cause of this change?

   A. Dressler's syndrome

   B. Mitral regurgitation

   C. Tricuspid regurgitation

   D. Cardiogenic shock

67. Nine days after a myocardial infarction a patient returns to his cardiologist for a checkup. When the nurse performs an ECG on the patient, which of the following findings would be expected?

   A. Large-peaked T waves

   B. ST elevations

   C. Q waves

   D. T-wave inversions

68. A patient in the emergency department is being prepped for a cardiac catheterization for suspected inferior myocardial infarction. When assessing the ECG, the nurse would notice changes in which leads?

    A. II, III, aVF
    B. V1, V2, V3, V4
    C. V5, V6, I
    D. V1, V2

69. After surgery, a patient with a psychiatric history is admitted to the ICU for close monitoring. As the anesthesia wears off and the patient becomes more alert, they begin stating aliens abducted him. He also admits to hearing voices. What diagnosis is likely in this patient's psychiatric history?

    A. Manic depression
    B. Schizophrenia
    C. Major depression
    D. Somatic symptom disorder

70. The nurse manager of a critical care unit decides to implement a 2-hour period of reduced noise to benefit the sleep of the patients on the unit. This policy was started in a committee reviewing the importance of sleep in the critically ill. Which of the following is not a correct understanding of managing the sleep of patients in the ICU?

    A. Group medication administrations together when appropriate
    B. Closing patient doors during sleeping hours
    C. Turning off alarms to the monitors at night
    D. Assessing for new onset delirium or changes in mental status

71. When a nurse acts as a representative for the patient and family in a meeting regarding the plan of care for the patient, the nurse is performing what ability?

    A. Moral judgment
    B. Moral justice
    C. Moral beliefs
    D. Moral agency

72. A team of nurses is reviewing the importance of assessing advance directives and DNR wishes at the time of admission. In which circumstance would it be appropriate to deviate from an advance directive of a patient?

    A. If the family wishes to alter certain components of the advance directive
    B. If the patient has implemented an advance directive, it should be followed
    C. If the patient becomes terminal and the healthcare team believes there is nothing left to be done
    D. If the nurse reviews the advance directive and finds conflicting information

73. An 18-year-old female patient is admitted to the intensive care unit after the ingestion of an unknown amount of acetaminophen. She states the ingestion was a suicide attempt and occurred 4 hours ago. Which of the following can be expected in the treatment of this patient?

    A. Performing gastric lavage with a large nasogastric tube
    B. Monitoring serum amylase and lipase levels
    C. Administering treatment of acetylcysteine
    D. Performing a fecal occult test on the stool

74. A patient in cardiogenic shock is receiving treatment with dobutamine and vasodilators. The healthcare team is considering implementing balloon pump therapy if the patient does not improve. Which hemodynamic parameters would indicate the best outcome of current treatment?

    A. Cardiac index 2.4, BP 105/60, urine output 25 mL/hr
    B. Cardiac index 1.5, BP 80/50, urine output 10 mL/hr
    C. Cardiac index 1.7, BP 90/60, urine output 15 mL/hr
    D. Cardiac index 2.4, BP 100/75, urine output 20 mL/hr

75. Albumin is a frequently used colloid in patients with large burns. What is the best explanation for this preference in treatment?

    A. Albumin will aid in the wound healing and preservation of the burned tissue
    B. Albumin does not contain potassium or electrolytes
    C. Colloids will maintain oncotic pressure of the intravascular space
    D. Colloids should replace crystalloids in the treatment of burn victims

76. After a spinal cord injury, a patient in the ICU is having difficulty maintaining their blood pressure. The nurse suspects neurogenic shock. What is the best explanation of the pathophysiology for neurogenic shock?

    A. Decreased innervation to the brain stem adversely affects the vital signs

    B. Neurogenic shock is a life-threatening type of hypovolemic shock

    C. Heightened stimulation to beta receptors decreases heart rate and contractility

    D. Lack of alpha innervation leads to decreased systemic vascular resistance

77. A patient in the ICU recently had an exploratory laparotomy performed for suspected internal bleeding. Part of the liver was removed, a cholecystectomy was performed, and part of the small bowel needed repair. When speaking with the dietician the following day, which considerations for tube feedings would the dietician and nurse agree on?

    A. Tube feedings should be high in protein, fat, and calories

    B. Tube feedings should be low in fat, adequate in carbs and protein

    C. Tube feedings should be administered in intermittent boluses

    D. Tube feedings are inappropriate at this time, total parenteral nutrition is best

78. When entering the room of a surgical patient, the nurse inspects the surgical wound and finds the dressing peeled back and the wound dehisced. In what position would the nurse immediately place the patient?

    A. Supine with the head flat and midline

    B. Legs flexed with the head slightly elevated

    C. Reverse Trendelenburg with the head flat

    D. High Fowler's with legs straightened

79. A 76-year-old patient is admitted to the ICU due to heat sickness. The patient was found in the park unconscious by a bystander. After stabilizing the patient, full inspection of the skin notes first degree burns. What would be appropriate care for the skin of these areas?

    A. Apply lotion and cover the area with light gauze

    B. Apply hydrocortisone cream as ordered

    C. Cleanse the area with diluted hydrogen peroxide

    D. Cover the wound with wet-to-dry dressings

80. After a prolonged ICU stay due to a serious viral respiratory infection, the patient wishes to ambulate out of bed. The patient was previously intubated for 2 weeks and now has a tracheostomy. What method would the nurse use to begin progressive mobility?

    A. Utilize a cardiac chair to begin

    B. Have a nursing assistant help the patient out of bed

    C. Keep the patient on bed rest until physical therapy can evaluate the patient

    D. Ambulate the patient as tolerated with oxygen

81. A 65-year-old patient in the ICU is recovering from a severe case of pneumonia. After prolonged intubation, the patient now has a tracheostomy. They remain bedridden. Which of the following will best reduce the chances of pressure ulcer development?

    A. Ensuring adequate oxygenation

    B. Providing nutrition high in protein

    C. Turn the patient every 2 hours

    D. Coordinate with physical therapy for range of motion exercises

82. After a fall down a flight of stairs, a patient is admitted to the emergency department. There are multiple injuries to the body, including abrasions on the face, swelling of the orbital socket, and a possible mandibular fracture. At the time of the fall the patient did not lose consciousness and the Glasgow Coma Score has been consistently 13 throughout the admission. Upon further inspection, the nurse notes clear liquid draining from the patient's nose. Which of the following is a priority concern at this time?

    A. Subarachnoid hemorrhage

    B. Nasopharynx laceration

    C. Infection of the brain or meninges

    D. Increased intracranial pressure

83. A 65-year-old male patient arrives at the emergency room via ambulance. For the past hour, the man states experiencing chest pain. The healthcare team suspects a myocardial infarction and immediately performs an ECG that displays ST depression with T-wave inversion. The patient is subsequently diagnosed with an NSTEMI. Which of the following is not included in the plan of care at this time?

    A. Reperfusion by cardiac catheterization

    B. Admit the patient for observation

    C. Follow trends of cardiac markers

    D. Administer oxygen for a pulse ox of 90%

GO ON TO NEXT PAGE ➤

84. An external ventricular drain (EVD) is inserted by the neurosurgeon for close monitoring of ICP. There is an order to keep the drain closed unless assessing ICP. When using the EVD, which action by the nurse is wrong and could potentially harm the patient?

    A. Leveling the transducer at the foramen of Monro

    B. Maintaining the collection bag in a closed system

    C. Placing the EVD on the bed during transportation

    D. Flushing the EVD if a clot is suspected

85. A patient in the intensive care unit is diagnosed with a COPD exacerbation. The patient was admitted on 2 L nasal cannula 2 hours ago. The patient is lethargic and weak. Given the following recently drawn ABG results, what recommendation would the nurse make involving the care of this patient?

    ABG RESULTS

    $pH = 7.25$
    $PaCO_2 = 80$
    $HCO_3 = 28$
    $PaO_2 = 65\%$

    A. Increase the oxygen to 4 L nasal cannula

    B. Administer PRN bronchodilators

    C. Initiate a bilevel positive airway pressure machine

    D. These results are expected, continue to monitor

86. During morning rounds, the physician requests a sedation vacation with a "wake up and breathe" trial. While performing these actions, which of the following parameters indicates the patient may be ready for extubation?

    A. HR 125, BP 155/80 mmHg, FiO_2 0.40

    B. Minute ventilation 5L, HR 95, FiO_2 0.40

    C. RR 32, tidal volume 250 mL, FiO_2 0.60

    D. PaO_2/FiO_2 ratio > 200, negative inspiratory pressure −10 cm H_2O

87. Bowel resection with anastomosis to a colostomy is often required for patients with colorectal cancer. The colostomy may be temporary or permanent. A patient had this surgery performed and does not engage with the nurse to learn during stoma care and colostomy bag changes. The nurse understands which of the following as most important?

    A. Leave the room and provide stoma care at a later time

    B. Perform the stoma care while explaining the steps

    C. Instruct the patient to hold the colostomy bag

    D. Tell the patient the colostomy is only temporary

88. A 22-year-old male trauma patient is admitted to the ICU after multiple gunshot wounds. One of the wounds was to the head. The Glasgow Coma Score is 3. The patient has no gag reflex. To the nurse's knowledge the family has not been contacted yet. What action by the nurse is best at this time?

    A. Attempt to contact the family and instruct them to come to the hospital

    B. Contact the chaplain and update them on the situation

    C. Instruct the unit secretary to contact the family

    D. Contact organ procurement services

89. During admission of a patient with a pulmonary embolism, the physician orders a heparin infusion. Upon completion of the initial assessment, the nurse finds a previous progress note describing a severe reduction of platelets after the patient received heparin. The nurse immediately calls the physician. Which professional nursing action has the nurse performed?

    A. Veracity

    B. Justice

    C. Moral agency

    D. Vigilance

90. A patient was extubated the previous day after an alcohol overdose. The patient states they are not a regular user, but since returning from active military service have had increasing difficulty focusing, describe being angry very fast and having images of gunfire. Which of the following actions would the nurse want to avoid with this patient?

    A. PRN lorazepam for anxiety or agitation

    B. Speaking with the patient and making eye contact

    C. Administering an IV push medication while the patient is sleeping

    D. Encourage the patient to discuss the experience

91. A woman with preeclampsia is started on magnesium sulfate therapy. Two hours later the patient develops respiratory depression and hyporeflexia. The current pulse ox reads 92%. What action by the nurse is the most appropriate?

    A. Initiate non-invasive ventilation (NIV)

    B. Request placement of a dialysis catheter

    C. Administer calcium gluconate

    D. Administer regular insulin and D50

92. While a patient is receiving hemodialysis, they develop a headache and confusion. The nurse suspects disequilibrium syndrome and stops the dialysis treatment. What is the pathophysiological reason for the patient's symptoms?

    A. Shifting fluid and increased cerebral edema

    B. Hypotension and decreased brain perfusion

    C. Increased urea and waste products in the blood

    D. Hypertension and intracerebral hemorrhage

93. In addition to the administration of lithium, the psychiatrist decides to add an additional pharmacological agent to a patient with severe bipolar disorder. The nurse recognizes the mediation as an anticonvulsant. Which of the following agents is most likely prescribed?

    A. Valproic acid

    B. Paroxetine

    C. Rivastigmine

    D. Risperidone

94. A patient is admitted with a hypercalcemic crisis. Serum results read as follows: calcium 16 mEq/L, creatinine 1.5, BUN 18. Which of the following treatments should begin immediately?

    A. Glucocorticosteroid therapy

    B. Furosemide therapy with potassium replacement

    C. Emergency hemodialysis

    D. IV fluid resuscitation

95. A patient with worsening ARDs requires increasing amounts of FiO_2, tidal volume, and PEEP via a mechanical ventilator. The patient suddenly becomes agitated, dyspneic, and hypoxic. Which of the following interventions should the nurse expect?

    A. Prone positioning with increased sedation

    B. Thoracostomy with tube suction

    C. Reduce the PEEP and tidal volume

    D. Administering a neuromuscular blocking agent

96. After administration of succinylcholine during intubation, a patient develops rapid onset hyperthermia and muscle rigidity. Which of the following agents should be administered at this time?

    A. Acetaminophen

    B. Lorazepam

    C. Rocuronium

    D. Dantrolene

97. When administering antihypertensive for a patient with hypertensive emergency, it is most important for the nurse to consider what sign as a potential adverse effect of treatment?

    A. Urine output 15 mL/hr with a BP 130/80 mmHg
    B. Headache and epistaxis
    C. Chest pain radiating to the left arm
    D. Creatinine 3.5 mg/dL, BUN 24

98. The nurse is discussing certain conditions that affect cardiac output. Which of the following is not a factor that may decrease cardiac output?

    A. Increasing age
    B. Sick sinus syndrome
    C. Sepsis and fever
    D. Hypocalcemia

99. Which of the following hemodynamic profiles is indicative of expected and effective treatment of pulmonary hypertension in a patient with right-sided heart failure?

    A. CVP 12 mmHg, PAP 35/17 mmHg, PAOP 18 mmHg
    B. CVP 3 mmHg, PAP 10/5 mmHg, PAOP 4 mmHg
    C. CVP 14 mmHg, PAP 22/10 mmHg, PAOP 12 mmHg
    D. CVP 6 mmHg, PAP 25/15 mmHg, PAOP 18 mmHg

100. When assessing a patient with suspected peripheral arterial disease (PAD) the nurse notes an ankle–brachial index of 1.20. How would the nurse interpret these results?

    A. The patient likely has borderline PAD
    B. The patient does not have PAD
    C. The patient likely has severe PAD
    D. The patient does not have PAD; however, the result is abnormal

101. Which of the following methods of assessing or treating pain is best for a patient diagnosed with dementia?

    A. Assess irritability and self-reported pain intensity
    B. Monitor patient behavior and body language
    C. Utilize a FLACC scale
    D. Administer medications based upon a RASS scale

102. After a motor vehicle accident resulting in multiple injuries, a patient is admitted to the ICU. When the nurse attempts to place an indwelling catheter for close monitoring of urine output, hard resistance is met. Which of the following actions are appropriate at this time?

    A. Obtain a smaller size catheter for placement; consider a coude

    B. Cease future attempts to place a catheter, call the physician

    C. Suspect kidney damage, assess for hematuria

    D. Assess for costovertebral tenderness

103. A patient in the ICU has complicated injuries requiring ventricular assistive devices, continuous renal replacement therapy and multiple titratable medications, and is intubated on mechanical ventilation. The nurse is providing a synergistic model of care when what occurs?

    A. Nursing advocacy is accepted by the healthcare team

    B. Care is providing regardless of cultural diversity

    C. The nurse participates in shared governance committee meetings

    D. Nurse competency matches patient needs

104. A 45-year-old patient is admitted to the ICU after a fall from a ladder. The tibia is protruding through the skin of the left lower leg. Gauze is dampened with sterile water to protect the wound until surgery. Which of the following is a priority intervention for the nurse at this time?

    A. Scheduling a V/Q scan

    B. Assessing pain intensity

    C. Apply compression at the site of injury

    D. Administering IV antibiotics

105. A wound care specialist has recently rounded on a number of patients in the intensive care unit. During a discussion about one of the nurse's patients, the wound care specialist states one of the wounds is healing by tertiary intent. How does the nurse interpret this process of healing?

    A. A laceration on the forehead was sutured closed

    B. A wound vac was applied to the surgical opening of the abdomen to stimulate granulation tissue

    C. The leg wound was cleaned and being kept open until inflammation decreases

    D. A pressure ulcer wound was packed with wet-to-moist dressings

106. A patient in the ICU has a questionable mental status. The nurse believes the patient to be confused, but the cause is likely multifactorial given the patient's history of substance abuse and medical conditions. Which of the following assessments indicates the patient might not be able to make their own decisions about their care?

    A. The patient nods yes or no when the physician is asking them about decisions for their care

    B. The patient indicates understanding of the diagnosis and potential consequences of treatment

    C. The patient toxicology report shows alcohol, cocaine, and methamphetamines in their system

    D. The patient mental capacity is ranked at the level of a 16-year-old

107. After signing an informed consent for surgery, the patient begins to ask questions regarding potential risks. The physician tells the patient they are busy and the nurse can answer those questions. What is the most appropriate response by the nurse?

    A. Answer the patient's questions to the best of his/her ability

    B. Speak with the physician at that moment about the informed consent

    C. Inform the physician about the patient's questions after they leave the unit

    D. Disregard the informed consent and do not add it to the patient chart

108. A patient has been in the ICU for 6 days for the treatment of multiple injuries. Upon assess this morning, the nurse finds the patient increasingly confused. Which of the following is not a method in reducing potential delirium in this patient?

    A. Assessing and treating pain accordingly

    B. Reorienting the patient to the time and situation of events

    C. Encouraging appropriate mentation by increasing sensory overload

    D. Exposing the patient to natural light from the outdoors

109. The healthcare team suspects brain death in a patient and begins testing for reflexes and other signs of higher brain function. Which of the following cranial nerves, if affected, results in a poor outcome on the Doll's eyes test and cold caloric test?

    A. Cranial nerve VIII

    B. Cranial nerve V

    C. Cranial nerve XII

    D. Cranial nerve IV

GO ON TO NEXT PAGE ➤

110. A patient in the ICU is recovering after a lumbar laminectomy. Vital signs have improved and the patient is ready to begin ambulation. The patient states they have not had a bowel movement in over 5 days now. Upon discussing this with the physician, a KUB is ordered, which displays dilated bowel loops and potential large bowel obstruction. Which other findings would the nurse note as being consistent with a large bowel obstruction?

    A. High pitched bowel sounds, abdominal distention, vomiting
    B. High pitched bowel sounds, abdominal pain, hyperkalemia
    C. Absent bowel sounds, flat abdomen, vomiting
    D. Low pitched bowel sounds, colicky abdominal pain, hypokalemia

111. A patient at risk for increased ICP after a craniotomy develops new onset lethargy, hypertension, and bradycardia. The nurse is concerned about increased ICP, but the patient does not have an EVD. The nurse administers mannitol as ordered. Which of the following vital signs displays effectiveness of the treatment?

    VITAL SIGNS

    BP = 108/70 mmHg
    HR = 55
    RR = 22
    SpO_2 = 94%

    A. Heart rate
    B. Respiratory rate
    C. Pulse ox
    D. Blood pressure

112. A patent with frequent episodes of pericarditis is admitted back to the intensive care unit after a previous admission 3 months ago. In addition to patient complaints of chest pain and shortness of breath, which other findings may the nurse assess?

    A. ST elevations on the ECG
    B. Muffled heart sounds and a narrowed pulse pressure
    C. Jugular venous distention and dependent edema
    D. Fever and friction rub upon breathing

113. During a cardiac stress test, a 70-year-old female patient develops angina pain. What is the closest association to anginal pain when described by the patient?

    A. A dull feeling over the left side of the chest
    B. A substernal pain that radiates to the jaw
    C. A throbbing pain over the left upper quadrant
    D. A squeezing feeling over the chest and abdomen

114. After a pancreaticoduodenectomy, commonly called a Whipple procedure, the patient develops a pancreatic fistula and leak. Which of the following changes may the nurse witness on arterial blood gas results?

    A. Respiratory acidosis
    B. Respiratory alkalosis
    C. Metabolic acidosis
    D. Metabolic alkalosis

115. A 36-year-old male patient is diagnosed with *Pneumonia jiroveci*. X-ray displays severe infection of the right lung. The patient has a history of HIV/AIDS, hypertension, CAD, and DM Type 2. After shift change, the monitor for the patient alarms displaying a decreasing pulse oximeter. Current vital signs are BP 155/80 mmHg, HR 125, RR 32, SpO_2 84%. Which of the following actions would the nurse perform first?

    A. Obtain a venturi mask and increase the FiO_2
    B. Raise the head of the bed and deep suction the mouth and trachea
    C. Place the patient on a left side-lying position with the head elevated
    D. Obtain a fingerstick glucose monitor, assess for hypoglycemia

116. An unconscious patient arrives at the emergency department and is immediately placed on 100% oxygen for suspected carbon monoxide poisoning. Which of the following ABG results would be expected in this situation?

    A. pH 7.25, $PaCO_2$ 65, HCO_3 22, PaO_2 60
    B. pH 7.25, $PaCO_2$ 40, HCO_3 18, PaO_2 85
    C. pH 7.35, $PaCO_2$ 30, HCO_3 24, PaO_2 80
    D. pH 7.55, $PaCO_2$ 25, HCO_3 24, PaO_2 90

GO ON TO NEXT PAGE ➤

117. After being thrown into the steering wheel during a motor vehicle accident, a patient arrives at the emergency department with an obvious flail chest. A chest x-ray is performed and a pneumothorax is also present. Which of the following treatments is not included in the plan of care for this patient?

    A. Insertion of a chest tube

    B. Intubation and mechanical ventilation

    C. Maintaining a supine position

    D. Sufficient pain management to reduce pain

118. A nurse in the cardiovascular surgical intensive care unit is concerned a patient is not adequately oxygenating organs and tissues due to cardiogenic shock. Which of the following provides the greatest amount of information regarding oxygen delivery and consumption for this patient?

    A. Urine output, serum lactate

    B. Mixed venous oxygen saturation

    C. VO_2 testing during appropriate treatment

    D. Blood pressure, heart rate, and SVR

119. A patent is being admitted to the intensive care unit by the nurse. Upon assessment, the patient is found to be hypotensive with dry mucous membranes and poor skin turgor. Based upon the below laboratory values, which of the following fluids is most appropriate for continuous administration?

    LABORATORY VALUES UPON ADMISSION

    Na - 155 mEq/L
    K - 3.8 mEq/L
    Cl - 110 mEq/L
    Ca - 11 mg/dL
    Glucose - 90 mg/dL
    Creatinine - 1.2 mg/dL
    BUN - 8 mg/dL

    A. 0.9 sodium chloride

    B. 0.45 sodium chloride

    C. 0.45 sodium chloride with 5% Dextrose

    D. 3% sodium chloride

120. After administration of an incorrect medication, the patient begins to develop orbital edema and tongue swelling. Which complication of anaphylaxis would lead to the need for immediate intubation?

    A. Laryngeal edema with stridor

    B. Pulmonary edema with crackles

    C. Bronchoconstriction with wheezing

    D. Pleurisy with pleural friction rubs

121. After administration of 1 unit of packed red blood cells the patient develops wheezing and shortness of breath. Current vitals include BP 165/90 mmHg, HR 125, and RR 32. Which of the following interventions would the nurse prioritize?

    A. Intubation and mechanical ventilation

    B. Fluid bolus of normal saline

    C. Administration of diphenhydramine

    D. Administration of furosemide

122. A 22-year-old patient is admitted to the critical care unit with a diagnosis of asthma exacerbation. Which of the following spirometry results is consistent with this diagnosis?

    A. FEV_1 2L

    B. Peak expiratory flow rate <40% of normal value

    C. Absolute peak flow >100 L/min

    D. Forced vital capacity 80% of normal value

123. Which of the following types of shock would result in a cardiac index of 1.8 $L/min/m^2$, tachycardia, and elevated left-ventricular filling pressure?

    A. Anaphylactic shock

    B. Septic shock

    C. Cardiogenic shock

    D. Neurogenic shock

124. An obese patient diagnosed with high cholesterol is being coached by the dietician about necessary dietary changes to avoid future coronary artery disease and potential myocardial infarction. The patient also has a history of diabetes and early signs of kidney failure. If the patient follows the recommended diet, what changes does the healthcare team hope to see?

    A. Low-density lipoprotein less than 250 mg/dL

    B. Total cholesterol less than or equal to 200 mg/dL

    C. High-density lipoprotein less than 40 mg/dL

    D. Low-density lipoprotein greater than 150 mg/dL

GO ON TO NEXT PAGE ➤

125. Which of the following changes to the oxyhemoglobin dissociation curve causes an increase in the release of oxygen from hemoglobin to the tissues?

A. Massive transfusion protocol of blood

B. Decreased levels of 2.3-DPG

C. Arterial pH of 7.25

D. Hypothermia

STOP. You have completed the practice test. Complete your answers before moving forward with the review and rationales.

Answer Key

Question 1

Answer: B

Rationale: The immediate and first priority is to identify each previous allergic reaction and the symptoms. This aids the healthcare team in avoiding allergens that are common triggers to the patient. A medication reconciliation will be part of the admission, but it is not the immediate priority at this time. An allergist may be consulted at a later time. The allergen is unknown at this time; assuming latex is an issue is premature.

Question 2

Answer: A

Rationale: Restraints should be used as a last resort and typically only if the patient is at risk for self-harm or harm to others. Using restraints during agitation will likely escalate and worsen the problem. The other answers are appropriate interventions for a patient with agitation.

Question 3

Answer: B

Rationale: The left ventricular end-diastolic pressure, also called left ventricular preload, is often estimated by using a Swan–Ganz catheter and the pulmonary artery wedge (occlusive) pressure (PAOP). This is an indirect measurement of left ventricular function. The other answers have to do with afterload rather than filling pressures (preload).

Question 4

Answer: D

Rationale: Cushing's triad includes bradycardia, hypertension (often with widened pulse pressure), and irregular breathing.

Question 5

Answer: C

Rationale: These ethical terms are not uncommon on the exam. Understand the major ethical terms. Paternalism is when healthcare opinions and advocacy are pushed over that of patient autonomy and wishes.

Question 6

Answer: C

Rationale: A priority of enteral feedings is the prevention of aspiration. The full list of interventions to prevent this includes anything from elevating the head of the bed to administration of a PPI (pantoprazole). Whenever manipulating the patient position or a supine (flat) position is expected, the tube feeding should be stopped.

The other answers are not appropriate for enteral feedings. Tube placement must be confirmed. Feeding rate begins at the lowest amount, typically 10 mL/hr. There is no need to decompress before feedings.

Question 7

Answer: A

Rationale: The patient is exhibiting signs of dehydration. Priority is fluid resuscitation with isotonic fluids, typically normal saline. An NG tube is not necessary at this time; the patient is alert and able to swallow. A urine culture may be appropriate down the line if urine displays signs of infection or a urinalysis is positive for infectious markers. Anti-diarrheal medication may be indicated; however, it would be of secondary importance behind addressing the dehydration and hypovolemia.

Question 8

Answer: C

Rationale: Hypoglycemic unawareness (HU) is a condition where neurological problems manifest before any compensatory mechanisms occur and before the patient becomes aware of the hypoglycemia. Adrenergic responses, like the release of epinephrine, cause tachycardia and potentially diaphoresis, which alert the diabetic of impending hypoglycemia. This mechanism does not occur in HU.

Question 9

Answer: B

Rationale: Orthostatic hypotension appears to be the culprit for the syncope. The reduction in BP and reflex tachycardia is indicative of this orthostasis and general hypovolemia. Correcting preload will aid in cardiac output and orthostasis. A tilt-test may be ordered if the syncope continues without a known cause. Increasing digoxin may be indicated, but at this time the likely underlying problem should be corrected. Beta blockers may help the heart pump more effectively, but similar to digoxin, a less invasive method should be applied first. Least invasive to most. Administering fluids is simpler.

Question 10

Answer: B

Rationale: When blood pressure or cardiac output decreases, the body compensates to increase perfusion to tissues and organs. This happens through the endocrine and neurological systems. Catecholamine release will cause the increase in HR and oxygen consumption as well as vasoconstriction. The RAAS system is also activated (increased renin).

Question 11

Answer: D

Rationale: Early stages (1 and 2) in status asthmaticus the ABG will display respiratory alkalosis and mild to moderate hypoxia. In the early stages, the patient is hyperventilating; however, as the asthma progresses the patient will tire and respiratory acidosis ensues (stage 4).

Question 12

Answer: A

Rationale: The full clinical picture of a PE is rather large, but dyspnea, tachypnea, tachycardia, and hypoxemia are standard across the board. Crackles, cough, and hemoptysis are not uncommon. An atrial gallop, otherwise known as an S4 heart sound is also possible in PE.

Question 13

Answer: D

Rationale: The ABG is showing respiratory alkalosis without compensation and mild hypoxemia. The tidal volume or respiratory rate will likely be decreased and the FiO_2 increased to correct the hypoxemia.

Question 14

Answer: A

Rationale: Certain factors predispose a thrombus (plaque) to rupture. Increased turbulence such as the location of plaque on the edge of a vascular tree or hypertension increases the risk of rupture. Increased macrophages and unstable fibrous caps increase this risk as well.

Question 15

Answer: C

Rationale: One hallmark of hemorrhagic stroke treatment is correcting any underlying coagulopathy issues. This may include administration of FFP, platelets, vitamin K, protamine sulfate, etc. Opioids or benzodiazepines may mask advancing symptoms of the stroke and should be avoided. Tissue plasminogen activator (tPA) is contraindicated in hemorrhagic stroke. Blood thinners, such as heparin or clopidogrel, will also worsen the bleeding and should be avoided.

Question 16

Answer: D

Rationale: The moment intubation is performed, $ETCO_2$ is measured by observing color change from purple to yellow or tan. This is an immediate and primary intervention. Following this measurement, the nurse typically inspects for bilateral chest expansion, auscultates for bilateral breath sounds, notes absence of sounds over the stomach (epigastric). Once completed, a portable x-ray will confirm absolute placement of the ETT. Generally speaking in a priority-type of question, documentation is the least important.

Question 17

Answer: B

Rationale: Given the excessive retching, Mallory–Weiss tears are not uncommon. This repeated increased pressure may tear the lining of the esophagus leading to hematemesis. This bleeding is not likely due to an ulcer or varices given the story of bulimia. Direct visualization of the sphincter of Oddi and the bile/pancreatic ducts is performed by ERCP.

Question 18

Answer: B

Rationale: A diastolic plateau occurs in cardiac tamponade. Patients with pulmonary artery catheters will show these pressures within 2 to 3 mmHg of each other. This includes the CVP, PAD, and PAOP. These numbers will also increase from baselines in cardiac tamponade.

Question 19

Answer: D

Rationale: The first thing noticed is two of these answers (A and B) are not representative of the respiratory system. Pneumothorax is known to happen in anaphylaxis, but is quite rare. Stridor, whether auscultated or audible naturally, is a symptom of airway obstruction. This along with hypoxemia is common with respiratory compromise due to anaphylaxis.

Question 20

Answer: A

Rationale: More research is needed around the premise of irrigating a catheter, but what is known is urinary catheters are best left in a closed system. Every access to the catheter opens up the risk for introduction of bacteria and infection. Most research points to the only legitimate reason to irrigate or flush a catheter is to break up visible clots. It should not be at random. The other answers are all appropriate protocols to prevent CAUTI.

Question 21

Answer: C

Rationale: Dialysate is clear or pale yellow normally. Changes in color reflect an underlying problem such as reddish for bleeding, dark yellowing for perforated bladder, brownish for perforated bowel, and purulent for infection.

Question 22

Answer: C

Rationale: Flumazenil is the reversal agent for benzodiazepines like midazolam. Naloxone is the reversal agent for opioids like fentanyl. Both of these agents are typically utilized during scope procedures (colonoscopy, EGD). This also means that both of these reversal agents could be used in a situation such as this; however, during opioid overdose, the pupils typically constrict not dilate. This makes the likely culprit of the current problem midazolam. If flumazenil did not work to correct this, naloxone would be a logical second step.

Question 23

Answer: C

Rationale: If a vasoactive agent is infusing through a peripheral line, infiltration of that line leads to extravasation and infusion of this material into the third space. When this happens, the agent will cause potent vasoconstriction and decreased perfusion to the tissues. Necrosis may follow. While a central line is preferred, using peripheral lines in the short term is not contraindicated.

Question 24

Answer: A

Rationale: Tumors are a potential cause of SIADH. In this case, there is an increase in secretion of the pituitary hormone, ADH. A decrease in serum osmolality shows fluid overload. Hypoosmolality begins at <275 mOsm/kg. The other answers would be seen in DI, not SIADH.

Question 25

Answer: B

Rationale: Tachycardia and diaphoresis are early signs of hypoglycemia. This would be seen in the range 55–79 mg/dL. As hypoglycemia worsens, so do the symptoms. By the point of severe hypoglycemia, less than 40 mg/dL, symptoms will include cognitive impairment and potential coma.

Question 26

Answer: D

Rationale: Compartment syndrome is a common complication of severe burns especially if they are circumferential in the area. Early numbness followed by severe pain is indicative of compartment syndrome. Worsening compartment syndrome will also lead to loss of pulses. Hypovolemic shock would show weak and thready pulses bilateral, not unilateral as in this case. Lumbar nerve damage does not explain pulse changes. Femoral artery perforation would show signs of bleeding.

Question 27

Answer: D

Rationale: One of the functions of the liver is glycogenolysis and gluconeogenesis, the production of glucose. In liver failure, these metabolic pathways are disrupted and may lead to severe hypoglycemia. Alcohol overdose is not possible given the current BAC of 0. Withdrawal typically causes restlessness and agitation, not lethargy. Wernicke's encephalopathy (WE) cannot be ruled out given the symptoms; however, there are usually ocular abnormalities such as nystagmus present in WE.

Question 28

Answer: A

Rationale: Epinephrine is the first-line as it will stimulate the natural body response of the sympathetic nervous system (fight or flight). It will cause vasoconstriction to help offset vasodilatory effects of histamine. It will bind to smooth muscle in the lungs causing bronchodilation.

Question 29

Answer: B

Rationale: As MODS worsens the neurological condition will follow. The LOC will worsen. Motor function and sensory ability worsens. In addition to LOC changes, mental status typically shifts to confusion and delirium. Diplopia and nystagmus are not commonly seen in neurological decline in MODS. Urine output and lactate levels are not neurological issues.

Question 30

Answer: A

Rationale: The patient is hypothermic as shown by the vital signs. As hypothermia normalizes, vasodilation will occur further exacerbating any hypotension. Because this patient has received a fluid bolus, it is likely the patient will require more norepinephrine until stabilized. This is an expected need upon rewarming. Plasmalyte is a commonly used fluid in the OR (balanced crystalloid); there is no need to switch off of this fluid at this time.

Question 31

Answer: B

Rationale: The family is worried, and rightfully so. Having a family member in the hospital, especially the ICU, can be a frightening experience. The best solution is to help them through this process within our abilities. We can provide needed supplies such as a toothbrush, comb, possibly a shower. It is inappropriate to push them out of the hospital or make them leave. Reaching out to the chaplain would be more appropriate than a social worker to assist with family issues.

Question 32

Answer: C

Rationale: Regardless of what other people may say, the patient's wishes should be followed. A patient becoming unconscious or intubated and sedated does not change this fact. The nurse should advocate for the patient when they are unable to do so. The mother would be allowed to visit but not the brothers in this case.

Question 33

Answer: D

Rationale: Surgeries are typically not performed with a platelet count below 50,000. The surgeon may request a transfusion of platelets in a case such as this, but they must be notified first of the results. The surgery may be rescheduled, but this is not the job of the nurse. A platelet count less than 20,000 is associated with spontaneous bleeding.

Question 34

Answer: D

Rationale: The clinical picture of early septic shock involves vasodilation, increased cardiac output, and poor oxygen consumption. Vasodilation leads to decreased SVR. Poor oxygen consumption leads to increased SvO_2. As a reminder, a normal SvO_2 is roughly 65–75%.

Question 35

Answer: B

Rationale: With increased ventricular filling pressures and decreased ejection fraction, the heart is having difficulty pumping (ejecting) blood out of the heart due to increased afterload. Administering vasodilators will make the work of the heart easier. The other answers would worsen the current problem.

Question 36

Answer: A

Rationale: The case being described in this question is of HHS. In HHS (hot and dry), the serum osmolality will be greater than 320 mOsm/kg as the patient is dehydrated—hypovolemic. The pH is normal in HHS, so this is a point to disregard any answer that shows an abnormal pH, especially the acidotic answers that would point to DKA. Serum potassium is often elevated due to a lack of insulin production.

Question 37

Answer: D

Rationale: Myxedema coma may be triggered by infection. This dangerous decrease in thyroid hormone manifests with potential airway issues due to swelling of the neck, tongue, and throat. Intubation may be required if the airway is becoming occluded. Myxedema coma is associated with cold intolerance, not heat. Hypotension and decreasing levels of consciousness are also associated with myxedema coma.

Question 38

Answer: D

Rationale: High PEEP and airway pressures can lead to air leaks within the chest tube system. This may lead to infection such as pneumonia, empyema, and possibly pneumothorax if large enough. The other answers are correct actions by the nurse.

Question 39

Answer: C

Rationale: Because the change in blood pressure was caused by the position change, the best initial action is to reverse the potential cause. Place the patient back the way they were. If that does not correct the hypotension, norepinephrine may need to be increased temporarily. If the hypotension continues, the physician would be notified. A digital rectal exam may cause a vaso-vagal response causing the blood pressure to decrease further. This may be an appropriate intervention if autonomic dysreflexia was suspected.

Question 40

Answer: B

Rationale: The patient displays benefit to the presence of his mother. The mother wishes to spend the night. While policy and rules exist for reasons, barring any serious reason why the mother would not be allowed to stay, the nurse should arrange for the mother to spend the night as desired. Unrestricted access is proven to help emotional support of the patient.

Question 41

Answer: A

Rationale: Correct teaching follows a teach/teach-back mentality. Learned actions such as wound care may require multiple passes of education. Only after the nurse attempts repeated teaching should alternate options be considered (home health, wound care specialist). Providing alternate learning materials may be helpful while the nurse is providing teaching but it should not be the sole source of education.

Question 42

Answer: B

Rationale: Ascites when excessive enough can place pressure on the diaphragm and affect breathing and ventilation. This pressure against the large veins (vena cava) may also affect preload back to the heart thereby decreasing cardiac output and blood pressure. The other answers may occur in liver failure but do not explain hypoventilation and low cardiac output.

Question 43

Answer: D

Rationale: Regardless of the question, and there are many that could be asked, following patient wishes is the priority. In this case, the patient would like to be left alone, so the appropriate action should be to leave them alone. If a patient is upset generally, asking open-ended questions around the feelings of the situation is appropriate, but not if the patient requests to be left alone. A chaplain may be appropriate if the patient requests it.

Question 44

Answer: D

Rationale: The ABG shown in this question is reflective of metabolic acidosis. There are multiple causes of metabolic acidosis, but in the options provided the only correct answer is excessive diarrhea. The bigger picture would be any large GI loss or bicarbonate loss. Status asthmaticus leads to respiratory acidosis. Frequent antacid consumption leads to metabolic alkalosis. Hyperventilation leads to respiratory alkalosis.

Question 45

Answer: C

Rationale: Metoprolol is the beta blocker of choice due to its cardioselective properties. Propranolol is noncardioselective and is used for many noncardiac conditions. The other answers are true statements regarding initial MI treatment.

Question 46

Answer: C

Rationale: V_2 should be at the fourth intercostal space on the left side. It is directly opposite of V_1 of the sternum. V_4 is at the fifth intercostal space, midclavicular line. The other electrode positions are correct.

Question 47

Answer: A

Rationale: Certain conditions may cause a decrease in either perfusion or ventilation; clinically what is referred to as a V/Q mismatch. Ventilation is affected by the movement of air such as in pneumonia, COPD, and pulmonary edema. A pulmonary embolism affects the perfusion of blood through the alveoli.

Question 48

Answer: C

Rationale: Fine crackles are associated with pneumonia, and at times CHF or pulmonary fibrosis. Coarse crackles, sometimes called rales, are heard in ARDS and pulmonary edema. The other answers are indicative of COPD.

Question 49

Answer: B

Rationale: There are two main considerations in this question: blood loss and DIC. With a blood loss of 1 L, cardiac output would be maintained, but other signs would be present such as tachycardia and respiratory rate. In the later stages of hemorrhagic shock, increasing amounts of blood loss would lead to decreased cardiac output and hypotension. A decreased hemoglobin would be expected with blood loss. Petechiae and thrombocytopenia are expected findings with DIC.

Question 50

Answer: A

Rationale: Patients with subarachnoid hemorrhage are maintained in a hypervolemic state. This is done to keep the vessels open and prevent vasospasms. Do not confuse hypervolemia with using a hypertonic solution; it is not the same thing. Hypervolemia is achieved by administering isotonic fluids. Remember, shifting sodium levels may cause further complications neurologically.

Question 51

Answer: D

Rationale: Psychogenic polydipsia is characterized as the excessive drinking of water without need or cause. This condition is typically seen in certain psychological conditions like dementia. As dilution and hyponatremia develop, cellular tissue swells. Severe hyponatremia can eventually lead to coma and death if not properly treated.

Question 52

Answer: B

Rationale: Benzodiazepines are the first-line anxiolytics utilized in the ICU. The medications lorazepam, clonazepam, and alprazolam are fairly common, with lorazepam being the most common across the board. Stronger benzodiazepines, such as midazolam, are utilized typically in procedures to induce moderate sedation. Opioids and barbiturates are utilized as secondary anxiolytics.

Question 53

Answer: B

Rationale: At times contrast is necessary even in the face of potential further kidney damage. The healthcare team will weigh the benefits versus the risks. Regardless of whether the patient has previous kidney damage (CKD), an acute kidney injury, or healthy kidneys, it is important to "flush" the kidneys after contrast. This is achieved with oral intake of fluid and intravenous fluids. Fluids administered will be isotonic. Serum creatinine and BUN will be expected to increase. A level will be obtained to assess the level of damage, but it is not a priority over the immediate correction. Consideration will be given to discontinue nephrotoxic medications; however, this decision is made by the physician not the nurse.

Question 54

Answer: C

Rationale: The most common complication of a bowel resection with anastomosis is an anastomotic leak. This complication is even more common when the patient is obese. The symptoms are indicative of early peritonitis due to the leak. As the leak worsens, the nurse may begin to see a stiff or board-like abdomen with rising leukocytosis and potential sepsis. A retained surgical towel would explain the symptoms but is far less common than anastomotic leak.

Question 55

Answer: D

Rationale: When food is dumped into the duodenum too quickly, hyperglycemia occurs. The pancreas responds by releasing insulin. The result is a reactive hypoglycemia. The symptoms the patient is experiencing is that of hypoglycemia. Remember the timing of the movement of food. In patients with an intact stomach, food chyme is passed into the duodenum slowly after 45 minutes to an hour. A gastrectomy patient would experience early versus late dumping syndrome. Early dumping syndrome (15–30 min) may lead to hypovolemia and hypotension. Late dumping syndrome may lead to hypoglycemia.

Question 56

Answer: B

Rationale: The most common DVT prophylaxis medications utilized in the ICU are low molecular weight heparin, unfractionated heparin, and fondaparinux. Other agents like aspirin or clopidogrel are typically used for outpatient reduction of clot risk. A heparin infusion would be used as treatment not prophylaxis; a similar mentality to the use of warfarin. Compression devices are preventive; however, a high-risk patient would require more than just this intervention.

Question 57

Answer: A

Rationale: Thrombocytopenia below 50,000/mm^3 increases the risk of bleeding. The word "mild" bleeding may also be used, whereas a platelet level below 20,000/mm^3 is associated with spontaneous bleeding such as intracranial hemorrhage.

Question 58

Answer: B

Rationale: There are two fairly reasonable answers to this question; however, the broadest explanation is the lungs "ability" expansion, elasticity, or ability to expand. The lung response to diaphragmatic movement also is in line with lung compliance, but there are more factors into compliance than simply the movement of the diaphragm. A ventilated patient, for example, may not be using much effort through the diaphragm since the machine is providing pressure, but the lung may still not be compliant.

Question 59

Answer: C

Rationale: Asthma is a reversible condition with the treatment of bronchodilators and steroids, whereas COPD is a chronic condition. Oxygen may assist both asthma and COPD patients; however, caution must be used in the oxygen use of a COPD patient. But that does not mean it is not helpful and should be wholly avoided. Sputum production is more common in COPD patients than asthma patients.

Question 60

Answer: D

Rationale: Inotropic therapy would help prevent an AKI, not cause it. A reduction of perfusion (prerenal AKI) is a potential risk. NSAID use, such as naproxen, is a risk. Nephrotoxic medications, such as vancomycin, are a risk.

Question 61

Answer: C

Rationale: Hypovolemia is a primary risk during and after dialysis due to the removal of fluid. Dysrhythmias are a risk, but the intention of the hemodialysis was to correct the hyperkalemia thereby fixing the underlying problem of the dysrhythmias. The patient will remain on telemetry for close monitoring, but the primary risk associated with the dialysis treatment is hypovolemia.

Question 62

Answer: B

Rationale: The best action in these situations is to assess patient feelings. Let the patient express how they feel with open-ended questions. Sit quietly and listen. If the patient requests family presence, the nurse would help facilitate that. At this time, there are no symptoms of anxiety or agitation, so an anxiolytic is not appropriate.

Question 63

Answer: D

Rationale: A pulmonary shunt exists when blood passes through the alveoli but does not participate in gas exchange. This may be due to pneumonia, ARDS, pulmonary edema, among many other conditions. Pulmonary embolism affects the perfusion, not the ventilation. Also do not confuse the difference between a cardiac and a pulmonary shunt. They occur in different locations (organs).

Question 64

Answer: A

Rationale: Myasthenia gravis crisis may be triggered by viral infections. It is crucial to rule out any diaphragmatic weakness that may be indicative of this crisis. Plethysmograph, or a pulse oximeter, will show oxygenation at the level of the hemoglobin. This would be a later sign of the crisis. The better solution is to analyze the source of the problem and catch it before it becomes an issue with oxygenation.

Question 65

Answer: D

Rationale: The clinical opioid withdrawal scale (COWS) will assess for additional symptoms of opioid withdrawal. The patient's vital signs in addition to agitation, yawning, and rhinorrhea indicate potential opioid withdrawal. Administering opioids may diminish these symptoms, but assessing the problem first is important. CIWA protocol is for alcohol withdrawal. Antihypertensives will not address the underlying problem.

Question 66

Answer: B

Rationale: Papillary muscle rupture with resulting mitral regurgitation is a potential risk with inferior wall MIs. Tricuspid regurgitation may lead to elevated CVP. Dressler's syndrome or post-MI pericarditis and cardiogenic shock do not cause a large V wave.

Question 67

Answer: C

Rationale: Q waves are seen hours to days after the initial infarct. It is due to scar tissue unable to conduct electrical signals. Peaked T waves occur at the onset of injury. ST elevations occur minutes to hours after the insult. T-wave inversions occur hours after the initial MI.

Question 68

Answer: A

Rationale: An inferior wall MI displays changes in leads II, III, and aVF.

Question 69

Answer: B

Rationale: Hallucinations with delusions are a hallmark of schizophrenia. In this case, it sounds like it may be paranoid in nature given the belief the surgery performed was by aliens. Somatic symptom disorder is that which cannot be explained by a medical condition, but the patient has symptoms regardless. Manic and major depression are not in line with the symptoms in this question.

Question 70

Answer: C

Rationale: Turning off the alarms completely is dangerous and inappropriate. Alarm parameters can at times be modified to reflect patient specifics, such as decreasing the pulse ox range on a COPD patient; however, this should be done very carefully and with purpose. The other answers are correct actions to encourage substantive sleep.

Question 71

Answer: D

Rationale: Moral agency implies the ability for nurses to act as a moral representative for patients and family. This may include acting as the intersection between patient, family, and the healthcare team.

Question 72

Answer: B

Rationale: An advance directive, DNR, or living will is completed by a patient; their wishes have been explicitly explained to the healthcare team. These wishes should be followed regardless of family desire, healthcare belief, or nursing interpretation.

Question 73

Answer: C

Rationale: Treatment of acetaminophen overdose includes the administration of acetylcysteine. Liver enzymes would be primarily monitored, not pancreatic enzymes (amylase, lipase). Gastric lavage is only effective if performed within a 45 min to 1 hr window. A fecal occult is not appropriate in this situation.

Question 74

Answer: A

Rationale: Questions with large amounts of vitals, labs, or hemodynamic parameters can oftentimes be confusing, but stick to what you know. Oliguria is a known issue in all types of shock. If the kidneys are being perfused and urine output remains strong, it is understood that the current treatment is working. In this case, the best answer will be the outcome with the most improvement.

Question 75

Answer: C

Rationale: Colloids such as albumin will maintain the oncotic pressure within the intravascular space thereby decreasing the risk of unwanted third-spacing of fluid. The Parkland formula is still a widely used tool for initial crystalloid treatment; however, colloids such as albumin are often used to maintain the fluid in the intravascular space. Protein is a needed nutrient in wound healing, but it is not the reason for the use of IV albumin in the early stages of burns. It is true that albumin bottles do not contain potassium or electrolytes, but this is not the reason for their use.

Question 76

Answer: D

Rationale: Spinal cord injury may damage the innervation of alpha and beta dependent nerves. Alpha affecting vascular tone, and beta affecting heart rate and contractility. The resulting decrease in both leads to a distributive shock. The brain stem is not the cause of the pathophysiological changes in neurogenic shock; in this case, the cause was stated as a SCI.

Question 77

Answer: B

Rationale: There is no reason tube feedings cannot be initiated on this patient as long as the GI surgeon has signed off. The starting point is generally considered to be when the patient has flatulence, passed stool, or has audible bowel sounds. A low-fat intake will be necessary for this patient while in the hospital and after discharge. Without an adequate supply of bile in the gallbladder, digestion of fatty acids is difficult. TPN is not indicated unless the patient cannot tolerate enteral feedings.

Question 78

Answer: B

Rationale: The primary goal is to not exacerbate the dehiscence further. Placing the patient in a slightly flexed position will decrease abdominal pressure. This is typically done supine with a slightly elevated head. The wound would be held with gentle pressure until the surgeon arrives to assess. Remember to avoid other pressure inducing actions such as coughing or sneezing.

Question 79

Answer: B

Rationale: Hydrocortisone creams and aloe vera may help reduce the pain associated with the burn. Harsh chemicals, however, should be avoided such as hydrogen peroxide, chlorhexidine, or alcohol. Oftentimes warm water and soap is best. First degree burns (sunburns) are generally left open to air since the epidermis is intact and infection risk is low.

Question 80

Answer: A

Rationale: A cardiac chair position is a safe first step for this patient. Many hospital beds are able to achieve this position. This allows progressive mobility without removing the patient from the bed. Progressive mobility, especially after such a long ICU stay, requires slow changes and consistent assessments of tolerance. Oftentimes patient wishes in this sense will not align with their physical ability.

Question 81

Answer: C

Rationale: All of the answers aid in the reduction of pressure ulcers, but the best method is to stick to a schedule for turning—minimum every 2 hours.

Question 82

Answer: C

Rationale: This case is describing a basilar skull fracture after a traumatic fall. If there is a break in the integrity of the meninges and the central nervous system, the risk of infection is high. This may lead to meningitis among other intracranial infections. A subarachnoid hemorrhage is not associated with cerebrospinal fluid drainage from the nose. A nasopharynx laceration would result in a bloody drainage, not clear. Increased ICP would result in changes to the GCS score among other symptoms.

Question 83

Answer: A

Rationale: Reperfusion is not necessary unless the symptoms worsen or the myocardial infarction develops ST elevation. At this time, the patient is diagnosed with an NSTEMI. Treatment follows similar pharmacological indications for STEMI, such as aspirin, beta blockers, and nitroglycerin. The patient would be admitted for observation and the cardiac markers monitored for trending downward. Oxygen may be applied if appropriate.

Question 84

Answer: D

Rationale: An EVD can be a foreign device to many ICU nurses if not exposed to severe neurological cases. There is a picture in the book to help familiarize yourself if need be. The catheter of an EVD is never flushed. It is a one-way flow—outward, if the EVD is open. In this case the order states to leave the EVD clamped unless assessing ICP. Flushing an EVD can increase ICP. The other actions are appropriate actions. Of note: Make absolutely sure the EVD is clamped when transporting.

Question 85

Answer: C

Rationale: This person is exhibiting severe acidosis with hypercapnia. A certain degree of acidosis is expected in a COPD patient; however, the acidosis combined with the severely elevated carbon dioxide requires intervention. The patient is also lethargic and weak; this will affect the respiratory drive. The best action at this time is to improve ventilation via a BiPAP machine. A PaO_2 greater than 60% is considered normal for a COPD patient. Remember oxygen toxicity in COPD patients decreases the respiratory drive further.

Question 86

Answer: B

Rationale: Weaning parameters or a successful trial is indicated by satisfactory vital signs (no tachycardia, no severe tachypnea, adequate oxygenation). In the best-case scenario, the patient should be calm and able to follow commands. Minute ventilation is best less than 10 l per minute; higher may indicate dyspnea and underlying pathophysiology (hypercapnia). The patient should be able to draw adequate tidal volumes, >5 mL/kg, typically 300 mL or higher per breath. A negative inspiratory force (NIF) around –25 to –30 cm H_2O is ideal. A PaO_2/FiO_2 ratio >200 is best.

Question 87

Answer: B

Rationale: It is not uncommon for patients to have abnormal feelings around devices that change their body appearance. These issues should be addressed with the patient if they ask questions or wish to speak about the psychological issues around this device. The stoma care does need to be performed and cannot be ignored, so the best action would be to gently, compassionately, provide the care while engaging the patient. The nurse is not aware of whether the colostomy is permanent or temporary; providing false hope is not appropriate.

Question 88

Answer: A

Rationale: The family should be contacted by the nurse themselves, not a unit secretary or chaplain. This is a delicate situation and the family needs to be present if possible. Organ procurement services will be called, but this is not the priority at this time.

Question 89

Answer: D

Rationale: Nursing vigilance is the anticipation of hazards of care and addressing them. In this case, the nurse anticipated heparin-induced thrombocytopenia and a potential complication due to the ordered heparin infusion. This is the right call and a very good catch by the nurse.

Question 90

Answer: C

Rationale: Patients with PTSD often experience hypervigilance or increased alertness to their surroundings. Approaching a PTSD patient without them having prior knowledge is dangerous. They can snap and potentially harm the nurse; granted they are likely unaware of what they are doing, but it is risky nonetheless. The other answers are appropriate actions for a PTSD patient.

Question 91

Answer: C

Rationale: The symptoms presented are in line with hypermagnesemia; a likely compilation given the current treatment for preeclampsia. Calcium is an antagonist to magnesium, so calcium gluconate or calcium chloride may be administered to correct the hypermagnesemia. NIV is not needed at this time; however, a small amount of oxygen via nasal cannula may be required. Dialysis will help filter out magnesium, but it will take too long to execute. Regular insulin with D50 is the intervention for severe hyperkalemia.

Question 92

Answer: A

Rationale: During dialysis, a fluid shift may occur in the brain causing cerebral edema and the associated symptoms (headache, nausea, restlessness, seizures). This results from removal of urea from the blood but not the brain. Treatment may include reducing the risk of intracranial pressure.

Question 93

Answer: A

Rationale: Valproic acid is a type of anticonvulsant that is also prescribed for patients with bipolar disorder. The medication helps regulate their mood. Paroxetine is an SSRI. Rivastigmine is a medication often used in dementia. Risperidone is an antipsychotic; it is sometimes used in bipolar disorder, but it is not an anticonvulsant.

Question 94

Answer: B

Rationale: Hypercalcemic crisis is a medical emergency that requires prompt treatment. If the patient has functioning kidneys and diuresis is possible, diuretic therapy is a first-line mainstay. If diuresis is not possible, hemodialysis is the next step. IV fluids will be included in any therapy but will not alone correct the calcium imbalance. Steroid therapy may lower serum calcium by inhibiting absorption, but this treatment is slow and reserved for very rare cases.

Question 95

Answer: B

Rationale: When high levels of PEEP and tidal volume are used, a potential complication is spontaneous pneumothorax. Alveolar rupture may also occur leading to increased bloody sputum and secretions. Sudden changes in oxygenation should lead the nurse to believe this has occurred. Immediate placement of a chest tube is required to equalize the pressure in the pleural cavity.

Question 96

Answer: D

Rationale: Dantrolene is a muscle relaxant commonly given in cases of malignant hyperthermia such as this. Fever and muscle rigidity are hallmark symptoms of malignant hyperthermia after administration of anesthesia. This is a medical emergency and administration of dantrolene should not be delayed.

Question 97

Answer: A

Rationale: During treatment of hypertensive crisis or emergency, too rapid a reduction in blood pressure may lead to symptoms of shock. Consider each patient body as unique; this patient is likely used to an elevated blood pressure where

120/80 mmHg is abnormal. Reduction of MAP should not be more than 25% in the first hour.

Question 98

Answer: C

Rationale: The topic is cardiac output; however, the question is asking about decreased cardiac output. Sepsis and fever increase the cardiac output. The other answers are all factors that may decrease the cardiac output.

Question 99

Answer: C

Rationale: If treatment has been effective, pulmonary artery pressure will be normalized. Normal pulmonary artery systolic pressure ranges between 18 and 25 mmHg. While the pulmonary hypertension would be corrected, the hemodynamic parameters would continue to show right-sided heart failure with an elevated CVP. Pulmonary artery occlusion (wedge) pressure is not affected by pulmonary hypertension or right-sided heart failure; this parameter would be normal. PAOP is also part of diagnosis for pulmonary hypertension; the PA pressures would be high, but the PAOP normal.

Question 100

Answer: A

Rationale: A normal range for an ankle–brachial index is 1.00–1.40. A decreased index is indicative of PAD. An elevated index is indicative of a noncompressible artery as may be seen in diabetes mellitus.

Question 101

Answer: B

Rationale: A dementia patient likely cannot self-report pain in a meaningful manner for assessment. It is best to monitor behavior, body language, breathing, and vocalization (moaning). A FLACC scale is used in children. A RASS scale is utilized for sedation, not pain management.

Question 102

Answer: B

Rationale: When genitourinary trauma is suspected, the general rule of thumb is one attempt and done. If an indwelling catheter cannot be placed, urethral trauma should be suspected and further attempts to place a catheter stopped. The physician or urologist may place a catheter themselves. Hematuria is the most common symptom of GU trauma; in this case urethral damage is suspected, not kidney damage (at this point). Costovertebral tenderness or flank pain is indicative of kidney trauma.

Question 103

Answer: D

Rationale: The framework of the Synergy Model is aligned when patient needs match nursing competency. This case is incredibly complicated and will require a high level of competency. For the Synergy framework to be realized, consideration should be placed on who can safety take care of this patient.

Question 104

Answer: D

Rationale: This case describes an open (compound) fracture of the tibia after the fall. Antibiotics should be immediately given to reduce the risk of osteomyelitis. The extremity should also be immobilized (priority) until surgically corrected. Pain management is a secondary priority. A V/Q scan may be warranted if symptoms of a fat embolism develop. Compressing the wound is contraindicated unless actively bleeding. This could otherwise cause further damage.

Question 105

Answer: C

Rationale: A tertiary intention of wound healing implies the wound was cleaned out (debridement, etc.) and purposefully left open until the inflammation subsides. At a later date, closure of the wound may be decided if it is clean, the tissue is adequately perfused, and inflammation has subsided. Sutures or staples that close a wound is healing by primary intent. Utilization of a wound vac to stimulate granulation tissue implies healing by a secondary intent. Wet-to-moist dressings that encourage mechanical debridement are also healing by secondary intent.

Question 106

Answer: A

Rationale: Decision-making capacity is assessed by a multitude of factors: comprehension, communication, expressing one's preference, and being informed, among many others. A patient, either vocalizing or by body language, simply agreeing with everything the physicians state at the bedside likely does not understand the implications for all of these medical decisions. Use of substances does not automatically remove patients' right to self-determination. If patients are under the influence of substances, however, they are not eligible to leave AMA. Mental capacity does not necessarily dictate decisional capacity as long as the deficit is not severe.

Question 107

Answer: B

Rationale: The most common appropriate reaction when something occurs that the nurse does not feel right about is to address it at that exact moment. This may be with a person, an IV pump, pretty much anything. Procrastination is not a virtue in a hospital setting. The physician is on the unit right now. The problem should be addressed right now.

Question 108

Answer: C

Rationale: Sensory overload should be minimized to encourage adequate sleep, not maximized or increased. The other answers will all help in reducing confusion and delirium in the ICU patient.

Question 109

Answer: A

Rationale: The vestibulocochlear nerve (VIII) is responsible for sound and equilibrium within the ear. Higher function of this cranial nerve may be tested by a Doll's eyes test or cold caloric test.

Question 110

Answer: D

Rationale: LBOs are associated with low-pitched bowel sounds, whereas SBIs associate with high-pitched bowel sounds. Both obstructions may result in abdominal distention and pain. Both result in dilated bowel loops, especially proximal to the obstruction. Hypokalemia is more common in bowel obstructions than hyperkalemia. Absent bowel sounds are more common in paralytic ileus.

Question 111

Answer: D

Rationale: The patient in this case is exhibiting signs of Cushing's triad in addition to level of consciousness changes; new onset lethargy. The blood pressure of 108/70 mmHg indicates an improvement in this patient given the new onset hypertension during the acute episode of increased ICP. A normalization of the Cushing's response indicates improvement. The heart rate remains bradycardic. The patient remains tachypneic. Pulse ox is not a parameter for a Cushing's response.

Question 112

Answer: A

Rationale: Pericarditis may result in ST elevations on an ECG and elevated cardiac markers, which is why it is important to rule out a myocardial infarction in these cases. A common hallmark of pericarditis is a pericardial friction rub. This is heard continuously regardless of breathing. Muffled heart tones and narrowed pulse pressure indicate cardiac tamponade. This is a potential complication of pericarditis, but not symptoms of the diagnosis itself. JVD and dependent edema indicate right-sided heart failure.

Question 113

Answer: B

Rationale: Angina pain is typically described as a substernal, squeezing (pressure), brutal type of pain that may or may not radiate to the arms, jaw, or neck.

Question 114

Answer: C

Rationale: When in doubt, choose the more obvious answer. Metabolic acidosis is far more common than metabolic alkalosis, the same way that respiratory acidosis is far more common than respiratory alkalosis. Metabolic acidosis, in this case, is caused by loss of bicarbonate in the pancreatic juices.

Question 115

Answer: C

Rationale: The patient is experiencing an episode of hypoxia. The easiest and most immediate intervention to perform is to change the patient position. If this does not rectify the matter, oxygen may be increased and titrated to effect. Suctioning may also be warranted at this time if crackles and auscultated or can be audibly heard. A hypoglycemic event is unlikely given the onset and nature of the symptoms, but it is not impossible. A fingerstick may be warranted after immediate stabilization.

Question 116

Answer: B

Rationale: The two main features on an ABG result in a patient with carbon monoxide poisoning include metabolic acidosis due to lactic acidosis (tissue ischemia) and a normal PaO_2 since hemoglobin is not adequately delivering oxygen to tissues.

Question 117

Answer: C

Rationale: A supine position is not necessary for flail chest. The head of the bed is elevated to encourage ventilation and appropriate oxygenation. Chest tube insertion, intuition with mechanical ventilation, and adequate pain management are all appropriate measures for management of flail chest with pneumothorax.

Question 118

Answer: B

Rationale: A mixed venous oxygen saturation, or SvO_2, is the gauge of how much oxygen is left in the blood as it returns to the lungs. This displays both delivery (DO_2) and consumption (VO_2). The mixed venous oxygen saturation will decrease when either delivery of oxygen decreases or consumption increases.

Question 119

Answer: B

Rationale: The patient is hypernatremic at 155 mEq/L. The crystalloid of choice in this matter would be hypotonic to sodium. The patient is not hypoglycemia, so dextrose is not needed. If the patient was hypernatremic and hypoglycemic, this would be an appropriate option.

Question 120

Answer: A

Rationale: The primary concern is a loss of airway due to angioedema (orbital and tongue swelling). This complication can be life-threatening if the airway is occluded. Immediate intubation would be indicated when this occurs. Many physicians choose to intubate before stridor may be present in anticipation of the complication and emergency.

Question 121

Answer: D

Rationale: The patient is exhibiting signs and symptoms of transfusion associated circulatory overload, or TACO for short. Correction of this fluid overload will be achieved by diuresis with furosemide. Oxygen supplementation may be required; however, this question does not state a current pulse ox. It is a bit of a leap to jump immediately to intubation. A fluid bolus will exacerbate the problem of fluid overload and diphenhydramine does not address the underlying problem.

Question 122

Answer: B

Rationale: An asthma exacerbation is due to rampant airway inflammation. As the occlusion worsens, the patient experiences increased shortness of breath and wheezing. Spirometry results will display a drastic reduction in peak expiratory flow (<40%), an absolute peak flow <100 L/min, and decreased forced expiratory volume (FEV_1 < 2L). The 80% function of forced vital capacity is adequate.

Question 123

Answer: C

Rationale: Decreased cardiac contractility is one of the causes of cardiogenic shock resulting in decreased cardiac output and cardiac index. Most shocks result in a reflex tachycardia as the body attempts to compensate for the decrease in tissue perfusion. Elevated left ventricular filling pressures also worsen the cardiogenic shock at times necessitating balloon pump therapy to reduce SVR.

Question 124

Answer: B

Rationale: Total cholesterol should be less than 200 mg/dL. LDL should be less than 150 mg/dL. HDL, the good cholesterol, is ideally greater than 40–60 mg/dL.

Question 125

Answer: C

Rationale: Acidosis causes a shift to the right in the curve, increasing the release of oxygen to tissues. Hypothermia, decreased 2.3-DPG, and massive transfusions of blood shift the curve to the left.

Practice Test 4

This is the fourth and final practice exam included in this book. The test contains 125 questions, the same as the CCRN exam. Questions are modeled after the blueprint in type and amount. A passing grade on the CCRN exam is 87 questions out of 125 questions. This is your benchmark for success.

1. A 22-year-old patient is being admitted to the ICU with a diagnosis of DKA. The ED report states she came in feeling nauseated but has been taking her insulin. Her roommate stated she has been ill the past few days with flu-like symptoms. The ED began a normal saline infusion post bolus, an insulin drip post bolus, and a 20 mEq KCL tablet. Which of the following would not be included in the plan of care at this time?

   A. Administer ondansetron PRN

   B. Assess an arterial blood gas with lactate

   C. Obtain a baseline serum glucose level

   D. Begin an ADA diet

2. A 50-year-old patient has been in the medical ICU for the past 3 days due to a severe pneumonia infection. He was initially on BiPAP and hydration IV therapy with antibiotics. Two days later he began showing symptoms of septic shock and deteriorating respiratory status. He was intubated and the need for pressors arose. Earlier this morning during assessment, the nurse noticed petechial spots over the torso. Which of the following complications and lab values may be expected in this patient?

   A. HIT: Platelet 40,000

   B. ITP: Platelet 75,000

   C. DIC: FSP 20 mcg/mL

   D. DIC: FSP 5 mcg/mL

3. A 48-year-old male patient has recently been admitted due to an episode of hematemesis at home and unstable vital signs. Upon admission, the patient is confused and agitated. An EGD is ordered to occur the following day. Two hours after admission the telemetry alarm is triggered. The monitor shows a low pulse ox at 90% and worsening rapid ventricular rate. Upon walking into the room, the patient is vomiting bright red blood. The following interventions would be appropriate for this patient EXCEPT for which answer?

   A. Oral suction with Yankauer

   B. Transfusion of platelets and FFP

   C. Perform endoscopy ASAP

   D. Administration of vasopressin

4. A 56-year-old Asian American female patient recently arrived at the emergency department complaining of pain in the right lower leg that has progressively been getting worse over the last couple days. She mentions recent travel to South America with hiking and a fall. Upon assessment of the leg, the nurse identifies a red blistering wound that is warm to the touch. Hours after admission the patient is moaning, stating the pain is now unbearable. Assessment of the wound shows it has increased in size. Which of the following conditions is consistent with the findings?

   A. Compartment syndrome

   B. Necrotizing fasciitis

   C. Cellulitis advancing to sepsis

   D. Osteomyelitis

5. Prescription drug abuse is a rapidly growing drug problem in the United States, much of which is associated with inappropriate/overprescription. Because of this, it is important for critical care nurses to be aware of any substance abuse issues separate from the admitting diagnosis. What signs and symptoms might the nurse expect in a patient withdrawing from prescription pain medication such as oxycodone?

   A. Yawning, piloerection, nausea

   B. Hypotension, pupillary constriction, tachycardia

   C. Hypertension, tachycardia, chest pain

   D. Respiratory depression, peripheral cyanosis

6. A patient with an upper GI bleed is admitted to the ICU for close monitoring with an expected emergency EGD by the gastroenterologist. Suspecting blood loss is greater than 1 L at this time. Upon admission the nurse draws blood, stool, and urine for a series of labs. Which of the following laboratory results would warrant an immediate phone call to the physician?

   A. Positive occult stool test
   B. Hemoglobin 8.6 g/dL
   C. Platelets 80,000
   D. aPTT 120 seconds

7. While reviewing the case of a patient with a creatinine of 3.5 mg/dL and a BUN of 32 mg/dL, the nurse notes factors that may be contributing to these laboratory abnormalities. Which of the following is not a likely contributing factor for this azotemia?

   A. Indomethacin toxicity
   B. Recent angiography
   C. Hepatitis A infection
   D. Excessive furosemide doses

8. An 80 kg patient in the ICU is in the refractory phase of shock after multiple injuries leading to internal bleeding. What clinical findings may the nurse witness at this moment?

   A. Normotensive and tachycardia
   B. Blood pressure improves with fluids
   C. Elevated troponin and alveolar edema
   D. BP 100/75 mmHg, urine output 80 mL over 2 hours

9. A 65-year-old male patient with a history of hypertension and hyperlipidemia presents to the emergency department with chest pain radiating to his left arm, diaphoresis, and dyspnea. The ECG reveals ST elevation in leads V5, V6, and I. What area of myocardial infarction is consistent with these findings?

   A. Anterior left ventricle
   B. Inferior left ventricle
   C. Lateral left ventricle
   D. Right ventricle

GO ON TO NEXT PAGE ➤

10. Physical barriers such as skin are part of innate immunity. The primary goal being to prevent the spread of pathogens immediately at the entry point. Which of the following is not an example of this innate immunity?

    A. Cilia in the respiratory tract

    B. Acidity of the stomach

    C. Mast cells in mucus

    D. Antibody development

11. Two hours after the admission of a patient with a hemorrhagic stroke of the frontal lobe, the patient begins to exhibit signs of increased intracranial pressure (ICP). Out of the following interventions, which of the following would the nurse do first?

    A. Elevate the head of the bed to 30 degrees

    B. Immediately perform a CT scan of the head

    C. Prepare for placement of Burr holes

    D. Administer antiepileptic medications

12. A 55-year-old patient is being prepared for a coronary bypass graft surgery. The patient will need cardiopulmonary bypass for the procedure. Which of the following is not a physiological change seen postoperative with the use of bypass?

    A. Decreased capillary permeability with third-spacing of fluid

    B. Changes in platelet count and clot formation

    C. Hyperthermia and activated inflammatory response

    D. Neurological and psychological disturbances

13. Four days after a left-sided stroke, an NG tube is removed so the patient may begin oral feedings. During the feeding of a dysphagia diet 1 day later, the nurse believes the patient may have aspirated. What assessment finding is most likely to be seen in this patient?

    A. Infiltrates over the left lung

    B. Crackles heard over the right lung

    C. Acute respiratory distress

    D. Bradycardia with hypertension

14. Which of the following ABGs would the nurse expect to see in a patient with diabetic ketoacidosis?

    A. pH 7.18, $PaCO_2$ 18, HCO_3 9.0 mmol/L, anion gap 16

    B. pH 7.30, $PaCO_2$ 33, HCO_3 22 mmol/L, anion gap 14

    C. pH 7.30, $PaCO_2$ 50, HCO_3 18 mmol/L, anion gap 10

    D. pH 7.10, $PaCO_2$ 50, HCO_3 30 mmol/L, anion gap 16

15. Thirty minutes after a patient with esophageal varices has stabilized, another episode of hematemesis occurs with bright red blood. The physicians decide to place a Sengstaken–Blakemore tube to temporize the situation. Three hours later the patient develops dyspnea; the monitor shows a pulse ox of 88%. Which of the following interventions is indicated at this time?

    A. Cut the tube with scissors at the bedside
    B. Prepare for emergency endoscopy with clipping
    C. Pull the tube back slightly to improve positioning
    D. Increase the oxygen through the nasal cannula

16. Which of the following statements regarding liver cirrhosis and portal hypertension is true?

    A. Alcohol abuse is the most common culprit for acute liver failure
    B. Portal hypertension causes collateral blood flow and an increase in ICP
    C. Jaundice commonly seen in the sclera of the eye is due to an increase in liver enzymes
    D. Spontaneous bacterial peritonitis is a risk for patients with ascites

17. Hours after the TIPS procedure is completed, the nurse returns to the room to find the patient difficult to arouse by noxious stimuli. Suspecting worsening encephalopathy, an ammonia level is drawn. Which of the following interventions would the nurse include at this time?

    A. Administer octreotide, place an NG tube and attach to suction
    B. Monitor sodium level, administer hypertonic solution if necessary
    C. Administer lactulose, monitor and prevent hypokalemia
    D. Suspect potential stent thrombosis, call the MD

18. A 45-year-old patient was admitted to the ICU for acute appendicitis. Recent assessment shows a dangerous change to vital signs. A pulmonary artery catheter was inserted for close monitoring. Given the information below, which of the following interventions would the nurse perform?

VITAL SIGNS	HEMODYNAMIC PARAMETERS
BP = 85/50 mmHg	PAP 20/8 mmHg
HR = 135 / min	PAOP 4 mmHg
RR = 26 / min	CVP 2 mmHg
SpO_2 = 94% on 2L NC	CO 7.5 L/min
Temp = 35°C	SVR 650 dynes/sec/cm^{-5}

    A. Fluid resuscitation, vasopressors, antibiotics
    B. Fluid resuscitation, dobutamine, sildenafil
    C. Fluid resuscitation, nitroglycerin IV, acetaminophen
    D. Fluid resuscitation, beta blockers, milrinone

19. A patient post thrombectomy is receiving a continuous heparin drip. A recent coagulation panel reveals an INR of 2.0 and an aPTT of 200 seconds. The patient is not exhibiting signs of bleeding at this time. Which of the following is indicated at this time?

    A. Maintain the heparin drip, continue to monitor for bleeding

    B. Decrease the heparin drip, draw a repeat aPTT in 12 hours

    C. Stop the heparin drip, contact the physician

    D. Administer protamine sulfate, continue to monitor for bleeding

20. The nurse is concerned about a patient admitted with Guillain–Barre syndrome. The patient is currently reporting numbness and bilateral paresis of the lower extremities up to the thighs. Which clinical changes are most important for the nurse to monitor in this patient?

    A. Paresis affecting the lower torso and back

    B. Decreases in vital capacity and tidal volume

    C. Changes in sensation and function of the upper extremities

    D. Increases in SpO_2 readings

21. A patient in the ICU has been intubated for over 7 days with a severe upper respiratory illness. The healthcare team believes the patient is ready for potential extubation. Once the patient is awake and following commands, which of the following changes to the ventilator and patient assessments reflect readiness for extubation?

    A. CPAP mode, RR 16/min, negative inspiratory force of >−25 cm H_2O

    B. CPAP mode, HR 110/min, vital capacity 1L

    C. SIMV mode, HR 80/min, FiO_2 60%

    D. AC mode, HR 60/min, FiO_2 40%

22. After the initiation of hemodialysis on a critically ill patient, the blood pressure decreases to 85/60 mmHg. The dialysis nurse immediately stops the treatment and returns the blood to the patient. The healthcare team decides the patient may require continuous venovenous hemofiltration (CVVH) therapy. What will be the primary goal of this treatment?

    A. Correct electrolyte imbalances

    B. Remove waste products

    C. Provide incremental fluid corrections

    D. Increase the blood pressure

23. A patient in the emergency department presents with a potential methamphetamine toxicity. Which of the following signs and symptoms would the nurse expect in this patient?

    A. Hypothermia, bradycardia, lethargy
    B. Hyperthermia, seizure activity, tachycardia
    C. Hyperthermia, hypotension, muscle pain
    D. Hypothermia, kidney failure, constricted pupils

24. Immediately upon arrival, the nurse calls a Code FAST (neuro) on a patient with suspected stroke. The patient is unable to answer questions at this time, but a family member is nearby who found the patient at home. Which of the following assessments is a priority?

    A. Pacemaker or cerebral clips
    B. DNR, advance directives
    C. History of anticoagulant use
    D. Onset of symptoms

25. A patient in ARDS is experiencing a V/Q mismatch due to the severity of the illness. When would the nurse suspect the patient has now developed a shunting of blood?

    A. A-A gradient 8 mmHg, PaO_2 90 on 40% oxygen
    B. A-A gradient 12 mmHg, P/F ratio < 200
    C. A-A gradient 6 mmHg, P/F ratio > 300
    D. A-A gradient 15 mmHg, PaO_2 65 on room air

26. The nurse is caring for a patient who immigrated to the United States from an Asian country. The patient has a diagnosis that is commonly associated with increased pain. What is best for the nurse to understand regarding this situation?

    A. This patient may become silent when in pain
    B. This patient may become angry and request to leave when in pain
    C. This patient may request pain medication when in pain
    D. This patient may experience more pain than a non-Asian patient

27. Which of the following correctly states the pathophysiology of an asthma exacerbation?

    A. Decreased vital capacity secondary to diaphragmatic dysfunction
    B. Decreased static compliance secondary to airway inflammation
    C. Decreased dynamic compliance secondary to bronchospasms
    D. Decreased peak flow secondary to inhibition of surfactant release

28. A 65-year-old male patient was admitted to the ICU with an anterior wall myocardial infarction. After admission, the nurse is assessing the patient and finds a loud murmur over the left ventricle. Which of the following complications is likely in this patient?

    A. Papillary muscle rupture
    B. Atrial septal defect
    C. Mitral valve regurgitation
    D. Ventricular septal defect

29. The nurse in a busy ICU is coordinating a CT scan on a complicated patient. Using systems thinking, the nurse would approach this difficult situation with what in mind?

    A. Speak with the physician about the need for the CT scan
    B. Consult with needed specialties to execute the CT order
    C. Refer the patient to radiology for management of the CT scan
    D. Use the situation as a learning opportunity to train a new nurse

30. A patient has received multiple doses of contrast for a series of CT scans. The patient will likely develop acute tubular necrosis (ATN) and which of the following changes?

    A. Azotemia, hypocalcemia
    B. Alkalosis, azotemia
    C. Acidosis, azotemia
    D. Oliguria, anemia

31. A patient with peripheral arterial disease (PAD) is not a candidate for surgical bypass. Which less invasive intervention may be indicated for this patient?

    A. Angiography
    B. Balloon angioplasty
    C. Endovenous laser ablation
    D. Doppler duplex scan

32. 15 minutes after the initiation of nitroprusside for hypertensive crisis, the most important assessment for the nurse is what?

    A. Thiocyanate levels
    B. Measurement of MAP
    C. Assessment of headache and mental status
    D. Capillary refill and paresthesias

33. A 75-year-old male patient presents with chest pain. ECG reveals ST elevation in leads II, II, and aVF. What area of myocardial infarction is consistent with these findings?

   A. Anterior left ventricle
   B. Inferior left ventricle
   C. Lateral left ventricle
   D. Right ventricle

34. After heart transplantation, a patient developed life-threatening bradycardia. They were immediately placed on transcutaneous pacing at the time. The current healthcare team goal is to wean the patient off the pacemaker and treat the bradycardia with medication. Which of the following agents would the nurse suspect to be ordered?

   A. Isoproterenol
   B. Atropine
   C. Epinephrine
   D. Dopamine

35. A patient in alcohol withdrawal develops seizure activity 4 hours after admission. Which of the following best describes a tonic-clonic seizure this patient may exhibit?

   A. Brief loss of consciousness followed by a period of lethargy
   B. Stiffening of muscles followed by rhythmic jerking of muscles
   C. Sporadic muscle jerking isolated to certain extremities
   D. Violent shaking of the body followed by paralysis

36. Six days after admission, an elderly patient begins to experience periods of delirium and agitation. Which of the following interventions will the nurse enact to encourage proper mentation?

   A. Contact the physician for a haloperidol order
   B. Keeping the room dark throughout the day, avoid noise
   C. Restrict family and healthcare staff to the room
   D. Reorientation when necessary, avoid sleep interruptions

37. A patient with a cerebrovascular accident exhibits abnormal eye movements. Which of the following cranial nerves would likely not be damaged in this case?

   A. Cranial nerve VI (abducens)
   B. Cranial nerve IV (trochlear)
   C. Cranial nerve VII (facial)
   D. Cranial nerve III (oculomotor)

38. The critical care nurse understands the importance of surfactant in the lungs for which of the following reasons?

    A. Prevention of alveolar collapse

    B. Encouraging the decrease of lung compliance

    C. Increasing the surface tension of the alveoli

    D. Prevention of ARDS

39. A patient in the intensive care unit has melena, abdominal cramping, and appears pale. Current vitals include BP 90/55 mmHg, HR 120/min, and RR 18/min. Which of the following laboratory changes might the nurse expect in this patient?

    A. Leukocytosis, decreased coagulation panel markers

    B. Thrombocytopenia, azotemia

    C. Elevated hematocrit, elevated PTT

    D. Hyponatremia, hypokalemia

40. A 45-year-old patient post coronary artery bypass surgery develops new onset hypotension 85/65 mmHg, and poor cardiac output. Given the below hemodynamic findings, which of the following interventions is likely?

    HEMODYNAMIC PARAMETERS

    CVP = 12 mmHg
    RAP = 16 mmHg
    PAOP = 18 mmHg
    CO = 1.6 L/min
    SVR = 1700 dynes/s/cm^{-5}

    A. Afterload reduction

    B. Pericardiocentesis

    C. Inotropes IV

    D. Balloon pump therapy

41. A patient in the early stages of hepatic encephalopathy is likely to exhibit which symptom?

    A. Asterixis

    B. Fetor hepaticus

    C. Sleep disturbances

    D. Somnolence

42. Liver failure is associated with increased serum ammonia leading to hepatic encephalopathy. Lactulose is typically ordered PO to aid in decreasing the ammonia level. Which assessment is the priority for a nurse prior to administration of lactulose?

    A. Mentation and LOC
    B. Presence of upper GI bleeding
    C. Diet
    D. Bowel habits

43. A psychiatric patient was admitted to the ICU with multiple episodes of fainting at home. ECG reveals a QT interval of 0.45 seconds. Which of the following treatments is a priority for this patient?

    A. Amiodarone
    B. Magnesium sulfate
    C. Calcium chloride
    D. Assessment of current medications

44. A 65-year-old male patient develops atrial fibrillation secondary to hypertension and valve dysfunction. Current vitals include BP 95/70 mmHg and HR 90/min. What intervention is likely indicated at this time?

    A. Digoxin and fluids
    B. Metoprolol and clonidine
    C. MAZE procedure
    D. WATCHMAN procedure

45. A patient with a heroin overdose is at increased risk of respiratory depression in the emergency department. Which of the following findings by the nurse would indicate impending respiratory distress?

    A. Respiratory rate 8/min
    B. pH 7.35
    C. Partial pressure of oxygen 65 mmHg
    D. End-tidal carbon dioxide 48 mmHg

GO ON TO NEXT PAGE ➤

46. A patient in the ICU was admitted due to an anterior-septal myocardial infarction. The patient develops the below ECG and dizziness with periodic losses of consciousness. Which of the following interventions is indicated?

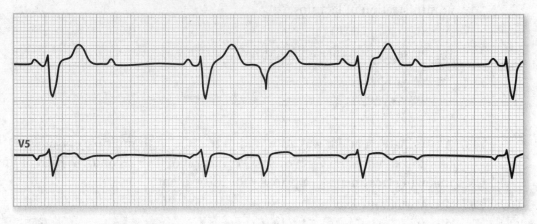

A. Transcutaneous pacing

B. Amiodarone IV bolus

C. Synchronized cardioversion

D. Atropine

47. A 70-year-old female patient was admitted to the ICU for close monitoring due to diagnosis of a subarachnoid hemorrhage (SAH). Which of the following would be included in the plan of care for this patient?

A. Administration of 0.45 NaCL

B. Administration of sedatives

C. Close monitoring of arterial pH

D. Administration of calcium gluconate

48. The nurse is caring for a patient in the ICU with DKA, the most recent glucose and labs are as follows following chronological time. The insulin has been titrated based on protocol. Dextrose 5% was added to the continuous solution at 1400. With the improvement in glucose and acidosis, which of the following would be most appropriate for the nurse at this time?

1300	1400	1500
Glucose = 300 mg/dL pH = 7.20	Glucose = 230 mg/dL	Glucose = 190 mg/dL pH = 7.30

A. Switch to 10% dextrose solution

B. Assess the need for sliding scale insulin

C. Assess the current potassium level

D. Reassess urine ketones

49. An anemic patient secondary to blood loss is receiving whole blood. During infusion, the patient developed a transfusion-related acute lung injury (TRALI). Which of the following assessments would be found in this patient?

    A. PaO_2 80 mmHg, P/F ratio 190
    B. PaO_2 55 mmHg, crackles, tachypnea
    C. $PaCO_2$ 45 mmHg, normal ejection fraction
    D. Hyperthermia, hypertension, new onset S3 murmur

50. A patient with a lateral wall myocardial infarction is at risk for left ventricular failure. Which of the following may potentiate left ventricular dysfunction in this patient?

    A. Ventricular septal defects (VSD)
    B. High blood pressure, arrhythmias
    C. Pulmonary embolism, pulmonary hypertension
    D. Papillary muscle rupture

51. A patient was recently told by the physician the terminal nature of their illness. The patient has decided to seek end-of-life care. All of the following would be included in this patient's plan of care EXCEPT for which?

    A. Improving the quality of life
    B. Encouraging spending time with family and friends
    C. Management and treatment of symptoms
    D. Care treatment and interventions

52. A 19-year-old female patient attempted to commit suicide by overdose of her prescribed tricyclic antidepressants (TCAs). Upon admission to the ICU, the patient was hypertensive with dilated pupils. What clinical findings would indicate a worsening condition in this patient?

    A. Tremors and seizure activity
    B. pH 7.55
    C. Hypothermia
    D. Respiratory rate 10/min

53. After the placement of a chest tube for a left pneumothorax, the nurse places the system to –20 mmHg suction. Assessment of the chest tube notes minimal serosanguinous output. The water seal chamber rises and falls with the breathing of the patient. How does the nurse interpret the function of the chest tube?

    A. Presence of air leak
    B. Functioning chest tube
    C. Improper placement of the tube
    D. Subcutaneous emphysema

GO ON TO NEXT PAGE ➤

54. A patient with multiple traumas is intubated, sedated on propofol, and paralyzed on cisatracurium. Morning ABG reveals the following: pH 7.30, $PaCO_2$ 55, HCO_3 30, PaO_2 65. How should the nurse interpret these results?

    A. Partial compensation, increase the FiO_2

    B. Partial compensation, increase the respiratory rate

    C. No compensation, decrease the paralytic

    D. No compensation, increase the sedation and paralytic

55. A patient in the ICU is not receiving a treatment the nurse believes may help them. The nurse is distraught because a patient on the same unit received the same treatment for the same diagnosis. What ethical principle is the nurse confronted with?

    A. Benefiscience

    B. Nonmaleficence

    C. Justice

    D. Fidelity

56. A family member approaches the nurse's station with a raised voice and visibly agitated. Which of the following would be an appropriate intervention?

    A. State their voice needs to be lowered while on the unit

    B. Explain the nurse will be in the patient room shortly to address their concerns

    C. Listen to the family member's concerns

    D. Call the charge nurse to explain the situation

57. A night-shift nurse is handing off a patient to a day-shift nurse but notices sluggish behavior with inappropriate slurring of words. What action should the night shift nurse perform at this time?

    A. Hand off patient, but remain on the unit until the nurse manager is present

    B. Continue the handoff, the nurse is likely tired

    C. Instruct the nurse to report to employee health

    D. Inquire with the nurse about the behavior

58. A patient is admitted to the ICU with a diagnosis of status asthmaticus. All of the following may be seen in this patient EXCEPT for what?

    A. Respiratory alkalosis is common in the early stages

    B. Development of auto-PEEP may occur

    C. Hyperresonance may be heard upon percussion over the lungs

    D. Anticholinergics are typically ineffective

59. Following a liver transplant, a patient is in the ICU for close monitoring and management of mechanical ventilation. A set of labs is drawn by the nurse, which includes a CBC, chemistry panel, and coagulation panel. Based upon the below results, what can the nurse indicate as the likely cause for abnormalities?

    LABORATORY RESULTS

    Hemoglobin = 9.4 g/dL
    Platelets = 120,000
    WBCs = 3000
    Sodium = 160 mEq/L
    Potassium = 3.6 mEq/L
    Glucose = 180 mg/dL

    A. Hypernatremia is likely due to methylprednisolone use
    B. Neutropenia is a likely indicator for liver rejection
    C. Metabolization in the liver may lead to hypokalemia
    D. Elevated liver enzymes may indicate liver rejection

60. The physician is choosing between administration of an angiotensin-converting inhibitor (ACEi) or an angiotensin receptor blocker (ARB). Regardless of the end prescription, what adverse effects of the medication are important for the nurse to monitor?

    A. Hypokalemia
    B. Hypernatremia
    C. Decreased preload
    D. Hyperkalemia

61. A 65-year-old patient arrives at the emergency department fatigued and nauseated. Fingerstick glucose assessment reveals a blood sugar of greater than 400 mg/dL. What serum assessment is best for the nurse to determine whether a diagnosis of DKA or HHS is likely?

    A. Serum chloride
    B. Serum sodium
    C. Serum osmolality
    D. Serum glucose

GO ON TO NEXT PAGE ➤

62. A patient with decompensated heart failure is admitted to the critical care unit. A pulmonary artery catheter is placed for close monitoring. Which of the following hemodynamic parameters would the nurse expect in this patient?

    A. CVP 12 mmHg, PAOP 22 mmHg

    B. RAP 2 mmHg, PAP 16/8 mmHg

    C. CI 3.0 L/min/m^2, SVR 800 dynes/sec/cm^{-5}

    D. PAP 20/10 mmHg, CVP 3 mmHg

63. After a crush injury to the right leg among other traumas, a patient is admitted to the ICU. Upon assessment, the left leg has +1 pulses distal to the femoral artery. The right leg has +2 pulses distal to the femoral artery. What symptom/s would the nurse monitor closely in anticipation of potential complications?

    A. Muffled apical pulse

    B. Stiffening right lower extremity

    C. Polyuria

    D. Pain relieved by morphine

64. An immunocompromised patient is at increased risk of infection and pneumonia. All of the following are additional risk factors for pneumonia EXCEPT:

    A. Decreased level of consciousness

    B. Damage to cranial nerve VI

    C. Chronic obstructive pulmonary disease

    D. CD4 count <200 cells/mm^3

65. A 65-year-old male has a history of diabetes and hypertension. Healthcare providers have instructed the patient over the past two years about his elevated risk for coronary artery disease. What additional risk factors place this patient at high risk for a myocardial event?

    A. LDL of 100, alcohol use

    B. Current use of metoprolol and losartan

    C. Diet including fiber, protein, and niacin

    D. Sedentary, obesity, total cholesterol of 220

66. A patient in renal failure develops hyperkalemia to 7.0 mEq/L. Which of the following changes on an ECG is likely present in this patient at this time?

    A. T-wave inversions

    B. Prolonged QT

    C. ST elevations

    D. Peaked T waves

67. A mechanically ventilated patient has a recent ABG as seen below. The patient is alert and calm, but a minute volume alarm is sounded on the ventilator. The patient is currently in SIMV mode at 10 breaths/min. Which of the following orders would the nurse question?

ABG ANALYSIS

pH = 7.28
$PaCO_2$ = 55
HCO_3 = 26
PaO_2 = 78

A. AC mode, RR of 14
B. CPAP mode, increase FiO_2
C. SIMV mode, increase tidal volume
D. AC mode, maintain FiO_2

68. The nurse is working in the ICU when an overhead code blue alarm is sounded for a patient in the same unit. As the nurse enters the room, they find the primary nurse using an ambu-bag to ventilate the patient. An endotracheal tube is sitting on the patient's abdomen. What action by the witnessing nurse should be done first?

A. Obtain the crash cart immediately
B. Turn off the code alarm as this is not a code blue
C. Have the unit secretary page overhead for anesthesia
D. Obtain a glidescope and replacement endotracheal tube

69. A patient has a temporary pacemaker via epicardial wires after an open-heart surgery. The past 4 hours the patient has been 100% paced at a rate of 70/min. Current assessment shows pacing spikes without depolarization. The current blood pressure is 80/60 mmHg. What intervention is appropriate at this time?

A. Gently pull at the epicardial wires
B. Increase the sensitivity of the pacemaker
C. Increase the milliamp output
D. Increase the demand rate to 100/min

70. A 50-year-old patient is warm and diaphoretic. A week-old surgical wound is purulent and painful. Based on the current vital signs below, what treatment protocol should be immediately started?

> **VITAL SIGNS**
>
> BP = 75/45 mmHg
> HR = 140/min
> RR = 32/min
> Temp = 103°F

   A. Antibiotics, IV fluid bolus and resuscitation, norepinephrine IV
   B. Norepinephrine IV, surgical wound irrigation, hypotonic fluid administration
   C. Acetaminophen, cooling blankets, beta blockers
   D. Dobutamine IV, fluid bolus and maintenance

71. Which chemistry panel derangements may be seen in a patient with chronic alcoholism?
   A. Elevated LFTs, hyperkalemia
   B. Transaminitis, hypomagnesemia
   C. Azotemia, hypermagnesemia
   D. Hyperglycemia, hyperkalemia

72. A male patient arrives at the emergency department with complaints of palpitations and anxiety. He admits to recent cocaine abuse. During the admission assessment, the nurse notes a history of hyperlipidemia with statin use, and hypertension with metoprolol use. During assessment, the patient requests a urinal to void. The nurse notes tea-colored urine. What further assessment should the nurse perform at this time?
   A. CBC and renal function
   B. ECG and chest pain assessment
   C. Patient history for chronic kidney disease
   D. Urinalysis and serum CK

73. An IV drug user was diagnosed with necrotizing fasciitis of the left arm. The patient is post aggressive surgical debridement. Hours later in the ICU, the patient continues to decline into severe sepsis. What intervention will this patient likely require?
   A. Placement of a wound vac
   B. Emergency amputation
   C. Drainage of surgical abscess
   D. Surgical arterial bypass

74. A patient scheduled for an appendectomy is visibly frightened and vocalizes this fear to the nurse. Upon questioning, the patient states he is afraid of becoming paralyzed like a family member of his who had surgery. What action by the nurse is the most appropriate?

    A. Notify the surgeon regarding the patient statements
    B. Explain anxiety is a common feeling prior to surgery
    C. Sit with the patient and explain the surgery
    D. Leave the room to provide privacy

75. A patient with a cerebellar tumor develops gait disturbances and frequent headaches. What intervention would the nurse include in the plan of care for this patient?

    A. Assessment of short-term memory
    B. Placement of object in dominant visual fields
    C. Keep sentences short and "yes" or "no" responses
    D. Bed in low position, activate bed alarms

76. A patient with advanced pneumonia is at risk for development of ARDS. Which of the following correctly explains the pathophysiology of acute respiratory distress syndrome?

    A. Increased pulmonary compliance → alveolar damage
    B. Increased capillary permeability → pulmonary edema
    C. Increased oxygen delivery → hypoxemia
    D. Increased surfactant release → endothelial damage

77. A patient with panic disorder is prescribed beta blockers. What is the purpose of using this medication in this patient?

    A. Avoid addictiveness of lorazepam
    B. Mimic effects of benzodiazepines
    C. Reduce symptoms due to catecholamines
    D. Decrease hypertension in states of panic

78. A 55-year-old male patient was brought to the emergency room by his wife after he shot himself in the leg while cleaning his gun. The wife believes the discharge of the gun was not a mistake and her husband was attempting to hurt himself. Assessment of what suicide risk is important for the nurse to include at this time?

    A. Method of suicide
    B. Intent of injury
    C. Access to community resources
    D. Relationship with his wife

GO ON TO NEXT PAGE ➤

79. A patient has a family history of hypercatabolic states after receiving anesthesia. The patient requires immediate intubation, and the anesthesiologist prefers to use succinylcholine and etomidate. Which findings would be of priority concern for the nurse after intubation?

    A. Tachycardia and hyperthermia

    B. Paralysis and loss of gag reflex

    C. Incontinence of bowel and bladder

    D. Muscle flaccidity and hypothermia

80. A patient with a severe upper respiratory illness due to an aggressive virus has been in the ICU for 9 days on high-flow nasal cannula. Patient ventilation is poor with current SpO_2 86%. End-tidal carbon dioxide and $PaCO_2$ are significantly elevated. The patient signed an advance directive stating their wish not to be intubated. After the patient becomes unresponsive, the family is pleading with the healthcare team to do everything they can. Which action is appropriate by the nurse?

    A. Rescind the advance directive, intubate the patient

    B. Allow the family to take over decision making for the patient

    C. Escort the family to a private area, explain the patient wishes

    D. Call a code blue and obtain a crash cart

81. A patient in cardiogenic shock is started on a dobutamine infusion with low-dose nitrate administration. What hemodynamic benefits should the nurse note as indicating effectiveness of the treatments?

    A. Increase in preload, decrease in cardiac output

    B. Decrease in pulmonary artery pressure, increase in central venous pressure

    C. Reduction of systemic vascular resistance, increase in cardiac index

    D. Increase in pulmonary artery wedge pressure, increase in right atrial pressure

82. A patient with severe burns to 35% of the body was recently admitted to the ICU for aggressive treatment. After 24 hours of following the Parkland formula, the nurse is assessing the effectiveness of fluid resuscitation. Which of the following best indicates success of treatment?

    A. CVP 2 mmHg

    B. Blood pressure 100/75 mmHg

    C. Heart rate 110/min

    D. VO_2 275 mL/min

83. While assessing a patient upon admission to the ICU, the nurse is inspecting the skin and notes bruising and discoloration to the left flank. The patient complains of pain in the upper left quadrant. What problem is most closely related to this skin discoloration?

   A. Kidney laceration

   B. Ectopic pregnancy rupture

   C. Hemorrhagic pancreatitis

   D. Large bowel perforation

84. A patient is suspect of a right ventricular myocardial infarction. While setting up for an ECG, where would the nurse understand to place the V_4?

   A. Fifth intercostal space, right midclavicular line

   B. Fourth intercostal space, right axillary line

   C. Fifth intercostal space, left midclavicular line

   D. Fourth intercostal space, right sternal border

85. During the recovery of an NSTEMI in the critical care unit, the nurse is closely monitoring lab values and trending cardiac markers. Given the below trended lab values, which of the following interventions is a priority?

DAY 2 – 0600	DAY 3 – 0600
HgB = 11.6 g/dL	Hgb = 11.4 g/dL
Plt = 140,000	Plt = 60,000
WBC = 6000	WBC = 5500
Na 135 = mEq/L	Na = 137 mEq/L
K = 4.0 mEq/L	K = 3.9 mEq/L
Trop = 0.45 ng/mL	Trop = 0.55 ng/mL

   A. Repeat an ECG

   B. Administer potassium chloride as ordered

   C. Obtain an order for platelet transfusion

   D. Discontinue heparin administrations

86. A 26-year-old male patient arrives at the emergency department with profound lethargy and recent worsening headaches and falls. A CT of the head reveals a meningioma. Which of the following patient signs or symptoms would indicate a worsening condition?

   A. Partial seizures lasting 15 seconds

   B. Ipsilateral pupillary dilation

   C. Changes in personality/behavior

   D. Dizziness and visual disturbances

GO ON TO NEXT PAGE ➤

87. Acute tubular necrosis is diagnosed in a patient with prolonged use of nephrotoxic medications. Urinalysis reveals proteinuria. In an effort to gauge potential for third-spacing of fluid, which of the following diagnostic assessments should be performed?

    A. Complete metabolic panel
    B. Complete blood count
    C. Renal ultrasound
    D. Serum osmolality

88. A patient is admitted to the intensive care unit with an acute kidney injury. Which of the following would indicate to healthcare professionals a diagnosis of a prerenal AKI instead of intrarenal?

    A. BUN–creatinine ratio 15:1
    B. Serum osmolality 320 mOsm/kg
    C. BUN–creatinine ratio 30:1
    D. Oliguria with elevated specific gravity

89. Magnesium sulfate is currently infusing for a patient with a serum magnesium of 1.4 mg/dL. During administration, when would the nurse consider requesting an order for calcium gluconate?

    A. Increased reflexes
    B. Positive Chvostek's sign
    C. Blood pressure 92/58 mmHg
    D. RR 12/min

90. A 60-year-old patient with heart failure has been on a strict regimen of beta blockers, calcium channel blockers, and loop diuretics. An acute exacerbation has warranted an ICU admission of this patient for monitoring of pulmonary edema and respiratory status. The patient is on a 2 L nasal cannula saturating at 94%. Which of the following acid–base imbalances would the nurse expect?

    A. pH 7.19, $PaCO_2$ 55, HCO_3 22, PaO_2 60
    B. pH 7.50, $PaCO_2$ 28, HCO_3 26, PaO_2 75
    C. pH 7.25, $PaCO_2$ 25, HCO_3 20, PaO_2 85
    D. pH 7.58, $PaCO_2$ 48, HCO_3 32, PaO_2 80

91. After a crush injury to a leg, a patient develops rhabdomyolysis and is admitted to the ICU. After reading the oncoming orders from the physician, which of the following would the nurse hold and clarify with the physician?

    A. Urinalysis

    B. 40 mg furosemide IV push

    C. Rapid infusion of hypertonic saline

    D. Serum electrolytes

92. Which of the following statements regarding the oxyhemoglobin dissociation curve is correct if the curve shifts to the left?

    A. Oxygen will release more readily from hemoglobin

    B. The cause may be hypothermia or increased pH

    C. Partial pressure of oxygen may decrease

    D. Pulse oximetry may display hypoxia

93. During the withdrawal of alcohol in the ICU, a patient develops delirium tremens. A seizure begins lasting longer than 5 minutes and the nurse immediately administers lorazepam. It has little effect and the seizure continues. The nurse would be concerned for the death of this patient due to what pathophysiology?

    A. Increased cerebral demand for oxygen

    B. Ventricular fibrillation and cardiac arrest

    C. Multiple system organ failure

    D. Destruction of muscle tissue

94. A patient with a respiratory illness is connected to pulse oximetry and telemetry for continuous monitoring. Which of the following statements regarding pulse oximetry is accurate?

    A. SpO_2 is a direct measurement of heart rate

    B. SpO_2 is an indirect noninvasive method for measuring SaO_2

    C. SpO_2 is a noninvasive method of obtaining PaO_2

    D. SpO_2 is an indirect measurement of oxygen consumption

95. A critical care nurse is caring for a 40-year-old patient admitted with a diagnosis of bowel obstruction. The patient has complained of incessant vomiting over the past 6 hours. In the emergency room, ondansetron was given with no relief. Which of the following findings would the ICU nurse likely see in this patient?

    A. Hyperkalemia and hypernatremia

    B. Hyperchloremia and serum hyperosmolality

    C. Increased urine specific gravity and serum hypoosmolality

    D. Hypokalemia and hypoosmolality

96. All of the following are examples of elder abuse EXCEPT:

    A. A family member using a parent's bank account without their knowledge

    B. A dementia patient who does not remember a sexual assault by a healthcare professional

    C. Placing an eloping patient with a GPS-tracking leg band

    D. Raising all four side rails and closing the door on an alert and oriented patient

97. Shortly after admission to the ICU, a patient with encephalopathy develops unequal pupils and withdraws to painful stimuli but has no eye opening or speech. What immediate actions by the nurse are necessary?

    A. Norepinephrine and lorazepam

    B. Osmotic diuretics and assessing potential acid–base imbalances

    C. Positioning of high-Fowler's and to the left side

    D. External ventricular drain placement

98. A patient in the neurological ICU has been admitted after being hit by a motorcycle. A CT of the spine shows cervical fractures. The nurse concerned for neurogenic shock would assess which of the following first?

    A. Systemic vascular resistance

    B. Cardiac output

    C. Pulmonary artery pressure

    D. Central venous pressure

99. A traumatic brain injury required a patient to be placed in an induced coma. The healthcare team is now attempting to reverse the coma. When arousing a patient such as this, what is a priority aspect of providing care?

    A. Monitoring for signs of pain and treating accordingly

    B. Assess potential bradycardia and hypotension

    C. Place the patient supine until movement is noticed

    D. Keeping a Yankauer suction device close by

100. Aside from liver dysfunction, what are additional common manifestations of acetaminophen overdose?

    A. Decreased levels of consciousness

    B. Abnormal behavior and mentation

    C. Decreased renal function

    D. Respiratory compromise

101. A terminally ill patient is unconscious in the ICU with family bedside. The family is concerned about a gurgling sound as the patient breathes. What action by the nurse may aid in addressing this concern?

    A. Administration of anticholinergics

    B. Suctioning of the airways

    C. Position the patient supine

    D. Administration of diuretics

102. The nurse is caring for a patient admitted to the ICU with a diagnosis of right-sided systolic cardiomyopathy. All of the following are expected findings for this diagnosis EXCEPT:

    A. Dependent edema and jugular venous distention

    B. Increased brain natriuretic peptide

    C. Frothy sputum with cough

    D. Atrial fibrillation with rapid ventricular response

103. A patient with multi-vessel disease of the coronary arteries requires a coronary bypass graft surgery. They will likely require a quadruple graft bypass. Which of the following are possible complications after the surgery?

    A. Hypermagnesemia, hyperkalemia

    B. Cardiac tamponade, tension pneumothorax

    C. Bleeding, bruising at the graft site

    D. Bleeding, dysrhythmias

104. The physician is placing an intra-aortic balloon pump (IABP) in a patient with cardiogenic shock. The nurse is assisting in setting up the device. The nurse knows that the IABP should inflate when?

    A. Ventricular systole

    B. End ventricular diastole

    C. Prior to ventricular systole

    D. At the point of the dicrotic notch

105. A 35-year-old female arrives at the emergency department with complaints of leg pain and swelling. A venous Doppler exam reveals a large thrombus. The patient ignores the nurses' request to stay in bed to walk to the bathroom and urinate. Ten minutes later the patient complains of shortness of breath. What additional findings would the nurse assess to confirm potential complications?

    A. Hypotension, bradycardia

    B. Tachycardia, hyperventilation

    C. Productive blood-tinged cough, hypothermia

    D. Syncope, bradycardia

106. An elderly patient is admitted directly to the ICU from a nursing home due to worsening fever and mentation. Upon admission the nurse notes a deep tissue injury to the sacrum. The wound appears infected with copious purulent drainage. What type of dressing would be indicated for this wound?

    A. Wet-to-moist

    B. Alginates

    C. 4 × 4 gauze

    D. Polyvinyl

107. Azotemia and oliguria are present in a new admission to the ICU. The healthcare team is attempting to assess potential causes. Which of the following will aid in the diagnosis for this apparent kidney injury?

    A. Administer a 1000 mL bolus of normal saline

    B. Administer low-dose dopamine IV

    C. Administer ibuprofen and steroids

    D. Hold all ACE inhibitors and ARBs

108. A patient at increased risk of blood clots develops nausea and vomiting. They are immediately admitted to the ICU from the emergency department. The ED nurse states the patient's abdominal pain is diffuse and out of control and is unrelieved by anything, including hydromorphone. Upon admission to the ICU, the nurse notes a still abdomen on palpation. What complication is this patient likely experiencing?

    A. Bowel obstruction with perforation

    B. Perforation of appendix

    C. Occlusion of mesenteric arteries

    D. Liver cirrhosis with portal hypertension

109. Mechanical ventilation is a common intervention in the ICU for acute respiratory distress. The nurse understands the primary purpose of the PEEP setting on a ventilator is what?

    A. Alveolar recruitment

    B. Prevention of pneumothorax

    C. Increase V/Q ventilation

    D. Improve function of surfactant

110. A patient receiving a neuromuscular blockade is intubated in the intensive care unit. The current ABG results show the following: pH 7.50, $PaCO_2$ 30, HCO_3 22, PaO_2 85. Which of the following changes to the ventilator would the nurse recommend?

    A. Increase the FiO_2
    B. Decrease the respiratory rate
    C. Increase the tidal volume
    D. Increase the PEEP

111. One common infection for patients with AIDS is of the upper respiratory tract. What specific pathogen is unique to severe immunosuppression, especially AIDS?

    A. *Haemophilus influenzae*
    B. *Streptococcus pneumoniae*
    C. *Klebsiella pneumoniae*
    D. *Pneumocystis jirovecii*

112. The critical care nurse is caring for a patient with anaphylactic shock. After administration of a fluid bolus and epinephrine IM, the nurse would expect which hemodynamic parameters to best indicate successful treatment at this time?

    A. Cardiac output 7.5 L/min
    B. PAOP 8 mmHg
    C. SVR 1200 dynes/sec/cm^{-5}
    D. Blood pressure 95/60 mmHg

113. While preparing for appropriate teaching to a patient and their family regarding post-op care. All of the following are components needed to consider when teaching EXCEPT:

    A. Readiness to learn of the patient and family
    B. Education level of the teaching materials
    C. Reinforced teaching by multiple nurses
    D. Obtain input by family

114. A nurse is caring for a patient with Hindu beliefs. What statement may the nurse encounter regarding the patient's feelings about their diagnosis and hospital stay?

    A. Accepting a plan of care may be based on karma beliefs
    B. Hinduism will likely interfere in many treatment protocols
    C. Opposite-sex nurses may not care for the patient
    D. Postmortem care must only be provided by a person of Hindu faith

GO ON TO NEXT PAGE ➤

115. A patient with suspected aortic aneurysm rupture is describing the chest pain they experience. Which of the following best describes patient reports of this chest pain?

    A. Sharp or burning
    B. Aching or throbbing
    C. Pulsating and severe
    D. Tearing and radiating

116. Which of the following findings would the nurse note upon the assessment of a patient who developed left-sided tension pneumothorax?

    A. Decreased chest expansion on the left, tracheal deviation to the right
    B. HR 95, BP 150/90, tracheal deviation to the left
    C. HR 135, BP 85/60, tracheal deviation to the left
    D. Decreased chest expansion on the right, jugular venous distention

117. A 26-year-old patient is in the ICU after a series of fractures to the lower extremities. The nurse is assessing current pain level. The patient is unable to vocalize their pain but shakes their head when asked. What is an appropriate action by the nurse at this time?

    A. Leave the room
    B. Document pain 0/10
    C. Administer morphine IV
    D. Utilize alternate pain scales

118. A patient in the ICU has a blood pressure of 90/65 mmHg. There is an order for an echocardiogram to assess current cardiac output. Cardiomyopathy is suspected with uncertainty of the type. All of the following medications may be appropriate at this time EXCEPT:

    A. Nifedipine
    B. Docusate
    C. Furosemide
    D. Metoprolol

119. A patient is receiving potassium chloride through a peripheral IV until central access can be obtained. The nurse suspects the IV has infiltrated due to patient complaints of discomfort at the site. Which of the following would the nurse perform first?

    A. Stop the infusion and apply a warm compress
    B. Discontinue the IV and apply a cold compress
    C. Flush the IV with normal saline
    D. Stop the infusion and aspirate contents with a syringe

120. The nurse is concerned about potential aspiration of food for a patient post-stroke. Which of the following cranial nerves would be assessed prior to PO intake?

    A. III, IV, V
    B. I, IV, VI
    C. VII, VIII
    D. IX, X, XII

121. A patient is admitted to the emergency department with suspected myocardial infarction. The patient reports chest pain during light activity such as walking. ECG reveals no ST elevations or abnormalities. What diagnosis is likely for this patient?

    A. Unstable angina
    B. NSTEMI
    C. Variant angina
    D. Lateral wall myocardial infarction

122. An anemic patient is to receive a blood transfusion for a hemoglobin of 7.6 g/dL. The patient develops tachycardia and peripheral cyanosis. What potential complication is this patient experiencing?

    A. Non-immune-mediated reaction
    B. Transfusion-associated circulatory overload
    C. Immune-mediated reaction (mismatched blood)
    D. Allergic reaction with urticaria and pruritus

123. A patient with a terminal illness decides they no longer want curative care. They appear visibly distraught and are tearful. Which action by the nurse is best at this time.

    A. Leave the room and provide privacy
    B. Stay with the patient and sit quietly
    C. Call the chaplain to see the patient
    D. Contact the family to come to the hospital

124. A patient in the ICU is diagnosed with acute tubular necrosis secondary to excessive NSAID use. Which of the following characteristics of the patient's urine would be expected?

    A. High urine sodium
    B. Low urine sodium
    C. High urine sodium
    D. Low urine sodium

125. A tensilon test is ordered for a patient with suspected myasthenia gravis. A lack of improvement in muscle strength after the injection of edrophonium would suggest what diagnosis?

    A. Myasthenia gravis
    B. Cholinergic crisis
    C. Guillain–Barre
    D. Huntington's disease

STOP. You have completed the practice test. Complete your answers before moving forward with the review and rationales.

Answer Key

Question 1

Answer: D

Rationale: A patient in active DKA will be NPO until stable. The patient in question is also nauseated and likely to vomit if given food. This patient should remain NPO for the time being. The other answers are correct interventions for this DKA patient upon admission to the ICU.

Question 2

Answer: C

Rationale: The patient is showing signs of DIC as well as sepsis and septic shock being a potential etiology for DIC. Increased fibrin split products is indicative of DIC. Look for values greater than 10 mcg/mL. Decreased fibrinogen less than 200 mg/dL, increased coag panel values, and increased D-dimer also all point to DIC.

Question 3

Answer: B

Rationale: The patient in this study is having repeated episodes of hematemesis. The initial suspected culprit is esophageal varices that have ruptured. A platelet count, hemoglobin, and coagulation panel are not listed here. Transfusion of platelets, FFP, or PRBCs are not indicated yet in this patient. Typically, an upper endoscopy is not emergent unless the bleeding is catastrophic. Because this is the second episode of bleeding now in this patient and the blood is bright red, performing an endoscopy ASAP makes sense. Regardless of the issue, ABCs take priority, aka suctioning the mouth to maintain an airway. Vasopressin is sometimes used in these situations to clamp down the splanchnic arterioles.

Question 4

Answer: B

Rationale: This patient is showing signs of necrotizing fasciitis (NF). The advancing wound is a big red flag. Compartment syndrome occurs due to trauma, casts, etc. Some cases of NF often look like cellulitis at first, making it difficult to diagnose NF in the beginning. The big difference here is the severe pain. Most cases of cellulitis are not associated with this unbearable severe pain. Osteomyelitis is unlikely here given the skin assessment of a spreading wound. It is absolutely possible for this infection to spread, but without radiographic evidence it would be hard to tell from straight observation of the wound.

Question 5

Answer: A

Rationale: Review the "Clinical Opiate Withdrawal Scale" for a full review of withdrawal signs and symptoms. This may be found in Chapter 11. Yawning, piloerection (goosebumps), and nausea or vomiting are symptoms of withdrawal. Pupillary constriction is associated with opiate use, dilation is expected in withdrawal.

Question 6

Answer: D

Rationale: An aPTT result of 120 seconds indicates hypocoagulability and a large risk for further bleeding. This patient may require protamine sulfate to reverse this dangerous elevation. The other answers would be expected findings for a patient who lost 1 L of blood. Nor the hemoglobin or platelet count are at the level of likely transfusion.

Question 7

Answer: C

Rationale: While considering the prerenal, intrarenal, and postrenal causes of acute kidney injuries, hepatitis A would not affect any of these. It is possible, with advanced liver failure, however, to cause what is known as hepatorenal syndrome leading to vasoconstriction in the kidneys and subsequent acute tubular necrosis. This would be seen in advanced liver cirrhosis and portal hypertension. The other answers are all known causes of AKI.

Question 8

Answer: C

Rationale: The refractory phase of shock is the final and irreversible stage before death. MODS and cellular death ensue, which may manifest with a number of organ dysfunctions; myocardial ischemia as witnessed by an elevated troponin, and ARDS as witnessed by alveolar edema may be seen.

Question 9

Answer: C

Rationale: ST elevations in leads V5, V6, and I are consistent with a lateral MI. The coronary artery affected in this situation is likely the circumflex.

Question 10

Answer: D

Rationale: Antibody development in response to an infection is performed by acquired immunity. All forms of innate immunity are either present at birth or inherent to a typical patient, from macrophages, to skin, to neutrophils. These components are innate to all humans. Acquired immunity, however, must be learned either by infection or vaccine.

Question 11

Answer: A

Rationale: By elevating the head of the bed (30 degrees) and maintaining a midline position of the head, this encourages drainage of cerebral venous blood. This is an immediate intervention the nurse can perform right now. The other options, while they may be performed, take time.

Question 12

Answer: A

Rationale: Pathophysiological changes with the use of cardiopulmonary bypass include INCREASED capillary permeability, not decreased. This increase leads to the third-spacing of fluid and edema. The other answers are also changes seen with the use of the pump.

Question 13

Answer: B

Rationale: It is more common for aspirated contents to enter the right lung given the vertical nature of the right main bronchus. This is not always the case, but it is the most common. Acute respiratory distress may develop if the aspirate is large enough; however it would not be the first thing assessed. Aspiration would cause tachycardia, not bradycardia.

Question 14

Answer: A

Rationale: Metabolic acidosis with an open anion gap >12 is indicative of diabetic ketoacidosis. The other answers reflect alternate types of acid–base imbalances.

Question 15

Answer: A

Rationale: If the balloon migrates upward from the stomach and esophagus, it is possible the Sengstaken–Blakemore balloon will place pressure against the airways, causing respiratory distress. In this circumstance, the scissors kept bedside will be used to cut the tube and release the air from the balloon. This patient certainly needs an upper endoscopy as soon as possible—remember that ABCs take priority. The endoscopy will happen as soon as we can get to it. The nurse does not manipulate a Sengstaken–Blakemore tube; it may also make the problem worse by moving the balloon even further toward airways. If the underlying problem of the balloon is corrected, the hypoxia currently experienced by this patient will resolve naturally and added oxygen will not be needed.

Question 16

Answer: D

Rationale: Spontaneous bacterial peritonitis is a risk factor for ascites due to the increased potential of the fluid becoming infected. Be cautious of potential signs and symptoms such as a rigid, board-like abdomen. Alcohol abuse is the main culprit for chronic liver failure, not acute, which is acetaminophen overdose. Portal hypertension does cause collateral blood flow, but remembering portal anatomy, the backup of blood goes to the esophageal and gastric veins, splenic veins, mesenteric veins, and hemorrhoidal veins, among others. The collaterals do not involve the brain and do not cause an increase in ICP. It is worth noting that ICP can be affected by liver failure; however, that thought is linked to hepatic encephalopathy, not portal hypertension. Jaundice is the result of an increase in bilirubin, not liver enzymes.

Question 17

Answer: C

Rationale: Hepatic encephalopathy whether present or worsening is a potential risk factor post-TIPS procedure. Because the procedure itself allows for blood to bypass the liver, less blood will be cleaned and detoxified. Close monitoring of ammonia levels is common in these patients. Treatment includes standard protocol for hyperammonemia like lactulose and neomycin. Hypokalemia is known to precipitate hepatic encephalopathy. It triggers an increase in ammonia production by the kidneys.

Question 18

Answer: A

Rationale: The patient is exhibiting signs and symptoms of septic shock. Initial treatment should include correcting preload (hypovolemia) with fluids. Vasopressors such as norepinephrine will correct the vasodilation as witnessed by the low SVR. Antibiotics should be immediately started, if not already. Appendicitis is a known risk factor for development of septic shock. The patient does not need inotropes—the CO is adequate. The patient should not receive a beta blocker, as it will further worsen the blood pressure. This patient does not have pulmonary hypertension, so sildenafil is not appropriate.

Question 19

Answer: C

Rationale: The aPTT is dangerously elevated in this patient. Correct actions that follow will be coordinated between the physician, pharmacy, and the nurse. In the meantime, an appropriate action is to stop the heparin drip and reevaluate with the team. It is likely the drip will remain off for an hour or more and a repeat aPTT drawn to indicate when the infusion should be restarted. Protamine sulfate may be indicated in this case, but the issue should be coordinated with the team first.

Question 20

Answer: B

Rationale: Guillain–Barre may eventually work its way up to the diaphragm and cause respiratory distress. This would be witnessed by acute changes in vital capacity or tidal volume. Changes in oxygenation reflected in a pulse ox would be a later finding once the ability to breath decreases. In that case it would also decrease, not increase.

Question 21

Answer: A

Rationale: Readiness for extubation and a weaning trial is performed by placing the patient on a CPAP mode. This will force the patient to do the lion's share of the work with a little pressure help. FiO_2 should be 50% or less. The HR and RR within normal limits and vital capacity greater than 3 L all indicate potential readiness.

Question 22

Answer: C

Rationale: Hemofiltration occurs due to changes in hydrostatic pressure and is mostly associated with correcting fluid imbalances. Dialysis, with the use of dialysate is very effective to remove waste products, electrolytes, and again correcting fluid imbalances. CVVH does remove a small degree of solutes through a semipermeable membrane, but this is not the main purpose of a hemofiltration. CRRT in general is used in the ICU for unstable patients that cannot tolerate hemodialysis; however, the primary goal is not to fix the blood pressure. Investigating and correcting the cause of the instability in the patient is warranted, but so does the indicated treatment reason for CVVH.

Question 23

Answer: B

Rationale: Signs and symptoms of methamphetamine overdose may include a wide variety of presentations. This is due to activation of the central and peripheral nervous system. There is an increase of serotonin which may affect temperature regulation. This leads to hyperthermia (similar to serotonin syndrome). Overdose increases the activity of neurotransmitters like dopamine (seizures) and norepinephrine. Overdose increases the release of epinephrine (tachycardia and hypertension) and histamines.

Question 24

Answer: D

Rationale: The "T" in FAST is time. When did the symptoms begin? The *Golden Window* goes up to 4.5 hours after the onset; however, tPA administration is best given under 3 hours after onset. If an ischemic stroke is identified, tPA may be indicated. At this time the nurse would assess for contraindications to its use, such as anticoagulant use, recent surgery, etc.

Question 25

Answer: B

Rationale: A shunt occurs when blood passes through the lungs without becoming oxygenated. This would lead to an increased A-A gradient; more than 10 mmHg is abnormal. A P/F ratio <200 is indicative of ARDS. A P/F ratio between 200 and 300 is indicative of ALI, not ARDS. The correct answer here has an abnormal A-A gradient and a P/F ratio in line with ARDS.

Question 26

Answer: A

Rationale: Pain is a subjective experience where it is what the patient says it is. A physiological response to pain does not differ from one human to another; however, the way the pain is interpreted and the behavior that may be seen is something that changes between people and cultures. A person of Asian descent may be silent and stoic in the face of pain. It is important to pay attention to questions that are clearly displaying a racial difference.

Question 27

Answer: C

Rationale: Asthma is a condition that affects the flow of air in the lungs. This is due to swelling, inflammation, and bronchospasms of the airways. This causes a reduction of peak flow and dynamic compliance. Asthma exacerbation is not affected by changes in surfactant production or the diaphragm.

Question 28

Answer: D

Rationale: Ventricular septal defect is a known complication of an anterior wall MI. This new onset murmur over the left ventricle would be systolic in nature as the abnormal blood movement shunts during contraction of the heart. This complication leads to shunting of the blood and potential oxygenation issues.

Question 29

Answer: B

Rationale: Systems thinking within the Synergy Model encourages the nurse to manage the environment and system resources to accomplish goals for patients, families, and staff. Coordination between specialties is needed in a complicated patient. It is not the responsibility of one specialty, nor radiology. Educating a new nurse is important, however not a part of systems thinking.

Question 30

Answer: C

Rationale: Acute kidney injury will manifest with oliguria, hyperkalemia, hypercalcemia, fluid retention, and acidosis. Anemia would be seen in chronic kidney disease or prolonged periods of kidney injury.

Question 31

Answer: B

Rationale: Angioplasty with or without stent placement is a potential treatment for PAD. This is not a surgery, as it is performed with an endovascular approach, similar to cardiac catheterization for the coronary arteries. Angiography and a Doppler duplex are diagnostic procedures, not curative. Laser ablation is performed for varicose veins, not arterial issues.

Question 32

Answer: B

Rationale: Nitroprusside is a potent vasodilator. The primary goal of treatment is to reduce the blood pressure slowly. MAP reduction should begin at 20–25%. Too quickly a reduction of blood pressure may lead to symptoms of shock. Cyanide toxicity is a possibility with long-term treatment, but this is shortly after initiation of the therapy.

Question 33

Answer: B

Rationale: ST elevations, Q waves, and T-wave inversion are indicative of myocardial infarction and damage. Changes in leads II, III, and aVF are indicative of an inferior MI.

Question 34

Answer: A

Rationale: A review of cardiac medications that affect certain receptors is found in the Chapter 2 (alpha, beta, dopamine). Isoproterenol is a beta-adrenergic agonist, meaning it will increase the heart rate and contractility of the heart. This medication is not often used, but this is a primary indication for this type of severe bradycardia. Remember with heart transplantation it is not uncommon for patients to exhibit bradycardia due to sympathetic denervation. Atropine is often used in symptomatic bradycardia, but again, due to denervation, the medication is not effective.

Question 35

Answer: B

Rationale: A tonic-clonic seizure, formerly known as a "grand mal" seizure, begins with a loss of consciousness, then stiffening of the muscles followed by jerking motions of the entire body. Seizures isolated to a singular area may be called a myoclonic or Jacksonian (focal) seizure. Paralysis is not seen in a tonic-clonic seizure postictal period although the patient may not be fully conscious or alert.

Question 36

Answer: D

Rationale: Delirium could be multifactorial in an elderly patient. The case presented does not point to the cause of the agitation and delirium, so looking at the bigger picture and inferring direction from the answers is important. This patient is likely experiencing delirium from sleep deprivation and sensory overload. Reorient and allow for uninterrupted sleep. The room should be kept dark at night, not during the day. Restricting family is not an appropriate intervention ever anymore. A haloperidol order is a bit of overkill at this point. Least invasive to most.

Question 37

Answer: C

Rationale: The facial nerve (VII) is responsible for facial expressions and sensation. Dysfunction may be exhibited by an inappropriate corneal reflex (blink). Do not confuse blinking or movement of the face with movement of the eyeball itself, as asked in this question.

Question 38

Answer: A

Rationale: Surfactant has three main functions: prevention of alveolar collapse, increasing pulmonary compliance by decreasing surface tension, and innate immunity by capturing pathogens and destroying them. Loss of surfactant may certainly lead to ARDS, but the purpose of surfactant alone is not to prevent ARDS. The clinical picture of ARDS is much larger.

Question 39

Answer: B

Rationale: Due to bleeding, the patient will likely be anemic and thrombocytopenic. The loss in volume may also cause a pre-renal AKI causing azotemia and potential oliguria. This patient will require fluids to correct these volume and electrolyte disturbances. Hypokalemia is possible given GI losses, but the patient would be hypernatremic given hyperosmolality and loss of excretion through the urine.

Question 40

Answer: B

Rationale: The clinical picture in this case is of cardiac tamponade. There is a narrowed pulse pressure with a dissociation between cardiac and thoracic pressures. This plateau comparison of filling pressures is commonly seen in cardiac tamponade. Once a pericardiocentesis is performed, the PAOP will immediately decrease and the left ventricle will begin to pump effectively again. The other answers are important components in fixing the hemodynamics seen here, but do not correct the underlying issue or the diagnosis here.

Question 41

Answer: C

Rationale: The early stages of HE are marked with agitation, mild confusion, sleep disturbances, and irritability. The other answers would be seen in the later stages of HE. Technically there are four stages of HE, with late stages including things like seizures and coma.

Question 42

Answer: D

Rationale: Prior to the administration of lactulose, it is crucial to assess bowel habits and if the patient is able to defecate appropriately. Constipation or a bowel obstruction will prevent the effectiveness of the medication since the patient is not able to pass stool. GI bleeding can exacerbate HE by increasing serum ammonia, but it is not a contraindication to the use of lactulose. It would, however, be used with extreme caution in a patient with a lower GI bleeding given the increase in peristalsis.

Question 43

Answer: B

Rationale: A prolonged QT can lead to torsades de pointe. Prevention of this is done by administration of magnesium sulfate. After this is complete, the nurse should assess the full medication profile for this patient and remove all medications that prolong QT. This may include antipsychotics, antibiotics, antiemetics, and more.

Question 44

Answer: A

Rationale: When patients revert into atrial fibrillation, they lose the atrial kick accounting for up to 20% of ejection fraction. The patient in this case became hypotension due to this loss of atrial kick. To increase the ejection fraction, digoxin may be administered. Fluids will also help stabilize any preload issues and optimize cardiac function. A beta blocker may help this patient, but a vasodilator (clonidine) is not indicated. A MAZE or WATCHMAN procedure may be indicated if the atrial fibrillation cannot be corrected with less invasive measures.

Question 45

Answer: D

Rationale: End-tidal CO_2 or a $PaCO_2$ is the first indicator of ineffective ventilation. Hypoxemia would be found later when the patient was already in full respiratory distress. A decreased respiratory rate is expected with a heroin overdose, but it does not necessarily imply hypoventilation. A dangerously decreased RR would be lower with associated shallow breathing.

Question 46

Answer: A

Rationale: The ECG strip shown displays second-degree heart block, type II. Symptomatic patients require immediate correction. This can be accomplished by transcutaneous pacing; atropine does not typically work in cases like this. The same applies to amiodarone, the medication is actually contraindicated in patients with advanced heart blocks who are not paced already. Synchronized cardioversion is not indicated here.

Question 47

Answer: C

Rationale: A patient with SAH is at increased risk of ICP-related issues. In cases such as these, the patient should not be acidotic or alkalotic as it may precipitate changes in ICP. Contrary to common belief, a patient should not be continuously alkalotic. That intervention is only used in emergency cases. Fluids and calcium channel blockers are often used to prevent vasospasms; however, that does not include hypotonic fluids or calcium itself. Sedative may mask symptoms the nurse is trying to assess, such as changes in mentation or LOC.

Question 48

Answer: C

Rationale: The patient has improved through the treatment of continuous fluids and an insulin drip. When acidosis is corrected, potassium decreases. This patient will require potassium replacement either PO or IV. Switching to 10% dextrose is not appropriate at this time, dextrose 5% was already added to the solution at 1400. Any subQ insulin is not initiated until acidosis is corrected and the anion gap closes. Reassessing for ketones in the urine is not needed; the diagnosis of DKA is already well established.

Question 49

Answer: B

Rationale: TRALI, a type of acute lung injury caused by a blood transfusion, is a potential precursor to ARDS. TRALI can be characterized by fever, hypotension P/F ratio between 201 and 300, crackles, dyspnea, and tachypnea. Hypercapnia would also be evident. A new onset S3 is associated with TACO.

Question 50

Answer: B

Rationale: The most common cause of left ventricular heart failure is hypertension and coronary heart disease. This patient already had an MI, so this is an obvious factor. Arrhythmias may worsen or potentiate the heart failure from loss of cardiac output. VSD is associated with an anterior wall MI. Papillary muscle rupture is associated with inferior wall MIs. Pulmonary embolism and hypertension would lead to right-sided HF.

Question 51

Answer: D

Rationale: Once a patient or family decides to engage end-of-life care or hospice care, the primary goal is no longer curative in nature. Palliative care, commonly included in end-of-life scenarios, are tailored to pain management and relief of symptoms. Family involvement with potential after death bereavement services are included.

Question 52

Answer: A

Rationale: Cardiovascular, cholinergic, and neurological abnormalities are seen in TCA toxicity. The most serious of which are ABC issues and seizure activity. Respiratory depression is common and may require intubation if the patient no longer protects the airway. Hypotension may occur due to dehydration, arrhythmias, and alpha-adrenergic blockade.

Question 53

Answer: B

Rationale: A functioning chest tube will tidal during inspiration and expiration. This is expected. An air leak would be noted with continuous bubbling. There is no reason to believe the chest tube was placed improperly, but this will be confirmed after a period of time by improvement in the pneumothorax. Subcutaneous emphysema occurs when air enters the tissue underneath the skin. As the skin is palpating, a crepitus can be felt.

Question 54

Answer: B

Rationale: The patient in this case is partially compensated for respiratory acidosis. The most common intervention for which is to increase either the respiratory rate or the tidal volume. The FiO_2 will self-correct when the patient begins to ventilate appropriately. There is no information to believe the sedation or paralytic are not working appropriately. If a patient, theoretically, was asynchronous with the ventilator and these ABG results were present, that would warrant further thought.

Question 55

Answer: C

Rationale: The ethical principle of justice states the needed fairness in nursing and healthcare. The same treatment should be offered to all patients who fit the criteria. By providing the treatment for one patient, but not another is intrinsically unfair. It should also not be based on any behaviors that may be interpreted as bad, such as smoking or alcohol abuse.

Question 56

Answer: C

Rationale: Address problems at the time of issue. Ignoring, delaying, or dismissing issues such as this is inappropriate. This family member may have legitimate or illegitimate concerns, but it doesn't really matter. Speaking with the family member directly will allow them to speak their mind. Listen more than speak. If necessary, escort the family member to a quiet area to speak. This will allow for privacy.

Question 57

Answer: D

Rationale: The nurse is exhibiting signs of substance use, possibly alcohol or benzodiazepines. If a nurse suspects potential substance abuse in a nurse, the problem needs to be addressed immediately. This can be done directly with the nurse or be reported to the nurse manager, which is often the better answer.

Question 58

Answer: D

Rationale: Anticholinergics like ipratropium bromide are a common mainstay in asthma treatment. Bronchodilators and steroids are also typically utilized. The other statements about status asthmaticus are true.

Question 59

Answer: A

Rationale: Corticosteroids are commonly given to patients after any transplant. Steroids, like methylprednisolone, are common until the patient may be transitioned to a PO prednisone. Steroids have side effects—hyperglycemia, immunosuppression, weight gain, and hypokalemia. Liver rejection would be indicated by fever, elevation of bilirubin and liver enzymes; however, these laboratory results are not in the exhibit given. It is a true statement but is not reflected in this question.

Question 60

Answer: D

Rationale: ACE inhibitors and ARBs affect renal function. The medications themselves increase renal excretion of fluid and sodium. Adverse effects therefore may include proteinuria, hyperkalemia, hyponatremia, and orthostasis, among others. Improvement by the medication use is seen in reduced preload, blood pressure, and work on the heart. Reduced preload is the effectiveness of the medication, however, not an adverse effect.

Question 61

Answer: C

Rationale: HHS is "hot and dry," typically brought on by severe dehydration. These changes would be seen in serum osmolality—an elevation. Serum glucose is not a great indicator for differentiation between DKA or HHS since there may be some crossover. Generally speaking, however, HHS has a higher serum glucose.

Question 62

Answer: A

Rationale: In cardiogenic shock (decompensated HF), a backflow of pressure will occur in the cardiac system. This leads to pulmonary edema and further worsening of hemodynamic numbers. The PAOP can reach numbers higher than 25 mmHg. The backflow will increase other pressures like PAP, RAP, and CVP. An SVR will likely be elevated in decompensated HF since hypertension is a likely culprit of worsening condition.

Question 63

Answer: B

Rationale: The patient is exhibiting potential signs of compartment syndrome of the right leg. Another potential risk factor could be rhabdomyolysis. A stiffening or "wood-like" limb is a potential sign of worsening compartment syndrome. A muffled apical pulse, polyuria, and pain relieved by morphine are not expected findings in compartment syndrome.

Question 64

Answer: B

Rationale: Cranial nerve VI (abducens) is responsible for extraocular movements of the eye. Damage to cranial nerves IX, X, and XII would potentially inhibit effective swallowing and lead to an aspiration risk for pneumonia. The other answers are risk factors for pneumonia.

Question 65

Answer: D

Rationale: The patient is diagnosed with hypertension and diabetes, placing them at increased risk of CAD and cardiac events. Obesity, sedentary lifestyle, smoking, and poor diet are all additional risk factors for CAD. Total cholesterol above 200 is considered high in adults. LDL levels should be 100 or less. Alcohol use does not necessarily predispose a patient to CAD unless it is moderate to heavy in use.

Question 66

Answer: D

Rationale: Peaked T waves are commonly seen in patients with severe hyperkalemia. This is due to increased action potential in the sodium–potassium pump. ST elevations and T-wave inversions are typically seen in myocardial infarctions. QT prolongation may be seen in relation to certain medications (haloperidol, antibiotics).

Question 67

Answer: B

Rationale: The ABG results, respiratory acidosis, and low minute volume alarm on the ventilator indicates the patient is not appropriately ventilating. Placing the patient on a CPAP mode offers no assistance to the patient in breathing. If the SIMV mode is not offering enough ventilation, the tidal volume or respiratory rate needs to increase. Changing the mode to AC will also give the patient time to recover energy.

Question 68

Answer: A

Rationale: The patient appears to have self-extubated and the primary nurse is ventilating until help arrives. As the secondary nurse, the first response would be to gather supplies to immediately help. This is the crash cart. The patient may not necessarily be in a medical code, but the situation is potentially dire. The crash cart will contain all necessary equipment at this time. Once the situation is assessed, if repeat intubation is necessary, anesthesia will be paged and a glidescope obtained.

Question 69

Answer: C

Rationale: Failure to capture occurs when the pacemaker fires, but it is not followed by depolarization (QRS). This can lead to bradycardia and hypotension if the intrinsic patient rhythm is not sufficient. Epicardial wires can cause slight scarring over time, requiring an increase in output. Repositioning the patient may also be warranted. Never pull on epicardial wires; it may cause them to dislodge. Increasing the sensitivity or demand rate will not correct the underlying problem.

Question 70

Answer: A

Rationale: The patient is exhibiting signs of severe sepsis with shock. Immediate blood cultures followed by antibiotics is warranted. Stabilization of hemodynamics will include isotonic fluid bolus and infusion, and norepinephrine infusion. Beta blockers will worsen the blood pressure. The patient in septic shock has increased cardiac output; dobutamine or dopamine is not warranted.

Question 71

Answer: B

Rationale: Poor nutrition in a chronic alcoholic tends to lead to low levels of most electrolytes—potassium, magnesium, phosphorus, and calcium. In addition to the electrolyte imbalances, chronic alcoholism may lead to elevated LFTs (transaminitis) and hypoglycemia.

Question 72

Answer: D

Rationale: Etiologies for rhabdomyolysis include statin and cocaine use. The onset of tea-colored urine is suspect for rhabdomyolysis. A full workup includes serum CK, urinalysis, and renal function. A CBC is not warranted at this time. With no complaints of chest pain, an ECG is not warranted; however, telemetry may be necessary with complaints of palpitations or concern for hyperkalemia.

Question 73

Answer: B

Rationale: After aggressive debridement and antibiotics, if necrotizing fasciitis continues to progress and patient condition continues to decline, amputation is likely. The goal is to immediately remove the insulting infection. Without prompt treatment, the infection can be life-threatening. Surgical arterial bypass is performed for poor perfusion due to arterial disease. A wound vac will not temporize the problem.

Question 74

Answer: A

Rationale: It appears the patient does not understand the nature of the appendectomy and risk factors. Paralysis due to appendectomy is unheard of. The surgeon will be needed to review the informed consent and review the surgery itself. The other answers are not appropriate at this time.

Question 75

Answer: D

Rationale: A patient with cerebellar dysfunction will exhibit gait and balance disturbances. Patient safety is a priority as they will be predisposed to falls. Keeping the bed in a low position with alarms will help prevent this. The other answers reflect dysfunction in alternate lobes of the brain.

Question 76

Answer: B

Rationale: Pathophysiology for ARDS includes increased capillary permeability leading to endothelial leakage, surfactant loss leading to poor compliance, alveolar edema, and eventual poor recruitment and decruitment.

Question 77

Answer: C

Rationale: The goal of beta blocker treatment in this patient is to decrease the heart rate and palpitations experienced during a panic attack. Catecholamines trigger a fight-or-flight reaction; the beta blocker attempts to stop this. If a patient had a previous history of addiction and substance abuse, it may warrant avoiding benzodiazepines all together. This, however, is not an initial thought.

Question 78

Answer: B

Rationale: The three pillars of suicide assessment are intent, injury, and lethality. It's possible this was indeed an accident, but the lethal nature of the injury warrants a full assessment. Asking the patient the nature of the injury and how it came to happen will offer more insight into the situation. Community resources and spousal relationships are not a priority at this time.

Question 79

Answer: A

Rationale: Malignant hyperthermia, a hypercatabolic state, is a reaction to certain anesthetics most commonly succinylcholine and volatile anesthetics (fluranes). This hypercatabolic state leads to tachycardia, tachypnea, hyperthermia, metabolic acidosis, and hypertension. When suspected, dantrolene is typically the first-line drug as a muscle relaxant.

Question 80

Answer: C

Rationale: When at all possible, patient wishes should be followed. The patient made clear in an advance directive their wish to not be intubated. These situations are difficult for all healthcare professionals, but the wishes of the patient must be followed. By escorting the family, this will allow an expression of feelings and a conversation with the nurse about the patient's wishes.

Question 81

Answer: C

Rationale: Benefit of this treatment should be seen with increased contractility (CO/CI) due to the dobutamine infusion, and a reduction in afterload (SVR) due to nitrate administration. The other answers do not reflex effective treatment by these medications.

Question 82

Answer: D

Rationale: Normal oxygen consumption (VO_2) is 250–350 mL/min. Proper oxygen consumption implies cellular metabolism (citric acid cycle) is utilizing oxygen appropriately for energy production. Anaerobic respiration and lactic acid buildup would indicate improper fluid resuscitation. The blood pressure, heart rate, and CVP in this case are not clear outcomes to the goals of fluid resuscitation.

Question 83

Answer: C

Rationale: Technically, any retroperitoneal bleeding may result in a Grey Turner's sign, the most common being hemorrhagic pancreatitis or necrotizing pancreatitis. This is usually in conjunction with Cullen's sign (periumbilical bruising). Given the stated pain in the left upper quadrant, the other answers do not correlate.

Question 84

Answer: A

Rationale: The patient is suspect for a right ventricular MI, meaning a right-sided ECG should be performed. This flips the expected placement of the leads and in this case, V_4 will now be at the fifth intercostal space at the *right* midclavicular line.

Question 85

Answer: D

Rationale: The reduction in platelet count from day 2 to day 3 is large—greater than 50% in 1 day. This is not expected or normal; it is indicative of HIT. All heparin needs to be discontinued and the patient transitioned to an alternate anticoagulant. A troponin is expected to peak anywhere between 12 and 48 hours. A continued rise in this case would be expected before it begins trending downward. Potassium will likely be given here, but it is not a priority comparatively.

Question 86

Answer: B

Rationale: In the context of a brain tumor, a space-occupying lesion, the main factor of signs and symptoms is dependent on the location of the tumor itself. A meningioma is a tumor of the lining of the brain, the meninges. The tumor can press on a variety of locations, but regardless of the type of tumor itself, increased intracranial pressure (ICP) is potentially life-threatening and a priority. Ipsilateral pupillary dilation manifests with increased ICP. The other answers are symptoms of the tumor itself.

Question 87

Answer: A

Rationale: In states of proteinuria, it is generally a good idea to assess serum albumin as well. Hypoalbuminemia may lead to increased third-spacing of fluid, hypovolemia, and edema. This is due to changes in oncotic pressure. A CBC will not change the nature of osmosis. Renal ultrasound is typically used for diagnostic purposes; the diagnosis for this patient has already been made. There would be no benefit to the question of third-spacing. Serum osmolality may indicate if third-spacing is happening, but the question is asking for the cause.

Question 88

Answer: C

Rationale: A BUN–creatinine ratio between 20:1 and 40:1 is indicative of a prerenal AKI. Less than 20:1 is indicative of an intrarenal AKI. Elevated serum osmolality, oliguria, and elevated specific gravity may be seen in all types of AKI.

Question 89

Answer: C

Rationale: Serious consequences, late signs of hypermagnesemia include hypotension and respiratory depression or arrest. An early sign of hypermagnesemia is hyporeflexia. A positive Chvostek's sign would indicate hypocalcemia and possible need for calcium gluconate; however, it has nothing to do with the infusion of magnesium sulfate.

Question 90

Answer: D

Rationale: Prolonged use of diuretics often leads to metabolic alkalosis. The other answers are alternate acid–base imbalances. The risk is especially high with loop and thiazide diuretics as they cause loss of hydrogen ions and potassium in addition to fluid.

Question 91

Answer: C

Rationale: Flushing of the kidneys involves 0.9% normal saline, not a hypertonic or hypotonic solution. These would further exacerbate sodium abnormalities likely present from the AKI. The other interventions are appropriate for patients with rhabdomyolysis.

Question 92

Answer: B

Rationale: States of a left shift cause hemoglobin to cling to hemoglobin, decreasing the readiness for cellular use. Because of this, a pulse ox, partial pressure of oxygen, and SaO_2 would all likely increase due to this shift. If the shift is drastic enough, the problem would be seen on the cellular level with anaerobic respiration and lactic acid production.

Question 93

Answer: A

Rationale: The cause of death due to status epilepticus is due to anoxic brain injury secondary to hypermetabolism of the seizure. The seizure activity itself drastically increases the oxygen consumption within the brain and without adequate supply massive cellular death occurs. There are several complications due to status epilepticus, such as breathing abnormalities, hyperkalemia due to muscle death, and potential cardiac arrest or MODS; however, all of these findings come later. The immediate concern and cause of death is cerebral hypoxia.

Question 94

Answer: B

Rationale: SpO_2 and SaO_2 oftentimes correlate with one another. This is what makes pulse ox so effective. There are certain conditions where this is not the case, however, as in carbon monoxide poisoning. Many pulse ox devices will estimate the heart rate based off of a waveform, but this is not an accurate or safe measurement. Oxygen consumption would be assessed on the venous side of circulation, not on the arterial side.

Question 95

Answer: B

Rationale: Excessive volume loss leads to dehydration, seen by an increase in hyperosmolality. Eventually the patient would become hypovolemic, with potential shock. Hyperchloremia is seen in these states of large amounts of fluid loss. Hypokalemia is likely due to prolonged GI losses. The patient would likely be hypernatremic due to the hyperosmolar state. An increased urine specific gravity is also likely given the dehydration.

Question 96

Answer: C

Rationale: There are certain interventions that at times may seem superfluous or unnecessary, but the safety of the patient must always come first. This is obviously within reason, but the use of a leg band is common among elopement patients. This typically causes the triggering of an alarm when they get near doorways or staircases. The other answers are examples of financial abuse, sexual abuse, and psychological abuse. Old age is not a guarantee for certain dysfunctions; it is abuse to assume so and place unneeded precautions.

Question 97

Answer: B

Rationale: The patient is exhibiting signs of increased ICP. Immediate interventions include a low Fowler's position with a midline head, osmotic diuretics (mannitol), and assessment of acid–base imbalances. Avoid acidosis or alkalosis. If respiratory status is encumbered, intubation may be necessary. An EVD placement may be necessary if these interventions fail.

Question 98

Answer: A

Rationale: Neurogenic shock is a type of distributive shock resulting from massive vasodilation. This would be seen with a decrease in SVR. The autonomic pathways are disrupted with neurogenic shock, so the patient may be tachycardic or bradycardic. Cardiac output would likely decrease due to potential bradycardia. Central venous pressure may be abnormally low due to decreased preload returning to the heart. The definitive hemodynamic, however, would be an SVR as this is specific to distributive shocks.

Question 99

Answer: D

Rationale: During arousement of a patient, regardless of situation (coma, drug overdose, etc.), nausea and vomiting is incredibly common. The priority risk here being airway obstruction or aspiration. Keep a Yankauer suction nearby, the head of the bed elevated, and antiemetics if necessary, among other appropriate interventions. A patient arousing from a coma would likely become tachycardic and hypertension. Pain is not a priority over airway.

Question 100

Answer: C

Rationale: In addition to liver toxicity, abnormal functioning of the cardiac and renal system may be seen. Eventually, if left untreated, these issues may lead to MODS. Acetaminophen overdose is the leading cause of liver transplant need in the United States.

Question 101

Answer: A

Rationale: Death rattle is a common manifestation at end of life. It can be disturbing to families who witness it. Repositioning of the patient and administration of anticholinergics may help reduce the sound. There is no proof that death rattle is uncomfortable for the patient themselves. Suctioning of the airways is inappropriate as it will likely cause discomfort or pain to the dying patient.

Question 102

Answer: C

Rationale: Frothy sputum with a cough indicated pulmonary edema associated with a left-sided failure, not right-sided. All of the other answers are seen in right-sided systolic failure. Atrial fibrillation is common when the right atria becomes dilated.

Question 103

Answer: D

Rationale: Bleeding is a common complication after open-heart surgery. Close monitoring of coagulation markers would indicate any severe increase in risk. The nurse will monitor surgical dressings and chest tube output. Dysrhythmias are also common given the close proximity of the surgery to the conduction pathway of the heart. These patients typically arrive at the ICU with epicardial wires and a temporary pacemaker in case this complication occurs. Hypomagnesemia and hypokalemia are risks. Bruising at the graft site is expected with the removal of the greater saphenous vein in the thigh.

Question 104

Answer: D

Rationale: IABP should inflate at the point of the dicrotic notch. Remember the dicrotic notch indicates the closure of the aortic valve and the beginning of ventricular diastole. A late inflation toward the end of ventricular diastole will not be effective. Inflation during ventricular systole would dramatically decrease cardiac output and potentially lead to cardiovascular collapse. IABP needs to be monitored very closely for appropriate use.

Question 105

Answer: B

Rationale: Dyspnea, tachycardia, and tachypnea are among the most common symptoms of a pulmonary embolism. Others may include hemoptysis, hypertension, and hyperthermia.

Question 106

Answer: B

Rationale: Copious amounts of drainage requires a dressing that is absorptive. Alginates and hydrofiber will serve this purpose. Polyvinyl dressings and wet-to-moist dressings will aid in autolytic debridement, but they offer little absorptive properties. Gauze is not appropriate for a deep wound.

Question 107

Answer: A

Rationale: The quickest and easiest way to differentiate a prerenal cause of AKI is to perform a fluid challenge with normal saline. If the AKI improves, the cause is prerenal. All nephrotoxic medications will be held, but this will take time to evaluate if they were the predominant cause.

Question 108

Answer: C

Rationale: The patient is at high risk for clots. The most likely explanation for the patient symptoms is mesenteric ischemia secondary to mesenteric artery occlusion. Peritonitis and "pain out of proportion" are commonly seen in mesenteric ischemia.

Question 109

Answer: A

Rationale: The primary purpose of PEEP is to prevent alveolar decruitment at the end of exhalation. By providing a small amount of pressure at the end of exhalation, the alveoli will stay open. In a patient with poor V/Q due to alveolar collapse, as with ARDS, increasing amounts of PEEP will help with alveolar recruitment. That, however, would be a different question.

Question 110

Answer: B

Rationale: The ABG displays respiratory acidosis. Decreasing the respiratory rate is an appropriate first step. Decreasing the tidal volume is another possible intervention, although typically not the first intervention. Changes in oxygen or PEEP are not warranted at this time.

Question 111

Answer: D

Rationale: *Pneumocystis jirovecii* is a fungal infection and opportunistic infection in the severely immunosuppressed, including AIDS patients. The other pathogens are fairly common across all populations of patients.

Question 112

Answer: C

Rationale: Anaphylactic shock, a type of distributive shock, is caused by massive vasodilation. Correction of this vasodilation with epinephrine IM is witnessed by normalization of SVR. Cardiac output is typically increased in distributive shocks as the body attempts to compensate. PAOP is not a good indicator in distributive shock. The blood pressure here remains low.

Question 113

Answer: C

Rationale: Teaching does not necessarily need to be performed by multiple nurses. Multiple disciplines, however, may need to be consulted depending on the teaching required. The other choices display appropriate concepts to include in teaching.

Question 114

Answer: A

Rationale: Hinduism has a strong component of karma and the acceptance of pain, but it will likely not interfere with treatment itself. Opposite-sex and postmortem considerations are more common in patients of Muslim faith.

Question 115

Answer: D

Rationale: Aortic aneurysm rupture or dissection is often reported as a tearing pain that radiates to the back.

Question 116

Answer: A

Rationale: Tension pneumothorax causes a contralateral deviation of the trachea. Hypotension and tachycardia are also expected due to compression of the great vessels resulting in poor cardiac output. This compression may be seen by distended jugular and neck veins. Chest expansion would be decreased on the affected side.

Question 117

Answer: D

Rationale: It is unclear if this patient is in pain. Because of the inability to vocalize, alternative scales should be used. Undertreatment of pain or overtreatment may result in further complications of care.

Question 118

Answer: C

Rationale: Given the hypotension bordering on shock, furosemide would be questioned. A diuretic may indeed be needed here, but a good idea would be to first question it until the blood pressure is stabilized. Docusate is appropriate in preventing a vaso-vagal response during defecation. The other medications are appropriate in heart failure.

Question 119

Answer: D

Rationale: The first act when infiltration is suspected is to stop the IV. Because potassium chloride is technically a vesicant, similar to dopamine or chemo, the IV line should be maintained to potentially aspirate out as much fluid as possible.

Question 120

Answer: D

Rationale: Assess the cranial nerves responsible for swallowing and gag. Dysfunction of these could lead to aspiration and pneumonia. The other cranial nerves listed involve other functions.

Question 121

Answer: B

Rationale: Out of the options provided, an NSTEMI correlates the best with the case. Stable angina may also describe the patient's pain if it is relieved by rest. Unstable angina is not relieved by rest and variant angina is typically triggered by stimulant abuse (cocaine).

Question 122

Answer: B

Rationale: A patient with TACO will present with symptoms typical of circulatory overload. Pulmonary edema is possible if cardiac output cannot be maintained. Tachycardia, cyanosis, and hypertension are among the symptoms of TACO.

Question 123

Answer: B

Rationale: Allow patients to express feelings in an open and nonjudgmental space. The nurse need not always be speaking. At times, the mere presence of the nurse can be relaxing to patients. The other answers are inappropriate unless the patient specifically asks for it.

Question 124

Answer: D

Rationale: When the kidneys have difficulty filtering water, solutes, and electrolytes, the result is more concentrated urine with decreased sodium. Concentrated urine may be reflected by dark color, a high specific gravity, or elevated urine osmolality.

Question 125

Answer: B

Rationale: When tensilon (edrophonium) is administered, if the muscle weakness improves the patient likely has myasthenia gravis. If the muscle weakness does not change or becomes worse, a cholinergic crisis is likely.

Notes

Notes

Notes

Notes

Notes

Notes

Notes

Notes